WF 100

MOLECULAR AND CELLULAR PEDIATRIC ENDOCRINOLOGY

CONTEMPORARY ENDOCRINOLOGY

P. Michael Conn, SERIES EDITOR

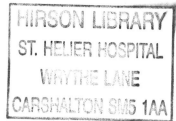
MOLECULAR AND CELLULAR PEDIATRIC ENDOCRINOLOGY

Edited by

STUART HANDWERGER, MD

Children's Hospital Medical Center, Cincinnati, OH

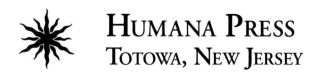

HUMANA PRESS
TOTOWA, NEW JERSEY

Molecular and cellular pediatric endocrinology/edited by Stuart Handwerger.
     p.   cm.—(Contemporary endocrinology; 10)
   Includes index.
   ISBN 0-89603-406-2 (alk. paper)
   1. Pediatric endocrinology. 2. Molecular endocrinology. 3.   Endocrine glands—diseases.   I.
Handwerger, Stuart. II. Series: Contemporary endocrinology (Totowa, NJ); 10.
   [DNLM: 1.   Endocrine Diseases—in infancy & childhood. WS930 M718 1999]
RJ418.M64   1999
618.92'4—dc21
DNLM/DLC
for Library of Congress   98-50918
                    CIP

PREFACE

During the past decade, there have been many advances in understanding the molecular and cellular basis of endocrine disorders. Many of these advances in molecular and cellular biology have resulted in new methods for diagnosis and better treatments of pediatric endocrine diseases. It is impossible to discuss all of these important advances in a single volume. The purpose of this volume is to focus on selected areas of endocrinology that have seen some of the most rapid changes. The first seven chapters of the book focus primarily on the members of the growth hormone/prolactin/placental lactogen gene family and the regulation of growth. The next five chapters deal primarily with steroid hormones, sexual development, and mineralocorticoid action; and the next two deal with the pathophysiology of diabetes mellitus. The remaining chapters focus on the molecular genetics of thyroid cancer, the molecular basis of hypophosphatemic rickets, and inherited diabetes insipidus.

I wish to express my gratitude to Dr. P. Michael Conn for his help and encouragement and to the staff at Humana Press for assisting me in the preparation of this volume. I am also grateful to the authors of the chapters for taking time from their busy schedules to write the chapters. I would also like to thank some very special people who have played critical roles in my career: Max Baum, Alsoph Corwin, Horace Hodes, Jesse Roth, Paul di Sant'Agnese, John Crigler, Louis Sherwood, and Samuel Katz.

Stuart Handwerger

*I would like to dedicate this volume to Bobbi, David, and Rachel.
Thank you for your love and support these many years.*

CONTENTS

CONTRIBUTORS

BARRY B. BERCU • *Department of Pediatrics, University of Florida College of Medicine, Tampa, FL, and All Children's Hospital, St. Petersburg, FL*

GARY D. BERKOVITZ • *Mailman Center for Child Development, University of Miami School of Medicine, Miami, FL*

MILTON R. BROWN •*Division of Pediatric Endocrinology, Emory University School of Medicine, Atlanta, GA*

STEVEN D. CHERNAUSEK • *Division of Endocrinology, Children's Hospital Medical Center, Cincinnati, OH*

JOY D. COGAN • *Department of Pediatrics, Vanderbilt University School of Medicine, Nashville, TN*

REGIS COUTANT • *Department of Pathology/Pediatrics, University of Florida College of Medicine, Gainesville, FL*

MICHAEL J. ECONS • *Department of Medicine, Indiana University Medical Center, Indianapolis, IN*

JAMES A. FAGIN • *Division of Endocrinology and Metabolism, University of Cincinnati College of Medicine, Cincinnati, OH*

MICHAEL FREEMARK • *Departments of Pediatrics and Cell Biology, Duke University Medical Center, Durham, NC*

STUART HANDWERGER • *Division of Endocrinology, Children's Hospital Medical Center, Cincinnati, OH*

PAUL L. HOFMAN • *James Whitcomb Riley Hospital for Children, Indianapolis, IN*

DAVID J. KLEIN • *Division of Endocrinology, Children's Hospital Medical Center, Cincinnati, OH*

NOEL K. MCCLAREN • *Department of Pathology/Pediatrics, University of Florida College of Medicine, Gainesville, FL*

WALTER L. MILLER • *Department of Pediatrics and the Metabolic Research Unit, University of California, San Francisco, CA*

HUGO W. MOSER • *John F. Kennedy Institute, Johns Hopkins Institute, Baltimore, MD*

JOHN S. PARKS • *Division of Pediatric Endocrinology, Emory University School of Medicine, Atlanta, GA*

O. H. PESCOVITZ • *James Whitcomb Riley Hospital for Children, Indianapolis, IN*

JOHN A. PHILLIPS, III • *Department of Pediatrics, Vanderbilt University School of Medicine, Nashville, TN*

CHERYL A. PICKETT • *Departments of Pediatrics and Internal Medicine, University of Colorado Health Sciences Center, The Children's Hospital, Denver, CO*

DAVID R. REPASKE • *Division of Endocrinology, Children's Hospital Medical Center, Cincinnati, OH*

RANDALL C. RICHARDS • *Division of Endocrinology, Children's Hospital Medical Center, Cincinnati, OH*

TOSSAPORN SEEHERUNVONG • *Mailman Center for Child Development, University of Miami School of Medicine, Miami, FL*

DOROTHY I. SHULMAN • *Department of Pediatrics, University of Florida College of Medicine, Tampa, FL, and All Children's Hospital, St. Petersburg, FL*

ERIC P. SMITH • *Division of Endocrinology, Children's Hospital Medical Center, Cincinnati, OH*

TIM M. STROM • *Abteilung für Pädiatrische Genetik, Ludwig-Maximilians Universität München, Munich, Germany*

LAURA WARD • *Division of Endocrinology and Metabolism, University of Cincinnati College of Medicine, Cincinnati, OH*

PERRIN C. WHITE • *University of Texas Southwestern Medical Center, Dallas, TX*

PHILIP S. ZEITLER • *Departments of Pediatrics and Internal Medicine, University of Colorado Health Sciences Center, The Children's Hospital, Denver, CO*

1

Molecular Basis of Disorders of Sexual Differentiation

Gary D. Berkovitz, MD
and Tossaporn Seeherunvong, MD

CONTENTS

NORMAL SEX DIFFERENTIATION *(1)*

Determination of Genetic Sex

Differentiation of the sex organs begins at fertilization when the combination of chromosomes from paternal and maternal gametes results in a karyotype that is 46, XX or 46, XY. In normal differentiation, the presence of a Y chromosome confers maleness, whereas the absence of the Y chromosome is associated with female development. However, the sex organs of the human male and female fetus are histologically identical until the fifth week of gestation. Up to that time, various bipotential and neutral structures form, each having the capacity to undergo sex-specific differentiation following the appropriate genetic signals.

Formation of the Bipotential and Neutral Structures

The bipotential gonad, also called the gonadal ridge, forms on the dorsal surface of the coelomic cavity close to the mesonephros. The gonadal ridge consists of mesenchymal cells, cells that are derived from the coelomic epithelium, cells that originated in the mesonephros, and germ cells that migrated from the yolk sac.

Two paired sets of sex ducts also form during the first 5 wk. The female or Müllerian ducts have the potential to become the upper two-thirds of the vagina, the uterus, and the fallopian tubes. The male ducts, called Wolffian ducts, have the capacity to become the seminal vesicles, vas deferens, and epididymis.

From: *Molecular and Cellular Pediatric Endocrinology*
Edited by: S. Handwerger © Humana Press Inc., Totowa, NJ

The neutral external genitalia comprise a genital tubercle, bilateral labio-scrotal folds, and a single urogenital sinus. Internally, the urogenital tract contains a utriculovaginal pouch that connects to both Müllerian and Wolffian structures.

Determination of Gonadal Sex

If the genome contains a Y chromosome, the bipotential gonad undergoes testis determination at about 5 wk. The first histologic sign is the appearance of Sertoli cells. As Sertoli cells increase in number, they surround germ cells to form seminiferous tubules. From the beginning of testis differentiation, Sertoli cells secrete antimüllerian hormone. About 1 or 2 wk later, Leydig cells appear and secrete testosterone. The biosynthesis of testosterone from its precursor cholesterol requires five principal enzymes.

In the absence of a Y chromosome, the bipotential gonad becomes an ovary. This so-called default process occurs somewhat later than testis determination. In the developing ovary, granulosa cells form and surround germ cells committing them to oocyte formation. It is thought that granulosa cells come from the same progenitors as Sertoli cells and that the origin of the theca-luteal cells is the same as that of Leydig cells.

Differentiation of External Genitalia and Sexual Duct Structures

In male sex determination, the regression of the Müllerian ducts is mediated by local secretion of antimüllerian hormone. Testosterone, also present in high, local concentrations, stimulates proliferation of the Wolffian ducts. This androgenic effect is dependent on interaction of testosterone with high-affinity receptors. Androgen binding activates receptors and results in translocation of receptors to the nucleus where they interact with regulatory elements of target genes. Whereas testosterone alone is sufficient for development of the Wolffian ducts, masculinization of the external genitalia requires conversion of testosterone to dihydrotestosterone. Testosterone and dihydrotestosterone interact with the same intracellular receptor.

Under the stimulation of androgen, the genital tubercle grows, incorporating the urethra to become the male penis. The labio-scrotal folds fuse to form the scrotum. The utriculovaginal pouch regresses and the prostate develops.

When an ovary develops, there is no antimüllerian hormone and no testosterone. Hence, the Müllerian ducts proliferate, the Wolffian ducts involute, and the external genitalia maintain their feminine form.

The past 10 years have seen extraordinary advances in our understanding of the molecular mechanisms that underlie the processes described above. The remainder of the chapter will focus on recent studies of two of these processes, namely, testis determination and androgen receptor function.

GENETIC CONTROL OF TESTIS DETERMINATION

Investigation of Subjects with Abnormal Gonadal Differentiation

Our current understanding of testis determination is built on the study of subjects with abnormal gonadal differentiation. The two most important groups of patients have been those with 46, XY gonadal dysgenesis and those with 46, XX sex reversal.

The 46, XY gonadal dysgenesis is characterized by a defect in testis determination in patients with a nonmosaic 46, XY karyotype *(2)*. When testis determination is absent, subjects develop bilateral streak gonads and have a completely female phenotype. If testis determination is incomplete, the gonads have a range of histologic appearance, but are generally characterized by disorganized seminiferous tubules. Müllerian structures are often present, Wolffian ducts are usually defective, and the external genitalia are generally ambiguous *(3)*.

The 46, XX reversal includes 46, XX maleness and 46, XX true hermaphroditism. The 46, XX maleness is characterized by normal male sex differentiation in subjects with a nonmosaic 46, XX karyotype *(4)*. Most affected subjects have a Klinefelter-like phenotype and present in their teens because of abnormal puberty. Approximately 10% of subjects have ambiguous genitalia and are evaluated in infancy. Other children come to attention because of multiple congenital anomalies.

When testicular tissue and ovarian tissue are both present in an individual with a 46, XX karyotype, the condition is termed 46, XX true hermaphroditism. The phenotype depends on the extent of testicular development.

Genes Involved in the Development of the Gonadal Ridge

Studies of normal sex determination suggest a role for various genes. First, there must be genes involved in the differentiation of the gonadal ridge, including those that mediate migration of cells from distant sites to the undifferentiated gonad. Second, there must be a gene that triggers testis determination. This gene has been termed the testis determining factor (TDF) and early karyotype studies made it clear that the TDF gene is encoded by the Y chromosome *(1)*. Finally, there must be target gene(s) for SRY and other downstream genes involved in the early steps of testis differentiation.

The syndrome of Wilms tumor, aniridia, mental retardation, and 46, XY gonadal dysgenesis *(1)* is associated with a deletion on chromosome 11. Analysis of this locus led to the isolation of the Wilms tumor suppressor gene (WT-1), which encodes a protein involved in renal development. The gene also has a role in gonadal differentiation. WT-1 is expressed in the gonadal ridge, prior to testis determination suggesting that its main role is in the development of the bipotential gonad. Nonetheless, there is some expression of WT-1 again after testis determination, suggesting a continuing role in Sertoli cell differentiation *(5)*.

The gene termed steroidogenic factor-1 has been of interest because of its involvement in the regulation of P-450 hydroxylase activity. Nonetheless, deletion of SF-1 in transgenic mice had several unexpected effects, namely, the absence of testis and ovary, as well as absence of adrenal glands and a portion of the hypothalamus. The failure to form either testis or ovary suggests that the gene plays a role in the development of the gonadal ridge before testis or ovarian determination takes place. Nonetheless, SF-1 also appears to play a role in testis differentiation as expression of SF-1 continues after testis determination. Recent evidence suggests that the SF-1 gene product is responsible for the induction of antimüllerian hormone *(6)*.

The "dosage sensitive sex reversal-adrenal hypoplasia congenita-critical region of human X chromosome 1" (DAX-1) has a pattern of expression in the gonadal ridge that is similar to that of SF-1. Although the role of DAX-1 in the development of the gonadal ridge is not completely clear, DAX-1 does probably have a specific function in ovarian differentiation. Two lines of evidence support this conclusion. First, DAX-1 expression declines when testis determination occurs and increases following ovarian determination. Second, overexpression of DAX-1 is associated with sex reversal in 46, XY individuals *(7)*.

Isolation of Sex Determining Region Y Gene

Identification of the TDF locus was based on determination of Y sequences missing in subjects with 46, XY complete gonadal dysgenesis but present in 46, XX males. Identification of overlapping sequences permitted the mapping of the TDF locus to a small region on the distal portion of the short arm of the Y chromosome. A gene termed sex determining region Y (SRY) was isolated from cloned sequences in this region on the basis of its conservation among mammals, presence in males, and absence in females *(8)*. Various lines of evidence support the role of SRY as TDF, the most compelling of which is the ability of SRY to convert XX transgenic mice into males *(9)*.

SRY is a transcription factor. It consists of a single exon and contains a DNA binding region similar to that of HMG proteins. The DNA-binding region is referred to as the HMG box *(8)*. SRY shows sequence specific DNA binding *(10)* and is also capable of bending DNA *(11)*.

Various mutations have been identified in the coding region of the SRY gene, but there have been several peculiarities *(12)*. First, almost all of the mutations occur in the HMG binding domain. Second, almost all of the mutations occur in subjects with 46, XY complete gonadal dysgenesis. Third, only about 20% of subjects with 46, XY *complete* gonadal dysgenesis have mutations in SRY.

Additional studies have investigated the possible role of sequences 3' and 5' to the coding region of the SRY gene in the pathogenesis of 46, XY gonadal dysgenesis. Only two patients were identified *(13–15)*. One subject had a deletion 5' to SRY *(13)* and another patient had a deletion 3' to SRY *(14)*.

The paucity of mutations in SRY among patients with 46, XY gonadal dysgenesis suggests that other genes must play a critical role in the development of the gonadal ridge or in the testis determining pathway.

Additional clues about the existence of such genes has come from investigating the role of SRY in the etiology of 46, XX maleness *(9)*.

Approximately two-thirds of 46, XX males have SRY sequences in genomic DNA, implicating translocation of SRY from the paternal Y chromosome to the paternal X chromosome. Subjects with SRY tend to have the Klinefelter phenotype *(4,16)*. Subjects who lack SRY are more likely to have sexual ambiguity or other congenital anomalies *(16)*.

The existence of 46, XX males who lack SRY raises questions about the mechanisms that underlie their sex reversal. Several investigators have proposed a model for the action of SRY based on these observations. According to this model the testis determination pathway is turned off prior to testis determination. SRY then acts by derepressing the testis determination pathway. Mutations in the putative repressor protein could permit testis development in the absence of SRY *(6)*. Recently, Graves suggested that derepression of such a downstream gene is likely to involve competition between SRY and an unknown gene for a DNA binding site *(17)*. This implies similarity in the DNA binding domain of the repressor and derepressor and suggests that the repressor is likely to be the product of a gene closely related to SRY. As such, it might be a member of the SOX family of genes *(17)*. The term "SOX gene" stands for "SRY-related HMG box" *(18)* and refers to genes that encode HMG proteins with DNA binding regions with significant homology (>50%) to that of SRY.

One of the SOX genes termed SOX-9 has both an HMG box and a transactivation domain *(19)*. Mutation of SOX-9 results in campomelic dysplasia and 46, XY gonadal dysgenesis *(20)*. SOX-9 appears to play a specific role in testis determination as expression of the gene increases after testis determination and declines after ovarian determination *(19)*. Graves has proposed that the SOX-9 gene may be the target gene of SRY *(17)*. Alternatively, it is possible that SRY acts primarily as a repressor of DAX-1 and directly or indirectly increases expression of both SF-1 and SOX-9.

There are also likely to be many other genes involved in the earliest stages of testis determination in addition to SRY, WT-1, SF-1, DAX-1 and SOX-9. Some clues to their identity come from studies of patients with 46, XY gonadal dysgenesis, and abnormalities of chromosome 9, whereas other indications come from analysis of kindreds with SRY-negative 46, XX maleness *(1)*. Continuing advances will depend on studies of such patients as well as on studies of sex differentiation in animal models.

ANDROGEN RECEPTOR FUNCTION

Structure of the Androgen Receptor Gene

The human androgen receptor gene is located on the long arm of the X chromosome close to the centromere *(21)*. The gene consists of eight exons that encode a protein of 910–919 amino acids *(22)*. The gene is a member of a superfamily that comprises the various steroid hormone receptor genes, as well as receptors for thyroid hormone, vitamin D, and retinoic acid. Like other steroid hormone receptors, the androgen receptor has a transcriptional activation domain, a DNA-binding domain, and a steroid-hormone binding domain *(23)*.

The transcriptional activation domain comprises the N-terminal portion of the receptor and is encoded by a single exon. The N-terminal portion may also mediate transcriptional repression of target genes. Within the N-terminal portion, there are two subregions with variable trimeric repeats. One region, consisting of (GGN) repeats, encodes 16–27 glycine residues. The second region consists of a variable number of (CAG) repeats and encodes 11–31 glutamine residues *(24)*.

The DNA binding region is encoded by exons 2 and 3 and is comprised of two cysteine-rich zinc fingers. Analysis of DNA sequences within the zinc-finger region indicates that the human androgen receptor has 80% homology with the DNA binding region of human glucocorticoid and progesterone receptors. Hence, the androgen, glucocorticoid, and progesterone receptors are considered to be members of a subfamily. In addition to including sequences involved in DNA binding, this region also encodes sequences necessary for the dimerization of androgen receptors and sequences for translocation of receptor into the nucleus *(25)*.

The steroid binding domain is encoded by exons 4–8 *(22)*. The inactive receptor is bound to heat-shock protein, but when androgen binds to the receptor, the heat-shock protein is released. Subsequently, there is a conformational change in the DNA binding domain, which permits dimerization of the receptor and interaction with androgen response elements *(26)*. In addition, phosphorylation of androgen receptor can occur and may play a role in receptor function *(24)*.

Androgen Insensitivity Syndrome

The study of subjects with androgen insensitivity syndrome (AIS) has provided information about the role of specific regions within the androgen receptor. This condition is defined by diminished androgen effect in an individual with a 46, XY karyotype despite normal secretion of testosterone and normal conversion of testosterone to dihydro-testosterone. The condition is inherited as an X-linked trait.

Complete androgen insensitivity syndrome is defined by absence of androgen effect. The external genitalia are completely feminine, but the vagina is short and blind-ending; Wolffian ducts do not proliferate. However, Müllerian structures are generally absent because the secretion of antimüllerian hormone is normal. The testes may be intra-abdominal or contained within an inguinal hernia. If the gonad is contained in a hernial sac, the condition may come to attention in infancy. In other cases, the condition remains undetected until puberty. At that time, the production of testosterone is normal, but the androgen has minimal or no effect. Conversion of testosterone to estradiol in extraglandular tissues results in sufficient estrogen for breast development. In this case, subjects come to attention because of lack of menses.

The syndrome termed partial AIS is characterized by incomplete androgen effect despite normal production of testosterone and dihydrotestosterone. The phenotypic appearance of affected subjects is quite variable. Most have ambiguous genitalia, partial development of Wolffian structures, but regression of Müllerian ducts. Some unusual patients with partial AIS present micropenis with subsequent gynecomastia at puberty.

Mutations in the Androgen Receptor Gene

Mutations of the androgen receptor gene have been identified in genomic DNA of subjects with both complete and partial AIS. Most are point mutations and mutations have been identified in all three domains. However, most of the abnormalities occur in the steroid-binding domain (24). Nonetheless, some subjects with AIS have apparently normal androgen receptor genes.

Relatively few mutations have been identified in the transcriptional activation domain of the androgen receptor gene. However, an unusual condition occurs if the number of CAG repeats is excessive. Specifically, if the number of polyglutamine repeats is over 42, the subject may develop a rare neuromuscular disorder termed Kennedy syndrome. Adults with the condition may have infertility and gynecomastia suggesting that the alteration of androgen receptor structure may also have a negative effect on androgen receptor function (27).

Several mutations of the DNA binding domain have been reported and are associated with both partial and complete AIS (24). The influence of amino acid substitutions in the steroid binding domain has recently been reviewed (24). Mutation in exons 4–8 are associated with both complete and partial AIS. Although correlation between the nature of the mutation and the phenotype of the patient have been made, one must be cautious in their interpretation. First, a given mutation may be associated with complete AIS in one subject and partial AIS in another (24). Second, subjects with AIS in the same kindred may have identical mutations, but one individual may have complete androgen insensitivity while another has partial androgen insensitivity (28).

The Role of Other Factors in Androgen Receptor Function

The existence of additional gene sequences that are necessary for complete androgen action is suggested by the observation of subjects who have androgen insensitivity but no defects in the coding region of the androgen receptor gene and by the recognition that identical mutations of the androgen receptor gene may result in very different pheno-types. In addition, the close similarity of the DNA-binding regions of the androgen, progesterone, and glucocorticoid receptors indicates that there ought to be other gene products that insure the specificity of these receptors *(29)*.

POSSIBLE INTERACTION OF ANDROGEN, PROGESTERONE, AND GLUCOCORTICOID RECEPTORS

With respect to additional genes that influence androgen receptor function, Yen et al. *(29)*. found that mutant androgen receptors influenced the ability of glucocorticoid and progesterone receptors to activate reporter gene transcription following binding of receptor to composite hormone response elements. More importantly, normal androgen receptor influenced the ability of the glucocorticoid receptor complex to activate transcription. Yen et al. *(29)* also proposed that androgen and glucocorticoid receptor may influence each other by interaction in tissues that contain receptors for both steroids. If glucocorticoid receptors also influence normal androgen receptor function, then glucocorticoids may also play a role in determining the phenotype of patients with mutant androgen receptors *(29)*.

Enhancer regions in target genes also play an important role in androgen receptor function. Several enhancer regions have been identified in sequences 5' to the transcription start site of the prostate specific antigen gene. The distal regulatory elements of this gene involve at least three regions *(30)*. It is likely that transcription of androgen-responsive genes involved in sexual differentiation also involves interaction of androgen receptor with similar regulatory elements, and that mutation of these putative response elements accounts for some cases of androgen insensitivity.

Steroid receptor coactivators are proteins that interact directly with steroid receptors and enhance their ability to influence androgen-dependent gene transcription. Several coactivators for steroid receptors have been isolated *(31,32)*. Recently, a specific coactivator for the androgen receptor in human prostate cells was isolated and termed androgen receptor-associated protein or ARA_{70} *(32)*. It is likely that similar or identical coactivators play a role in the androgen-mediated gene transcription of sex differentiation. It is also possible that mutation in these coactivators plays a role in the etiology of androgen insensitivity.

The target genes of the androgen receptor during male sex differentiation are not well known. Dean and Sanders have described a model for steroid hormone action that has relevance to understanding possible mechanisms for androgen action *(33)*. According to their scheme, a primary response to steroid is one in which interaction of the steroid receptor complex with the specific target gene results in the transcription of message. In a secondary response, the gene product of a primary response is itself a transcription factor that interacts with another gene to induce new protein synthesis. Finally, a delayed primary response is one in which the effect of the steroid receptor complex is enhanced by the binding of a primary response gene product, the two being necessary for complete androgen effect. It is clear from this schema that mutations of the genes involved in secondary and delayed primary responses to androgen could also result in some forms of androgen insensitivity.

One candidate for an androgen responsive gene in male sex differentiation is the gene for epidermal growth factor *(34)*. Support comes from observation that changes in quantity of epidermal growth factor mRNA in the Wolffian ducts of the fetal mouse is correlated with changes in testosterone concentration. Moreover, masculinization of a female fetus by exogenous androgen results in an increase in mRNA encoding epidermal growth factor.

In summary, the binding of the androgen receptor complex to target genes is likely to involve interaction with one or more enhancer sites and also involve the binding of one or several coactivators. In addition, other steroid receptors may also play a role in modulating androgen receptor function at the level of the target genes. Continued investigation of the various factors that influence androgen receptor function will help to elucidate the mechanisms involved in androgen action during male sex differentiation.

REFERENCES

1. Migeon CJ, Berkovitz GD, Brown TR. Sexual differentiation and ambiguity. In: Kappy MJ, Blizzard RM, Migeon CJ, eds. Wilkins The Diagnosis and Treatment of Endocrine Disorders in Childhood and Adolescence. 4th Ed. Charles C. Thomas, Springfield, IL, 1994, pp. 573–715.
2. Berkovitz GD, Fechner PY, Zacur HW, Rock JA, Snyder III HW, Migeon CJ, et al. Clinical and pathologic spectrum of 46, XY gonadal dysgenesis: Its relevance to the understanding of sex differentiation. Medicine 1991;70:375–383.
3. Migeon CJ. Male pseudohermaphroditism. Annales d'Endocrinologie (Paris) 1980;41:311–343.
4. de la Chapelle A. Nature and origin of males with XX sex chromosomes. Am J Med Genet 1972; 24:71–105.
5. Kriedberg JA, Sariola H, Loring JM, Meeda M, Pelletier J, Housman D, et al. WT-1 is required for early kidney development. Cell 1993;74:679–691.
6. Shen W-H, Moore CCD, Ikeda Y, Parker KL, Ingraham HA. Nuclear receptor steroidogenic factor 1 regulates the Mullerian inhibiting substances gene: a link to the sex determination cascade. Cell 1994;77:651–661.
7. Swain A, Zanaria E, Hacker A, Lovell-Badge R, Camerino G. Mouse Dax-1 expression is consistent with a role in sex determination as well as adrenal and hypothalamus function. Nature Genet 1996;12:404.
8. Sinclair AH, Berta P, Palmer MS, Hawkins J R, Griffiths BL, Smith MJ, et al. A gene from the human sex determining region encodes a protein with homology to a conserved DNA-binding motif. Nature 1990;346:240–244.
9. Lovell-Badge R, Hacker A. The molecular genetics of Sry and its role in mammalian sex determination. Phil Trans R Soc Lond B 1995;350:205–215.
10. Harley VR, Lovell-Badge R, Goodfellow PN. Definition of a consensus DNA binding site for SRY. Nucleic Acid Res 1994;22:1500,1501.
11. Pontiggia A, Rimini R, Harley VR, Goodfellow PN, Lovell-Badge R, Bianchi M. Sex-reversing mutations affect the architecture of SRY-DNA complexes. EMBO J 1994;13: 6115–6124.
12. Veitia R, Ion A, Barbaux S, Jobling MA, Souleyreau N, Ennis K, et al. Mutations and sequence variants in the testis determining region of the Y chromosome in individuals with 46,XY female phenotype. Hum Genet 1997;99:648–652.
13. McElreavey K, Vilain E, Abbas N, Costa J-M, Souleyreau N, Kucheria K, et al. XY Sex-reversal associated with a deletion 5' to the SRY "HMG box" in the testis-determining region. Proc Natl Acad Sci USA 1992;89:11,016–11,020.
14. McElreavey K, Vilain E, Barbaux S, Fuqua JS, Fechner PY, Souleyreau M, et al. Loss of sequences 3' to the testis determining gene, SRY, including the Y chromosome pseudoautosomal boundary, associated with partial testicular determination. Proc Natl Acad Sci USA 1996;93:8950–8954.
15. Kwok C, Tyler-Smith C, Mendonca BB, Hughes I, Bobrow M, Berkovitz GD, et al. Mutation analysis of the 2kb 5' to SRY in XY females and XY intersex individuals. J Med Genet 1996;33:465–468.
16. Fechner PY, Marcantonio SM, Jaswaney V, Stetten G, Goodfellow PN, Migeon CJ, et al. The role of the sex determining region Y gene (SRY) in the etiology of XX maleness. J Clin Endocrinol Metab 1993;76:690–695.
17. Graves JAM. Two uses for old SOX. Nature Genet 1997;16:114,115.
18. Goodfellow PN, Lovell-Badge R. SRY and sex determination in mammals. Ann Rev Genet 1993;27:71–92.
19. Cameron FJ, Sinclair AH. Mutations in SRY and SOX-9: Testis-determining genes. Hum Mutat 1997;9:388–395.
20. Foster JW, Dominguez-Steglich MA, Guioli S, Kwok C, Weller PA, Stevanovic M, et al. Campomelic dysplasia and autosomal sex reversal caused by mutations in an SRY-related gene. Nature 1994;372: 525–530.

21. Kuiper GG, Faber PW, van Rooij HC, van der Korput JA, Ris-Stalpers C, Klaassen P, et al. Structural organization of the human androgen receptor gene. J Mol Endocrinol 1989;2:R1–R4.
22. Lubahn DB, Joseph DR, Sar M, Tan J, Higgs HN, Larson RE, et al. The human androgen receptor: complementary deoxyribonucleic acid cloning, sequence analysis, and gene expression in prostate. Mol Endocrinol 1988;2:1265–1275.
23. Evans RM. The steroid and thyroid receptor superfamily. Science 1988;240:889–895.
24. Brown TR. Androgen receptor dysfunction in human androgen insensitivity. Trends Endocrinol Metab 1995;6:170–175.
25. Zhou Z-X, Sar M, Simental JA, Lane MV, Wilson EM. A ligand-dependent bipartite nuclear targeting signal in the human androgen receptor. Requirement for the DNA-binding domain and modulation by NH2-terminal and carboxyl-terminal sequences. J Biol Chem 1994;269:13,115–13,123.
26. Wong C-I, Zhou Z-X, Sar M, Wilson EM. Steroid requirement for androgen receptor dimerization and DNA binding. Modulation by intramolecular interactions between the NH2-terminal and steroid-binding domains. J Biol Chem 1993;268:19,004–19,012.
27. LaSpada AR, Wilson EM, Lubahn DB. Androgen receptor gene mutations in X-linked spinal and bulbar muscular atrophy. Nature 1991;352:77–79.
28. Rodien P, Mebarki F, Mowszowicz I, Chaussain J-L, Young J, Morel Y, et al. Different phenotypes in a family with androgen insensitivity caused by the same M780I point mutation in the androgen receptor gene. J Clin Endocrinol Metab 1996;81:2994–2998.
29. Yen PM, Liu Y, Palvimo JJ, Trifiro M, Whang J, Pinsky L, et al. Mutant and wild-type androgen receptors exhibit cross-talk on androgen-, glucocorticoid-, and progesterone-mediated transcription. Mol Endocrinol 1997;11:162–171.
30. Cleutijens KBJM, van der Korput HAGM, van Eekelen CCEM, vanRooij CJ, Faber PW, Trapman J. An androgen response element in a far upstream enhancer region is essential for high, androgen-regulated activity of the prostate-specific antigen promoter. Mol Endocrinol 1997;11:148–161.
31. Onate SA, Tsai SY, Tsai MJ, O'Malley BW. Sequence and characterization of a coactivator for the steroid hormone receptor superfamily. Science 1995;270:1354–1357.
32. Yeh SJ, Chang C. Cloning and characterization of a specific coactivator, ARA$_{70}$, for the androgen receptor in human prostate cells. Proc Natl Acad Sci USA 1996;93:5517–5521.
33. Dean DM, Sanders MM. Ten years after: reclassification of steroid-responsive genes. Mol Endocrinol 1996;10:1489–1495.
34. Gupta C, Singh M. Stimulation of epidermal growth factor gene expression during the fetal mouse reproductive tract differentiation: role of androgen and its receptor. Endocrinology 1996;1:705–711.

2

Insulin-Like Growth Factor Control of Growth

Insights from Targeted Disruption of Murine Genes and from Human Disease

Steven D. Chernausek, MD

CONTENTS

INTRODUCTION

It is common knowledge that the adult height of healthy children reared in modern times reflects their parents' heights, yet we have no certain knowledge of which genes are passed through the generations to effect this phenomenon. It seems logical that some of the genetic determinants of stature reside in the terminal regions of the short arm of the X chromosome because patients with Turner syndrome caused by deletions of this region are short. A recent report *(1)* purports to have identified a novel and important growth regulating gene within this region. This gene was termed SHOX, for short stature homeobox-containing gene, because of its homeodomain structure and because mutations of the gene were found in a number of children with idiopathic short stature. The implication is that SHOX might regulate the expression of an array of other genes more directly involved regulation of growth and thus serve as a master growth determinant. However, at this point, the precise function and downstream targets of SHOX are not known and more study and evidence are needed before its exact role in growth control can be appreciated.

Though much remains to be learned about the genetics of growth control in general, there is abundant evidence that the insulin-like growth factor (IGF) axis plays a critical

From: *Molecular and Cellular Pediatric Endocrinology*
Edited by: S. Handwerger © Humana Press Inc., Totowa, NJ

role in growth control in vertebrates. A wealth of biologic data that ranges from studies in diseased and healthy humans to experiments involving the targeted disruption of the murine genes encoding the important elements for IGF expression and action clearly demonstrate the pivotal role of the IGFs in growth control and begin to define the function of the specific components. This chapter will review molecular aspects of growth regulation via the IGF system, primarily focusing on the lessons learned from humans with specific genetic defects that influence IGF action and from studies of experimental "knockouts" of IGF axis genes. A brief overview of the elements of the IGF axis, beginning with the GH receptor, is provided as background.

THE IGF AXIS

Growth Hormone Receptor (2,3)

The GH receptor is a large (620 amino acid) single chain transmembrane protein that mediates the action of pituitary GH. The hormone is bound to the extracellular domain, but dimerization with another GH receptor is required for normal function of the receptor. Following dimerization, there is intracellular activation of the JAK-2 kinase which, in turn, stimulates other intracellular signaling pathways and ultimately results in the increased gene transcription for IGF-1, IGF binding protein 3 (IGFBP-3), and the acid labile subunit (ALS). These last three elements combine to form a ternary complex which contains the majority of circulating IGF in mature species.

The IGFs (4–7)

The IGFs are two related peptides: IGF-I and IGF-II. They are structurally similar and relatively small (7.5 kDa) molecules that are approx 50% homologous with proinsulin. IGF-I was initially identified as the primary mediator of GH's growth-promoting action. Hence, the IGFs have been termed "somatomedins." The somatomedin hypothesis states that the growth-promoting actions of GH are indirect and mediated by the somatomedins (principally IGF-I), which are secreted in response to GH and act on target tissues to evoke growth (8). A competing theory of GH action is termed the dual effector theory (9,10). In this model, the IGFs and GH both exert direct actions on growing tissues. Cells, such as prechondroblasts, require an exposure to GH which induces the capacity to respond to the mitogenic effects of IGF-I. Whichever theory is correct, both acknowledge the critical role of the IGFs in somatic growth control.

Because GH's role is predominately one that manifests postnatally, it was initially speculated that IGF-I was principally involved in the control of postnatal growth. IGF-II, being highly expressed during fetal life in rodents (11), was thought to acts as the "fetal IGF." Although GH is a dominant regulator of IGF-I plasma concentration during postnatal life, it is now clear that the IGFs also act as paracrine/autocrine growth factors in a variety of tissues and under many circumstances are controlled by factors other than GH. In its role as a growth factor, IGF-I frequently exerts dual actions by stimulating cell division and DNA synthesis and by promoting protein synthesis, amino acid uptake, and cell differentiation. Both the molecular biology of the IGF genes and the regulation of their expression are quite complex. Furthermore, the components that link GH receptor activation to IGF gene expression are incompletely delineated. Detailed analysis of IGF gene regulation is beyond the scope of this chapter and the reader is referred to several reviews.

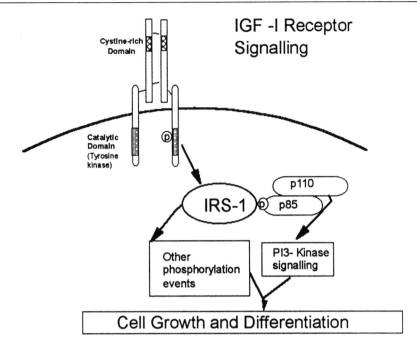

Fig. 1. Schematic of the IGF-I receptor and initial signaling pathway. IRS-1 = insulin receptor substrate 1. Adapted from LeRoith et al. *(13)*.

Type I IGF Receptors and Signal Transduction (12,13)

The IGFs, either IGF-I or IGF-II, exert their actions by first binding to cell surface IGF-I type receptors. Because IGF-II binds to the IGF-I type receptor, and likely exerts its growth-promoting actions through that receptor, it may take the place of IGF-I in some situations. The IGF-I receptor (Fig. 1) is a disulfide linked heterotetramer that contains extracellular ligand-binding domains (α-subunit) and intracellular catalytic domains (β-subunit). Both subunits are derived from a single gene and are generated by proteolytic processing. When IGF binds to the α-subunit, phosphorylation of the β-subunit occurs, activating an intrinsic tyrosine kinase. This leads to phosphorylation of insulin receptor substrate-1 (IRS-1), a key component in the signal transduction pathway for the IGFs. Activation and phosphorylation of other intracellular proteins follows and, ultimately, the activation of specific genes and cell growth.

The IGF-I receptor is homologous with the insulin receptor and, indeed, shares the IRS-1 signal transduction pathway with the insulin receptor. It is likely that this homology is in part responsible for the insulin-like properties of the IGFs and the capacity of the IGFs to alter insulin sensitivity when given to diabetic humans *(14)*.

IGF-2 Receptor (15)

The IGF-II/manose-6-phosphate receptor is a single chain, transmembrane protein that binds both manose-6-phosphate and the IGFs (although at different sites). It does not have the intrinsic protein kinase machinery like the receptors for IGF-1 and insulin and is structurally unrelated to those. It appears to be involved in the transport of manose-6-phosphate, however its function in terms of IGF action, remains somewhat obscure.

Table 1
Phenotypes of IGF Axis Deletion Mutants

Gene(s)	Prenatal growth	Postnatal growth	Neonatal lethality	Other	Refs.
IGF-I	60%	Very slow	±	Pulmonary hypoplasia	23,24
IGF-II	60%	Normal	No	Most of growth retardation before E14	29
IGF-I and IGF-II	30%	NA	Yes		30
IGF-I R	45%	NA	Yes		23
IGF-II R	145%	NA	Yes	Polydactyly, cardiac abnormalities	31–33
IGF-II R and IGF-II			No		31
IGF-II R and IGF-I R	100%		No		31
IRS-1	80%	Near normal	No	Glucose intolerant	34
Insulin R	90%		No	Ketoacidosis after birth	35

Early experiments suggested that it might be involved in IGF trafficking or regulation of extracellular IGF concentrations. More recent physiologic experiments described below support this notion. One particularly interesting aspect of the expression of the IGF-2 receptor (and the IGF-2 gene, as well) is that these elements are genetically imprinted in the mouse *(16,17)*. For IGF-2, the paternal gene is expressed, whereas it is the maternal IGF-2 receptor gene that is expressed. The physiologic relevance of this is not known, but may serve as a mechanism for more maternal/paternal specific control of fetal growth.

IGF Binding Proteins

The actions of the IGFs are modulated by a group of distinct, but related, proteins known as the IGF binding proteins (IGFBPs). The IGFBPs 1–6 bind both IGFs specifically and with high affinity. They are believed to influence IGF bioactivity within tissues by complexing with the ligands and to serve as transport proteins for the IGFs. More recently, other IGFBP-like molecules (termed IGFBP-7, and so forth) have been identified principally by searching gene sequence databases for homologous species *(18)*. Whether these homologs function similarly to IGFBPs 1–6 or serve other purposes is unknown. Although the IGFBPs are certainly involved in integrating the response of cells to the IGFs, their specific roles and breadth of actions remains largely unclear. It is well beyond the scope of this chapter to detail IGF/IGFBP physiology and the reader is referred to several reviews *(19–22)*.

GENE "KNOCKOUTS" ALONG THE IGF AXIS: PHENOTYPES AND IMPLICATIONS FOR FUNCTION (TABLE 1)

IGF-I (23–25)

The effect on somatic growth is perhaps the most striking feature observed in mice with primary deficiency of IGF-I. The animals are small at birth and have increased perinatal lethality, depending somewhat on the background strain. Those animals that do survive have severe and persisting growth failure, consistent with the evidence for IGF-I being a dominant factor in the regulation of postnatal growth. Fertility is impaired in both sexes and is associated with reduced spermatogenesis and androgen secretion in males and reduced ovulation and severe uterine hypoplasia in females *(26)*. The latter observation supports prior work suggesting that IGF-I acts as a paracrine factor to mediate estrogen-induced uterine growth. Other features found in murine models of IGF-I deficiency include reduced brain size and myelinization *(27)* and, curiously, hypertension and increased cardiac contractility *(28)*.

IGF-II (29)

The phenotype in null mutants for the IGF-II gene is less severe than for those lacking IGF-I. The degree of growth retardation noted at birth is similar, but the animals are healthier and postnatal growth is better. Although the animals remain smaller than normal, the proportionate growth (e.g., the percentage increase in body weight) they experience postnatally is normal. The growth retardation appears to occur exclusively prior to embryonic d 14 (E14), supporting the notion that IGF-II is particular important in the control of fetal growth.

IGF-I Receptor (IGF-I R) and IGF-I/IGF-II Double Deletion Mutants

If the IGF-I R indeed mediates significant growth-promoting effects of both IGF-I and IGF-II, then it stands to reason that animals lacking the IGF-I R would manifest a greater degree of growth attenuation than mutants lacking either single ligand. This is exactly what has been observed. IGF-I R deletional mutants are approx 45% of normal birthweight, have significant organ hypoplasia, muscular and osseous underdevelopment, and usual die shortly following birth *(23)*. The phenotype of IGF-I and IGF-II mutants is roughly similar with even greater fetal growth retardation [30% of normal] *(30)*. These data are all consistent with the concept that IGF-I and IGF-II have overlapping functions, exerting common effects via the IGF-I receptor.

IGF-II/M6P Receptor (IGF-II R)

A curious phenotype arises when the IGF-II R is "knocked out." Fetal overgrowth occurs with animals reaching an average birth weight 145% of normal *(31–33)*. However several other morphologic changes, such as edema, polydactyly, and marked cardiac enlargement, occur as well and the animals usually die perinatally apparently because of the heart abnormalities. It was postulated that the phenotype might be the result of an overabundance of IGF-II since one of the putative functions of the IGF-II R is to "clear" local IGF-II. To test this hypothesis, the IGF-II R deletional mutants were crossed with IGF-II null mutants *(31)*. These double mutants were small at birth (presumably because of the lack of IGF-II), but they were rescued from the lethal phenotype. Similarly, when mice lacking the IGF-I R are crossed with the IGF-II R deficient mice, neonatal lethality was avoided suggesting that overstimulation of the IGF-I R by IGF-II is the problem. Of further interest is the observation that IGF-II R/IGF-I R double mutants have normal birthweights. Thus, the overgrowth found in the IGF-II R null mutants appears to be damped out when the mutation is combined with the IGF-I R deficiency.

Insulin Receptor Substrate-1 (IRS-1) and Insulin Receptor (IR)

Mice deficient in IRS-1, the phosphoprotein mediator of insulin receptor and IGF-I receptor signals, are about 80% normal size at birth and have minimal postnatal growth failure *(34)*. The fact that the IRS-1 deficient phenotype is relatively mild implies that other signal transduction pathways for the IGF-I R and/or other IGF-I R actions are important for the stimulation of cell growth. This is of little surprise since the IGF-I R is known to stimulate multiple intracellular pathways and intracellular mediators elements continue to be discovered (e.g., IRS-2). These data also indicate that the role of the insulin receptor (and probably insulin as well) in the control of rodent fetal growth is limited. In support of this notion, the fetal growth is near normal in rodents lacking the IR; they are about 90% of normal birthweight *(35)*. However, shortly after birth, the animals develop severe failure to thrive and ketoacidosis.

THE IGF AXIS IN HUMAN GROWTH

The phenotypes observed following the gene deletions described above are dramatic and yield clear insights into the mechanisms of growth control. Yet there are presently very few human clinical correlates to these murine experiments and even those disclose some significant differences. For example, babies born with grossly disruptive mutations in the insulin receptor (or insulin deficiency) have severe intrauterine growth retardation *(36)*, unlike the murine models. Perhaps this is explained by the fact that humans are developmentally much more mature at birth than rodents and thus the third trimester of human development is affected by the lack of insulin action much like the infant rodent. However, the possibility that this reflects interspecies differences cannot be discounted.

Substantive abnormalities of the GH receptor gene result in severe GH resistance and produce Laron syndrome *(37)*. These patients have extremely poor postnatal growth, osseous immaturity, and metabolic abnormalities such as hypoglycemia *(38,39)*. As noted in a previous chapter, most of the patients with this rare condition have gene mutations that either severely attenuate the expression of the entire GH receptor gene or vastly reduce binding of GH by the GH receptor molecule. However, the syndrome is occasionally produced by mutations that allow normal GH binding but disrupt the function of the intracellular domain or interfere with dimerization of the GH receptors *(40)*.

Recent evidence suggests that milder forms of GH resistance may not be so rare. Functionally important mutations in the GH receptor gene may be responsible for inherited short stature in some situations and may explain deficits in stature in some patients previously thought to have idiopathic short stature. Ayling et al. *(41)* showed that an intracellular mutation of the GH receptor gene produced the phenotype of Laron syndrome in successive generations and that it appeared that the mutation, which was in the intracellular signal transduction region, had a dominant negative effect on GH action. Also, Goddard et al. *(42)* found mutations in the extracellular domain of the GH receptor in four of 14 patients screened from a larger pool of patients with idiopathic short stature. They postulated that some of these children had a relative insensitivity to GH as a result of this mutation and that this produced the short stature.

Human genetic defects in the IGFs or the IGF receptors have been described rarely. Lack of a single copy of the IGF-I R has been postulated to be the cause of fetal growth retardation in patients with abnormalities of chromosome 15 *(43,44)*. The described patients are missing small portions of chromosome 15 known to contain the IGF-I R gene. The patients have been developmentally delayed as well. It is difficult to know which effects are caused by the lack of IGF-I R and which might be explained by the loss of contiguous genes. Nonetheless, potentially important implications are the possible confirmation of the phenotype for the human as well as the apparent gene

Table 2
Comparison of GH Receptor Deficiency (Laron Syndrome)
with Primary IGF-I Deficiency (IGF-I Gene Deletion)

Feature	GH receptor deficiency	IGF-I deficiency (n = 1)
GH secretion	Increased	Increased
IGF-I	Markedly decreased	Markedly decreased
Postnatal growth	Markedly decreased	Markedly decreased
IGF-II	Depressed	Normal or increased
IGFBP-3	Markedly decreased	Normal
Prenatal growth	Near normal	Markedly decreased
Bone age	Very retarded	Mildly retarded
Hypoglycemia	Yes	No
Mentation	Normal	Retarded
Head growth	Appropriate	Deficient
Hearing	Normal	Deficient
Dysmorphism	No	Yes

Discordant features are in italics.

dosage effect (i.e., IUGR in the heterozygous deletion), something that does not occur in the rodent models.

A recent case study reported by Woods et al. *(45)* provides important insights into the effects of primary IGF-I deficiency in humans. The patient was homozygous for deletion of exons 4 and 5 in the IGF-I gene, which ablated the translation of any functional IGF-I. Intrauterine growth retardation was severe (birth weight and length 4 and 5 SDs below average) and postnatal growth failure was persistent, mirroring the phenotype of the IGF-I murine knockout. Contrasting the clinical features of this patient with those found in GH receptor deficiency (Table 2) is valuable in beginning to understand the differing roles of GH *per se* and the IGFs. Although, all have short stature, high circulating GH concentrations, and extremely low levels of IGF-I during childhood, there is discordance in several areas. Patients with Laron syndrome typically have birth weights in the normal range, implying that GH and GH R mediated effects have little to do with the control of fetal growth. Though IGF-I sufficiency is necessary for normal fetal growth, the expression must be controlled by other factors. That growth is so attenuated in the patient with the IGF-I gene deletion despite normal to supranormal IGF-II concentrations suggests that IGF-II offers poor compensation for loss of IGF-I in man. Furthermore, the degree of skeletal retardation (measured by bone age) is relatively mild compared to patients with GH resistance or GH deficiency. The reason for this is not clear, but perhaps it indicates that GH is capable of exerting effects on the skeleton in the absence of IGF-I as postulated by the dual effector theory of GH action.

Another important difference is the apparent effects on brain growth and mentation. Though some reports have described suppressed IQ in patients with Laron syndrome, most are normal. The patient with the IGF-I gene deletion had delayed development, hyperactivity, microcephaly, sensorineural hearing loss, and apparent mental retardation. Although it is possible that these features are caused by some factor other than lack of IGF-I (the parents were consanguineous and other recessive diseases may have manifest), a wealth of experimental evidence supports a role of IGF-I in brain cell growth and function. For example, the IGF-I receptor is widely distributed within the CNS *(46,47)*, suggesting that the IGFs exert specific effects on nervous tissue *(48)*. In support of this notion, the IGFs have been shown to promote proliferation and differentiation of neural cells *(49–51)*, enhance neurite outgrowth *(52–54)*, and support the repair and survival of neuronal cells *(53,55,56)*. Furthermore, the brains of transgenic mice overexpressing IGF are enlarged *(57)*. Thus, it is plausible that the microcephaly and developmental delay found in IGF-I in the patient with the defective IGF-I gene may truly reflect the effects of CNS deficiency of IGF-I during critical periods of brain development. However, confirmation by additional cases is needed.

SUMMARY AND FUTURE DIRECTIONS

The role of the GH/IGF axis in the control of growth is beginning to be clarified. The IGFs and the IGF-I R are deeply involved in the regulation of somatic growth and this likely represents their most important function. In this regard, IGF-I probably plays a greater role than IGF-II. Growth during the postnatal period is largely controlled by GH and its influence on IGF-I expression.

Though the above conclusions seem secure, important questions remain. It is curious that the fetal growth phenotype of the mice lacking both IGFs is more severe than those lacking the IGF-I R, suggesting that the IGF-I R is not mediating all IGF action. Baker et al. *(30)* have postulated that there are other receptors, possibly yet undiscovered, that transduce the IGF signal. Additional support for this concept is evident from mice lacking both IGF-II R and IGF-I R *(31)*. If the IGF-I R were the sole pathway for IGF growth-promoting effects, then it seems these animals should be born small. Yet, the animals have normal birthweights. The extent to which a yet undescribed receptor may contribute to the normalization of such growth or whether nonreceptor-mediated actions of the IGFs could be involved remains to be determined.

What is the extent and form of integration between the insulin receptor and its signal transduction pathway with the IGF-I R mediated actions? Perhaps the insulin R acts to stimulate growth in the double IGF R null mice described above. Also, it is possible for α- and β-subunits of the IGF-I R to combine with the homologues from the insulin R to form receptor hybrids *(58,59)*. Such a hybrid might bind an IGF but direct the signal along the insulin action pathway. Finally, there appear to be many opportunities of "crosstalk" among the various intracellular signaling molecules shared by the IGF-I R and the insulin R.

The role the IGFBPs play in the regulation of growth also remains to be determined. Though a wealth of circumstantial evidence implies they serve important functions, deletion of the IGFBP-2 gene appears to be largely harmless *(60)* and preliminary evaluation of IGFBP-4 null mutant mice shows only modest reduction in growth *(61)*. These somewhat negative results do not necessarily indicate the IGFBPs are superfluous, but may be in keeping with roles as local modulators of IGF bioactivity. Given the complexity of the IGF axis and the multiplicity of IGFBPs, it would not be surprising that the system could compensate for the deletion of a single IGFBP species. The physiological importance may only be revealed when disease or injury stresses the animals, when animals lacking multiple IGFBPs are bred, or when another component of the IGFBP axis is disrupted.

The extent to which the abnormalities of IGFs, the IGFBPs, and the IGF Rs are involved in the expression of human disease remains enigmatic. Though lack of IGF-I secretion is certainly an important part of the pathogenesis pituitary dwarfism and Laron syndrome, there are surprising few descriptions of disease caused by primary (e.g., genetic) abnormalities of the IGF axis. Only a single case of IGF-I insufficiency owing to a genetic lesion of the IGF-I gene has been reported, evidence that the IGF-I R is involved in intrauterine growth retardation is circumstantial, and there are no reports of diseases attributable to abnormalities of any IGFBP. Despite this, it seems inevitable that more extensive involvement of the IGF axis in human disease will become evident with time. This is because the data are so compelling for an important and broad role for the IGFs in the control of growth of multiple tissues from embryogenesis into adult life. Presently, we are limited partly by lack of understanding of physiologic roles that leads to inability to postulate the phenotype. For example, what phenotype will be produced by diseases of the IGFBPs? In other cases, technical limitations have precluded study; IGF-I receptor dysfunction is a plausible cause of in some cases IUGR, but examination of IGF-I receptor abundance, structure and function is complex. Thus, our present understanding of the involvement of the IGF axis in human disease has been restricted by the lack of appropriate tools and incomplete exploration. Future investigation seems bound to reveal new insights into the role of the IGF axis in a wide variety of pediatric conditions.

REFERENCES

1. Rao E, Weiss B, Fukami M, Rump A, Niesler B, Mertz A. Pseudoautosomal deletions encompassing a novel homeobox gene cause growth failure in idiopathic short stature and Turner syndrome. Nature Genet 1997;16:54–63.
2. Goffin V, Kelly PA. Prolactin and growth hormone receptors. Clin Endocrinol 1996;45:247–255.
3. Carter-Su C, Schwartz J, Smit LS. Molecular mechanism of growth hormone action. Ann Rev Physiol 1996;58:187–207.
4. Daughaday WH, Rotwein P. Insulin-like growth factors I and II. Peptide, messenger ribonucleic acid and gene structures, serum, and tissue concentrations. Endo Rev 1989;10:68–91.
5. Cohick WS, Clemmons DR. The insulin-like growth factors. Ann Rev Physiol 1993;55:131–153.
6. Spagnoli A, Rosenfeld RG. The mechanisms by which growth hormone brings about growth: the relative contributions of growth hormone and insulin-like growth factors. Endocrinol Metab Clin North Am 1996;25:615–631.
7. D'Ercole AJ. Insulin-like growth factors and their receptors in growth. Clin Endocrinol Metab 1996;25:573–590.
8. Daughaday WH, Hall K, Raben MS, Salmon WD Jr, Van den Brande JL, Van Wyk JJ. Somatomedin: proposed definition for sulphation factor. Nature 1972;235:107.
9. Isaksson OGP, Lindahl A, Nilsson A, Isgaard J. Mechanism of the stimulatory effect of growth hormone on longitudinal bone growth. Endocr Rev 1987;8:426–438.
10. Moats-Staats BM, Brady JL, Jr., Underwood LE, D'Ercole AJ. Dietary protein restriction in artificially reared neonatal rats causes a reduction of insulin-like growth factor-I gene expression. Endocrinology 1989;125:2368–2374.
11. Moses AC, Nissley SP, Short PA, Rechler MM, White RM, Knight AB, Higa OZ. Increased levels of multiplication-stimulating activity, an insulin-like growth factor, in fetal rat serum. Proc Natl Acad Sci USA 1980;77:3649–3653.
12. Nanto-Salonen K. Insulin-like growth factors, their receptors and binding proteins: Increasing complexity. Ann Med 1993;25:507,508.
13. LeRoith D, Werner H, Beitner-Johnson D, Roberts CT Jr. Molecular and cellular aspects of the insulin-like growth factor I receptor. Mol Endocrinol 1995;16:143–163.
14. Moses AC, Morrow LA, O'Brien M, Moller DE, Flier JS. Insulin-like growth factor I (rhIGF-I) as a therapeutic agent for hyperinsulinemic insulin-resistant diabetes mellitus. Diabetes Res Clin Pract 1995;28(suppl):S185–194.
15. Kiess W, Yang Y, Kessler U, Hoeflich A. Insulin-like growth factor II (IGF-II) and the IGF-II/manose-6-phosphate receptor: the myth continues. Hormone Res 1994;41:(suppl 2):66–73.

16. DeChiara TM, Robertson EJ, Efstratiadis A. Parental imprinting of the mouse insulin-like growth factor II gene. Cell 1991;64:849–859.

17. Polychronakos C. Parental imprinting of the genes for IGF-II and its receptor. Adv Exper Med Biol 1997;343:189–203.

18. Oh Y, Nagella SR, Yamanaka Y, Kim HS, Wilson E, Rosenfeld RG. Synthesis and characterization of insulin-like growth factor binding protein (IGFBP)-7. Recombinant mac25 protein specifically binds IGF-I and -II. J Biol Chem 1996;271:30,322–30,325.

19. Baxter RC, Martin JL. Binding proteins for the insulin-like growth factors: structure, regulation and function. Prog Growth Factor Res 1990;1:49–68.

20. Clemmons DR. IGF binding proteins and their functions. Mol Reprod Dev 1993;35:368–375.

21. Baxter RC. Insulin-like growth factor binding proteins in the human circulation: A review. Horm Res 1994;42:140–144.

22. Clemmons DR, Jones JI, Busby WH, Wright G. Role of insulin-like growth factor binding proteins in modifying IGF actions. [Review]. Ann NY Acad Sci 1993;692:10–21.

23. Liu J, Baker J, Perkins AS, Robertson EJ, Efstratiadis A. Mice carrying null mutations of the genes encoding insulin-like growth factor I (Igf-1) and the type 1 IGF receptor (Igf1r). Cell 1993;75:59–72.

24. Powell-Braxton L, Hollingshead P, Warburton C, Dowd M, Pitts-Meek S, Dalton D, et al. IGF-I is required for normal embryonic growth in mice. Genes Dev 1993;7:2609–2617.

25. Wharburton C, Powell-Braxton L. Mouse models of IGF-I deficiency generated by gene targeting. Receptor 1997;5:35–41.

26. Baker J, Hardy MP, Zhou J, Bondy C, Lupu F, Bellve AR, Efstratiadis A. Effects of an Igf1 gene null mutation on mouse reproduction. Mol Endocrinol 1996;10:903–918.

27. Beck KD, Powell-Braxton L, Widmer HR, Valverde J, Hefti F. Igf1 gene disruption results in reduced brain size, CNS hypomyelination, and loss of hippocampal granule and striatal parvalbumin-containing neurons. Neuron 1995;14:717–730.

28. Lembo G, Rockman HA, Hunter JJ, Steinmetz H, Koch WJ, Ma L, et al. Elevated blood pressure and enhanced myocardial contractility in mice with severe IGF-I deficiency. J Clin Invest 1996; 98:2648–2655.

29. DeChiara TM, Efstratiadis A, Robertson EJ. A growth-deficiency phenotype in heterozygous mice carrying an insulin-like growth factor II gene disrupted by targeting. Nature 1990;345:78–80.

30. Baker J, Liu J, Robertson EJ, Efstratiadis A. Role of insulin-like growth factors in embryonic and postnatal growth. Cell 1993;75:73–82.

31. Ludwig T, Eggenschwiler J, Fisher P, D'Ercole AJ, Davenport ML, Efstratiadis A. Mouse mutants lacking the type 2 IGF receptor (IGF2R) are rescued from perinatal lethality in the Igf2 and Igf1r null backgrounds. Dev Biol 1996;177:517–535.

32. Wang Z-Q, Fung MR, Barlow DP, Wagner EF. Regulation of embryonic growth and lysosomal targeting by the imprinted IGF2/Mpr gene. Nature 1994;372:464–467.

33. Lau MMH, Stewart CEH, Liu Z, Bhatt H, Rotwein P, Stewart CL. Loss of the imprinted IGF2/cation-independent mannose 6-phosphate receptor results in fetal overgrowth and perinatal lethality. Genes Dev 1994;8:2953–2963.

34. Tamemoto H, Kadowaki T, Tobe K, Yagi T, Sakura H, Hayakawa T, et al. Insulin resistance and growth retardation in mice lacking insulin receptor substrate-1 [see comments]. Nature 1994;372:182–186.

35. Accili D, Drago J, Lee EJ, Johnson MD, Cool MH, Salvatore P, et al. Early neonatal death in mice homozygous for a null allele of the insulin receptor gene. Nature Genet 1997;12:106–109.

36. Accili D. Molecular defects of the insulin receptor gene. Diabetes/Metab Rev 1995;11:47–62.

37. Berg MA, Argente J, Chernausek S, Gracia R, Guevara-Aguirre J, Hopp M, et al. Diverse growth hormone receptor gene mutations in Laron syndrome. Am J Hum Genet 1997;52:998–1005.

38. Rosenfeld RG, Rosenbloom AL, Guevara-Aguirre J. Growth hormone (GH) insensitivity due to primary GH receptor deficiency. Endocr Rev 1994;15:369–390.

39. Laron Z, Klinger B. Laron syndrome: Clinical features, molecular pathology and treatment. Horm Res 1994;42:198–202.

40. Amselem S, Sobrier ML, Dastot F, Duquesnoy P, Duriez B, Goossens M. Molecular basis of inherited growth hormone resistance in childhood. Ballieres Clin Endocrinol Metab 1996;10:353–369.

41. Ayling RM, Ross R, Towner P, Von Laue S, Finidori J, Moutoussamy S, et al. A dominant-negative mutation of the growth hormone receptor causes familial short stature. Nature Genet 1997;16:13,14.

42. Goddard AD, Covello R, Luoh SM, Clackson T, Attie KM, Gesundheit N, et al. Mutations of the growth hormone receptor in children with idiopathic short stature. N Engl J Med 1995;33:1093–1098.

43. Roback EW, Barakat AJ, Dev VG, Mbikay M, Chretien M, Butler MG. An infant with deletion of the distal long arm of chromosome 15 (q26.1—>qter) and loss of insulin-like growth factor 1 receptor gene. Am J Med Genet 1991;38:74–79.

44. Tamura T, Tohma T, Ohta T, Soejima H, Harada N, Abe K, Niikawa N. Ring chromosome 15 involving deletion of the insulin-like growth factor 1 receptor gene in a patient with features of Silver-Russell syndrome. Clin Dysmorphol 1993;2:106–113.

45. Woods KA, Camacho-Hubner C, Savage MO, Clark AJL. Intrauterine growth retardation and postnatal growth failure associated with deletion of the insulin-like growth factor I gene. N Engl J Med 1996;335:1363–1367.

46. Sara VR, Hall K, Misaki M, Frykland L, Christensen N, Wetterberg L. Ontogenesis of somatomedin and insulin receptors in the human fetus. J Clin Invest 1983;71:1084–1094.

47. Ocrant I, Valentino KL, Eng LF, Hintz RL, Wilson DM, Rosenfeld RG. Structural and immunohistochemical characterization of insulin-like growth factor I and II receptors in the murine central nervous system. Endocrinology 1988;123:1023–1034.

48. Sara VR, Carlsson-Skwirut C. The role of the insulin-like growth factors in the regulation of brain development. Prog Brain Res 1988;73:87–99.

49. McMorris FA, Furlanetto RW, Mozell RL, Carson MJ, Raible DW. Regulation of oligodendrocyte development by insulin-like growth factors and cyclic nucleotides. Ann NY Acad Sci 1990;605:101–109.

50. Shinar Y, McMorris FA. Developing oligodendroglia express mRNA for insulin-like growth factor-I, a regulator of oligodendrocyte development. J Neurosci Res 1995;42:516–527.

51. Aizenman Y, de Vellis J. Brain neurons develop in a serum and glial free environment: effects of transferrin, insulin, insulin-like growth factor-I and thyroid hormone on neuronal survival growth and differentiation. Brain Res 1987;406:32–42.

52. Recio-Pinto E, Ishii DN. Insulin and insulin-like growth factor receptors regulating neurite formation in cultured human neuroblastoma cells. J Neurosci Res 1988;19:312–320.

53. Bozyczko-Coyne D, Glicksman MA, Prantner JE, McKenna B, Connors T, Friedman C, et al. IGF-I supports the survival and/or differentiation of multiple types of central nervous system neurons. Ann NY Acad Sci 1993;692:311–313.

54. Torres-Aleman I, Naftolin F, Robbins RJ. Trophic effects of insulin-like growth factor-I on fetal rat hypothalamic cells in culture. Neuroscience 1990;35:601–608.

55. Recio-Pinto E, Rechler MM, Ishii DN. Effects of insulin, insulin-like growth factor-II, and nerve growth factor on neurite formation and survival in cultured sympathetic and sensory neurons. J Neurosci 1986;6:1211–1219.

56. Mozell RL, McMorris FA. Insulin-like growth factor-I stimulates regeneration of oligodendrocytes in vitro. Ann NY Acad Sci 1988;540:430–432.

57. Behringer RR, Lewin TM, Quaife CJ, Palmiter RD, Brinster RL, D'Ercole AJ. Expression of insulin-like growth factor I stimulates normal somatic growth in growth hormone-deficient transgenic mice. Endocrinology 1990;127:1033–1040.

58. Moxham CP, Duronio V, Jacobs S. Insulin-like growth factor I receptor beta-subunit heterogeneity. Evidence of hybrid tetramers composed of insulin-like growth factor I and insulin receptor heterodimers. J Biol Chem 1989;264:13,238–13,244.

59. Siddle K, Soos MA, Field CE, Nave BT. Hybrid and atypical insulin/insulin-like growth factor I receptors. Hormone Res 1994;41(Suppl 2):56–64.

60. Pintar JE, Schuller A, Cerro JA, Czick M, Grewel A, Green B. Genetic ablation of IGFBP-2 suggests functional redundancy of the IGFBP family. Prog Growth Factor Res 1995;6:437–445.

61. Pintar JE, Schuller A, Bradshaw S, Cerro J, Wood T. Genetic analysis of IGFBP function. Proc Endocrine Soc Ann Meet 1997; pp. 59(Abstract).

3

Molecular Defects in the Growth Hormone Axis

Joy D. Cogan, PhD and John A. Phillips III, MD

CONTENTS

BACKGROUND

Growth Hormone Synthesis

Growth hormone (GH) consists of a single polypeptide chain of 191 amino acids and two disulfide bridges that is produced by the somatotropic cells of the anterior pituitary (Fig. 1). GH is a multifunctional hormone which promotes postnatal growth of skeletal and soft tissues through a variety of effects. Controversy remains about the contribution of the various direct and indirect actions of GH. On one hand, the direct effects of GH have been demonstrated in a variety of tissues and organs and GH receptors have been documented in a number of cell types. On the other hand, substantial data indicate that a major portion of the effects of GH are mediated through the actions of GH-dependent insulin-like growth factor-I (IGF-I). While IGF-1 is produced primarily by the liver, it is also synthesized by many tissues. IGF-1 acts through its own receptor to enhance the proliferation and maturation of many tissues including bone, cartilage, and skeletal muscle. In addition to promoting growth of different tissues through these various effects, GH has also been shown to exert a variety of other biological effects including lactogenic, diabetogenic, lipolytic, protein-anabolic, and sodium/water-retention *(1)*.

From: *Molecular and Cellular Pediatric Endocrinology*
Edited by: S. Handwerger © Humana Press Inc., Totowa, NJ

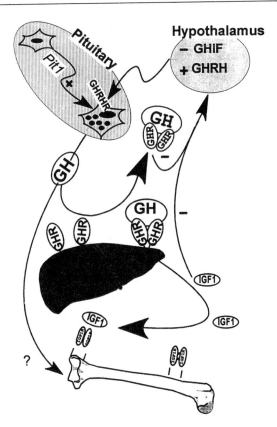

Fig. 1. Pathway of GH biosynthesis showing sites of expression of component genes whose products regulate GH secretion.

At the cellular level, following cleavage of its 26 amino acid signal peptide and secretion into the circulation, a single mature GH molecule initially binds a single GH receptor (GHR) molecule (Fig. 1). This binding causes conformational changes that result in binding of a second (GHR) molecule as a dimer. Dimerization of the two GHR molecules bound to GH is thought to be necessary for signal transduction which also requires the tyrosine kinase JAK-2. It has been suggested that the diverse effects of GH may be mediated by a single type of GHR molecule which can possess different cytoplasmic domains and/or phosphorylation sites in different tissues. When activated by JAK-2, these differing GHR cytoplasmic domains can lead to distinct phosphorylation pathways, some resulting in growth effects whereas others cause the various metabolic effects attributed to GH *(1,2)*.

Derangements of the GH Pathway

Deficiencies of synthesis, secretion, or action of GH causes short stature as well as multiple metabolic changes. The frequency of GH deficiency (either isolated or concomitant with other pituitary hormone deficiencies) is estimated to range from 1/4000 to 1/10,000 in various studies. Most cases are sporadic and are assumed to arise from central nervous system insults or defects that include cerebral edema, chromosome anomalies, histiocytosis, infections, radiation, septo-optic dysplasia, trauma or tumors affecting the hypothalamus or pituitary. For perspective, ~12% of patients who have isolated GH deficiency (IGHD) also have hypothalamic or pituitary anomalies that are detectable by magnetic resonance exams.

Interestingly, estimates of the proportion of GH deficient cases having an affected parent, sib, or child range from 3 to 30% in different studies. This occurrence of familial clustering suggests that a significant proportion of GH deficiency cases may have a genetic basis. The current understanding of the genetic basis and molecular pathophysiology of familial isolated GH deficiency and combined pituitary hormone deficiency will be discussed in the following sections.

Clinical Features

Adequate amounts of GH are needed throughout childhood to maintain normal growth. Most newborns with GH deficiency are usually of normal length and weight, whereas those with complete deficiency because of GH gene deletions can have birth lengths that are shorter than expected for their birth weights. The low linear growth of infants with congenital GH deficiency becomes progressively retarded with age and some may have micropenis or fasting hypoglycemia. In those with isolated GH deficiency (IGHD), skeletal maturation is usually delayed in proportion to their height retardation. Truncal obesity along with a facial appearance that is younger than that expected for their chronological age and delayed secondary dentition and a high-pitched voice are often present. Puberty may be delayed until the late teens, but normal fertility usually occurs. The skin of adults with GH deficiency appears fine and wrinkled, similar to that seen in premature aging. Concomitant or combined deficiencies of other pituitary hormones (LH, FSH, TSH, and/or ACTH) (OMIM#s 262600 and 312000) in addition to GH is called combined pituitary hormone deficiency (CPHD) or panhypopituitary dwarfism. The combination of GH and these additional hormone deficiencies often causes more severe retardation of growth and skeletal maturation and spontaneous puberty may not occur.

Diagnosis

Although short stature, delayed growth velocity, and delayed skeletal maturation are all seen with GH deficiency, none of these symptoms or signs is specific for GH deficiency. Therefore, patients should be evaluated for other, alternative systemic diseases before doing provocative tests to document GH deficiency. Provocative tests for GH deficiency include postexcercise, L-Dopa, insulin-tolerance, arginine, insulin-arginine, clonidine, glucagon, and propranolol protocols. Inadequate GH peak responses (usually <7–10 ng/mL) differ from protocol to protocol. Importantly, additional testing for concomitant deficiencies of LH, FSH, TSH, and/or ACTH should be done to provide a complete diagnosis and thus enable planning of optimal treatment.

FAMILIAL ISOLATED GH DEFICIENCY

Genetic Basis and Molecular Pathophysiology of Disease

Familial IGHD is associated with at least six different Mendelian disorders. These include four forms (IGHD IA and IB; Biodefective GH and a GH releasing hormone receptor or GHRHR defect) (OMIM#s 262400, 139250, 262650, and 139191), all of which have autosomal recessive modes of inheritance. In addition, there is a form with

Table 1
Mutations in the GH Genes of GH-Deficient Subjects

IGHD type	Location	Nucleotide change[a]	Effect of mutation	Refs.
IA		Deletion	7.6-kb deletion of GH gene	7
		Deletion	7.0-kb deletion of GH gene	7
		Deletion	6.7-kb deletion of GH gene	7
	Exon II	5536 del C	Frameshift after 17th aa of signal peptide	9
	Exon II	5543 G → A	Stop codon after 19th aa of signal peptide	10
IB	Intron IV	6242 G → C	Donor splice site mutation; frameshift	11
	Intron IV	6242 G → T	Donor splice site mutation; frameshift	12
	Intron IV	6246 G → C	Donor splice site mutation ; frameshift	13
	Exon III	5938-39 del AG	Frameshift after 55th aa of mature GH	14
II	Intron III	5955 G → A	Donor splice site mutation; exon 3 skip	15
	Intron III	5955 G → C	Donor splice site mutation; exon 3 skip	17
	Intron III	5960 T → C	Donor splice site mutation; exon 3 skip	11
	Intron III	5982-99 del	Splicing mutation; exon 3 skip	18
	Intron III	5982 G → A	Splicing mutation; exon 3 skip	18
	Exon V	6664 G → A	Amino acid change (Arg → His)	19

[a]Nucleotide numbering according to ref. 30.

an autosomal dominant (IGHDII, OMIM# 173100) and another with a X-linked (IGHD III, OMIM# 307200) mode of inheritance. Recently, a variety of molecular defects have been detected that cause these various disorders (Table 1). These defects will be reviewed based on the type of inheritance (IGHD I-III) that they cause.

IGHD IA

The most severe form of IGHD, called IGHD IA (OMIM# 262400), has an autosomal recessive mode of inheritance. Affected neonates occasionally have birth lengths that are shorter than expected for their birth weights and hypoglycemia in infancy, but uniformly develop severe dwarfism by 6 mo of age. In response to replacement therapy with exogenous GH subjects with IGHD IA have a strong initial anabolic and growth response that is frequently followed by the development of anti-GH antibodies in sufficient titer to block their continued and/or future response to GH replacement.

GH GENE DELETIONS

Phillips et al. *(3)* showed that IGHD IA is caused by a deletion of the growth hormone (GH1) genes. Initially, all individuals with IGHD IA were found to be homozygous for GH1 gene deletions and because of ascertainment they had all developed anti-GH antibodies following treatment with exogenous GH preparations. Subsequently, additional cases with GH1 gene deletions were described which contrasted to the initial cases in their good response to GH replacement and lack of anti-GH blocking antibodies. These included reports by Laron et al. *(4)* of four cases with homozygous GH1 deletions, all of whom had good growth responses to exogenous GH and Matsuda et al. *(5)* in their study of four Japanese patients with IGHD IA. Thus, variations in the clinical outcomes of subjects with IGHD IA having the same molecular findings were observed due to

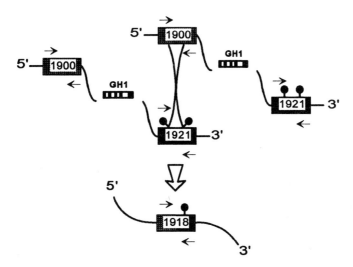

Fig. 2. Illustration of the unequal homologous recombination that can occur because of the presence of homologous sequences flanking the GH gene.

the inconsistent occurrence of anti-GH antibodies following GH replacement in different cases.

At a molecular level, Southern blot analysis showed heterogeneity in the genomic DNA deletions of ~ 6.7, 7.0, or 7.6 kb with most (~75%) being 6.7 kb. DNA sequence analysis of the fusion fragments associated with GH1 gene deletions have shown that homologous recombination between sequences flanking the GH1 gene cause these deletions (Fig. 2) *(6)*. Currently, GH1 gene deletions are detected using polymerase chain reaction (PCR) amplification of the homologous regions flanking the GH1 gene and the fusion fragments associated with GH1 gene deletions (Fig. 3) *(7)*. Since the fusion fragments associated with 6.7 kb deletions differ in the size of fragments produced by certain restriction enzymes (*see Sma*I sites indicated by solid circle in Fig. 3), homozygosity or heterozygosity for these deletions can be easily detected by enzyme digestion of PCR products. A variety of studies suggest that ~15% of subjects with severe IGHD (>–4.5 SD in height) have GH1 gene deletions *(8)*. Recently, frameshift and nonsense mutations have also been found in subjects with the IGHD IA phenotype so that this disorder may be best described as complete GH deficiency caused by GH1 gene defects, rather than gene deletions alone.

GH GENE DELETION AND FRAMESHIFT MUTATIONS

Two affected sibs diagnosed with IGHD IA have been reported who are compound heterozygotes for deletion and frameshift mutations of the GH1 gene *(9)*. Southern blot analysis showed the patients to be heterozygous for the 6.7 kb GH gene deletion. DNA sequence analysis of the retained GH1 gene showed it had a cytosine deleted in the 18th codon of the prohormone sequence. This single base deletion results in a frameshift within the signal peptide coding region, which prevents the synthesis of any mature GH protein. These patients presented with severe growth failure and, following an initial growth response to treatment with exogenous GH, developed high titers of anti-GH antibodies.

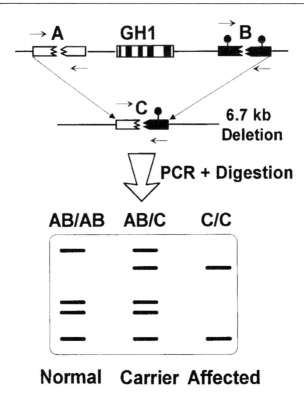

Fig. 3. PCR amplification of homologous sequences flanking the GH1 gene. Flanking sequences are distinguished from GH-deletion fusion fragments by restriction enzyme digestion (●), shown above, and gel electrophoresis, shown below.

GH Gene Nonsense Mutations

A G → A transition in the 20th codon that converts a Trp codon (TGG) to a termination codon (TAG) of the GH signal peptide was reported in a consanguineous Turkish family with IGHD IA *(10)*. This transition results in termination of translation after residue-19 of the signal peptide and no production of mature GH. Patients homozygous for this Trp20Stop mutation have no detectable GH and produce anti-GH antibodies in response to exogenous GH treatment. Interestingly, this mutation generates a new *Alu*I site that can be readily screened for by PCR amplification of the GH gene followed by *Alu*I digestion and gel electrophoresis.

IGHD IB

IGHD IB is characterized by an autosomal recessive mode of inheritance; low, but detectable levels of GH, stature more than 2 SD below the mean for age and sex, and a positive response and immunological tolerance to treatment with exogenous GH. Some IGHD IB patients have been clinically diagnosed as IGHD 1A, because of their apparent lack of endogenous GH. The GH gene defects in some of these patients produce a mutant GH protein that cannot be effectively measured by RIA. The presence of this mutant protein may explain their good response to GH therapy and lack of anti-GH antibodies. A diagram showing all of the IGHD IA and IB mutations is shown in Fig. 4.

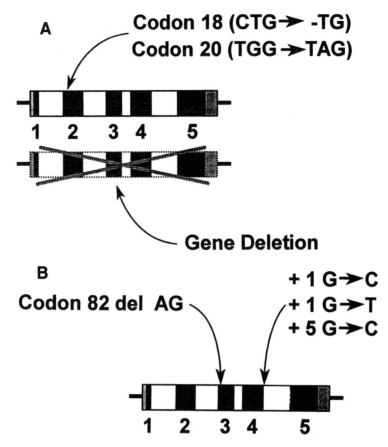

Fig. 4. Schematic representation of the GH1 gene showing the locations of various IGHD IA **(A)** and IB mutations **(B)**, respectively.

GH GENE SPLICING MUTATIONS

A G → C transversion in the first base of the donor splice site of intron 4 (IVS4 +1G → C) has been detected in a consanguineous Saudi Arabian family *(10)*. The effect of this mutation on mRNA splicing was determined by transfecting the mutant gene into cultured mammalian cells and DNA sequencing of the resulting GH cDNAs. The mutation was found to cause the activation of a cryptic splice site 73 bases upstream of the exon 4 donor splice site. This altered splicing results in the loss of amino acids 103 → 126 of exon 4 and creates a frameshift that alters the amino acids encoded for by exon 5 *(11)*. Such changes in the amino acids encoded by exons 4 and 5 may not only affect the stability and biological activity of the mutant GH protein, but as studies with bovine GH mutants have shown, also derange intracellular targeting of GH protein products to the secretory granule.

A G → T transversion (IVS4 +1G → T) has been identified at the same site in another consanguineous Saudi family *(12)*. Analysis of GH mRNA transcripts from the lymphoblastoid cells of affected patients confirmed that the G → T transversion had the same effect on splicing as the G → C transversion. Both of these mutations destroy an *Hph*I site that enables their detection by restriction digestion of GH gene PCR products followed by gel electrophoresis. Patients homozygous for these defects responded well to exogenous GH treatment and did not make anti-GH antibodies.

A G → C transversion of the fifth base of IVS 4 (IVS4 +5G → C) was identified in a consanguineous family diagnosed with IGHD I *(13)*. This mutation created a new *Mae*II site which was used to screen all family members for the mutation. RT-PCR analysis of GH mRNA transcripts from the lymphoblastoid cells of an affected patient demonstrated that the mutation destroyed the intron 4 donor splice site and had the same overall effect on splicing as the IVS4 +1G → C transversion described above.

GH GENE DELETION AND FRAMESHIFT MUTATIONS

An IGHD patient with severe growth retardation was found to have two GH gene defects. The first GH allele was a 6.7 kb deletion and the second had a 2 bp deletion in exon 3 *(14)*. This 2 bp deletion results in a frameshift within exon 3 and generates a premature stop codon at the position of amino acid residue 132 in exon 4. The patient had a positive response to GH replacement therapy and did not produce anti-GH antibodies again suggesting that some GH-related protein is produced.

IGHD II

IGHD II has an autosomal dominant mode of inheritance. Patients diagnosed with IGHD II have a single affected parent, vary in clinical severity between kindreds, and respond well to GH treatment *(11,15,16)*. Almost all IGHD II patients with GH gene defects reported to date have mutations in intron 3 that alter splicing of GH transcripts resulting in skipping of exon 3 (Fig. 5A). The mechanism by which the mutant, truncated GH protein inactivates the normal GH protein is not proven, but is thought to be through disruption of normal intracellular protein transport or the formation of GH hetero-dimers (Fig. 5B).

GH GENE DOMINANT-NEGATIVE MUTATIONS

A T → C transition of the sixth base of the donor splice site of IVS 3 (IVS3 +6 T → C) was the first mutation found to be associated with IGHD II *(11)*. The mutant GH gene was transfected into cultured mammalian cells and the GH mRNA transcripts analyzed by direct sequencing of their corresponding cDNAs. The mutation was found to inactivate the IVS3 donor splice site causing deletion or skipping of exon 3 and the loss of amino acids 32 → 71 from the corresponding mature GH-N protein products (Fig. 6). All of the affected patients in this family were heterozygous for the IVS3 +6 T → C change and had low, but measurable GH levels following provocative stimulation. Affected subjects responded well to treatment with exogenous GH without forming significant levels of anti-GH antibodies.

Two additional IGHD II mutations have been identified that both alter the first base of the IVS 3 donor splice site. One is a G → C transversion (IVS3 +1G → C) and the other is a recurring G → A transition (IVS3 +1G → A) (Fig. 5A) *(15,17)*. The latter has been identified in three nonrelated kindreds and is believed to arise as a result of the high mutation frequency of CpG dinucleotides. Both mutations were shown to cause exon 3 skipping in lymphoblastoid cells and transfection studies, respectively.

Subsequently, other IGHD II mutations that alter splicing but do not occur within the branch consensus, donor, or acceptor sites have been identified *(18)*. The first deletes 18 bp (IVS3 del+28-45) and the second is a G → A transition (IVS3 +28G → A) of IVS 3 (Fig. 5A). These mutations segregated with autosomal dominant GH deficiency in both

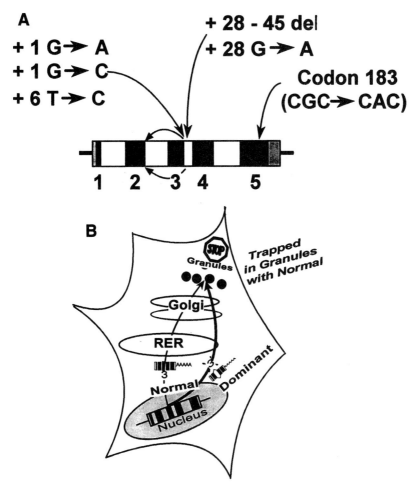

Fig. 5. Schematic representation of **(A)** the GH1 gene showing the locations of various IGHD II mutations and **(B)** hypothesized intracellular processing steps corresponding to the normal and IGHD II mutant allele products.

IGHD II kindreds and no other allelic changes were detected in their GH genes. RT-PCR amplification of transcripts from expression vectors containing the IVS3 del+28-45 or IVS3 +28G → A alleles yielded products showing a >10-fold preferred use of alternative splicing similar to findings previously reported by Cogan et al. 1996 for IVS3 donor site mutations. Examination of the mutations revealed they perturb an intronic XGGG repeat similar to the repeat found to regulate mRNA splicing in chicken β-tropomyosin.

Recently, Wajnrajch et al. *(19)* reported a family with IGHD II in which all affected family members were heterozygous for a G → A transition which results in an Arg → His substitution at residue 183 (Arg183His) of the GH molecule (Fig. 5A). They hypothesize that this substitution may alter the intracellular processing of the GH molecule by binding to zinc, thereby deranging the zinc-associated presecretory packaging of GH.

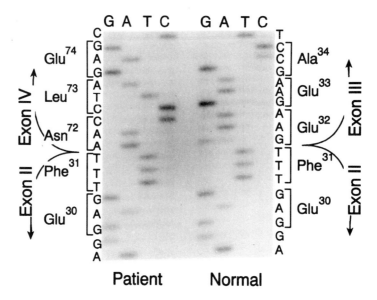

Fig. 6. DNA sequence analysis of normal **(A)** and IGHD II mutant **(B)** GH cDNAs showing exon III skipping in the latter.

IGHD III

IGHD III has an X-linked mode of inheritance, but distinct clinical findings in different families. Affected individuals in some kindreds have agammaglobulinemia associated with their IGHD, but others do not. This suggests that contiguous gene defects of Xq21.3 → q22 may occur in some cases. Interestingly, other cases of IGHD have been found to have an interstitial deletion of Xp22.3 or duplication of Xq13.3 → q 21.2 suggesting that multiple loci may cause IGHD III.

BIODEFECTIVE GH

Genetic Basis and Molecular Pathophysiology

Kowarski et al. *(20)* studied two unrelated boys, with growth retardation, delayed bone ages, low levels of somatomedin but normal GH levels after stimulation. Unlike those with Laron syndrome, exogenous human GH-induced normal levels of somatomedin and a significant increase in growth rate. While the family data did not support a specific mode of inheritance a mutation resulting in a biologically ineffective GH molecule was speculated. Valenta et al. *(21)* described a similar case and confirmed a structural abnormality of the GH molecule: 60–90% of circulating GH was in the form of tetramers and dimers (normal, 14–39% in plasma) and the patients' GH polymers were abnormally resistant to conversion into monomers by urea.

Subsequently, Takahashi et al. *(22)* reported a boy who was short at birth (39 cm at 41 wk gestation) and –6.1 SD below the mean at 4.9 yr when his bone age was 2 yr. He had normal body proportions except for a prominent forehead and a saddle nose. His IGF-I was 34 ng/mL (normal 35–293). Basal GH levels were 7–14 ng/mL and peak levels after insulin-induced hypoglycemia; arginine and levodopa administration were 38, 15, and 35 ng/mL, respectively. Nocturnal urinary GH excretion ranged from 58.8 to 76.7 pg/mg creatinine (normal, 7.1–41.1). Serum IGF-I were unchanged after 3 d of daily sc infections of 0.1 U of recombinant human GH/ kg of body weight (0.035 mg/kg). During prolonged treatment with GH (0.18 mg/kg/wk) his serum IGF-I was 200 ng/mL and his rate of linear growth increased to 6.0 cm/yr from 3.9 cm/yr before treatment. Assay of the bioactivity of his GH was below the normal range and isoelectric focusing of his serum showed an abnormal GH peak in addition to a normal peak, while serum from his father and normal controls contained only one peak. The proband was heterozygous for a C → T transition that encodes an Arg → Cys substitution at codon 77 (Arg77Cys) of his GH1 gene. Inexplicably, his father, who was also heterozygous for this mutation, was of normal height, had a peak GH level of 23.7 and normal isoelectric focusing results.

LARON SYNDROME

Genetic Basis and Molecular Pathophysiology

Laron syndrome is an autosomal recessive disorder caused by resistance to the action of GH because of proven defects at the growth hormone receptor (GHR) locus (OMIM# 262500) or theoretical postreceptor defects (OMIM# 245590). Laron syndrome is characterized by clinical GH deficiency manifest by short stature, delayed bone age, and occasionally blue sclera and hip degeneration. However, at the biochemical level, Laron syndrome subjects have low levels of IGF-1, despite their having normal or increased levels of GH (Fig. 1). This contrasts with the low levels of both IGF-1 and GH that are seen in GH deficiency and exogenous GH does not induce an IGF1 response or restore normal growth in Laron syndrome subjects. Whereas plasma levels of GH binding proteins (GHBP), which are derived from the extracellular domain of GHR, are usually low in Laron syndrome subjects, Woods et al. *(23)* described a homozygous point mutation in the intracellular domain of the GHR that caused Laron syndrome with elevated GHBP levels. They predicted that the mutant GHR would not be anchored in the cell membrane but would be measurable in the serum as GHBP, thus explaining the phenotype of severe GH resistance combined with elevated circulating GHBP.

Molecular analyses (OMIM# 262500) have identified heterogeneous exon deletions and base substitutions in the GHR genes of a large number of Laron syndrome patients. Berg et al. *(24)* reported ten different GHR mutations; one of which was a recurrent mutation involving a CpG dinucleotide hot spot. While treatment with exogenous GH is ineffective in those with GHR dysfunction replacement therapy with recombinant IGF-I has been shown to be effective.

GHRH RECEPTOR MUTATIONS

Genetic Basis and Molecular Pathophysiology

Lin et al. *(25)* demonstrated that the molecular basis for the "little" *(lit)* mouse phenotype, characterized by a hypoplastic anterior pituitary gland, is a point mutation in the growth hormone releasing factor receptor (GHRHR) gene that results in an Asp → Gly substitution at residue 60 (Asp60Gly). Anterior pituitaries of mutant mice showed spatially distinct proliferative zones of GH-producing stem cells and mature somatotrophs, each regulated by a different trophic factor.

Wajnrajch et al. *(26)* found a nonsense mutation in the human GHRHR gene in two first cousins, a boy and a girl, of a consanguineous Indian Moslem family with profound GH

Table 2
Mutations in the Pit-1 Genes of Subjects with Panhypopituitary Dwarfism

Mode	Codon[a]	Nucleotide change	Effect of mutation	Refs.
AR		del	Deletion of Pit-1 gene	30
	143	G → A	Amino acid change (Arg → Gln)	29
	158	G → C	Amino acid change (Ala → Pro)	30,31
	172	C → T	Generates a stop codon	28
AD	24	C → T	Amino acid change (Pro → Leu)	29
	271	C → T	Amino acid change (Arg → Trp)	34,35

[a]Codon number from the translation start site.

deficiency. The phenotypes of the 3.5-yr-old girl and her 16-yr-old cousin were poor growth since infancy and both were extremely short. They were prepubertal with frontal bossing and predominantly truncal obesity. While both failed to produce GH in response to standard provocative tests and to repetitive stimulation with GHRH, they responded to administration of GH. The affected individuals were homozygous for a G → T transversion at position 265 of their GHRHR genes resulting in a premature termination mutation (Glu72Stop). The mutation introduced a *Bfa*I restriction site into the amplified fragment that could be used for tracing the gene through the family. Wajnrajch et al. *(26)* noted that, since both GH releasing peptide, a synthetic hepapeptide, and nonpeptidyl benzamines can stimulate GH release without involvement of the GHRH receptor, they might be useful in therapy of this disorder. Subsequently, Maheshwan et al. *(27)* found the same GHRHR mutation in a isolate from the Indus valley of Pakistan.

COMBINED PITUITARY HORMONE DEFICIENCY

Genetic Basis and Molecular Pathophysiology

Combined pituitary hormone deficiency (CPHD) is a clinically and etiologically heterogeneous disorder characterized by deficiency of one or more of the other pituitary trophic hormones (ACTH, FSH, LH, or TSH) in addition to GH deficiency (OMIM# 262600). Although the great majority of cases are sporadic, there are also autosomal recessive, autosomal dominant, and X-linked forms. To date only the Pit-1 gene, in a small number of cases, has been associated with familial CPHD. Pit-1 is an anterior pituitary-specific transcription factor that regulates the expression of GH, PrL, and TSHβ. Pit-1 has also been shown to play an important role in pituitary cellular differentiation. Pit-1 is a member of the POU domain family of transcription factors and has three functional domains. The first domain is responsible for transactivation, whereas the other two domains, POU-specific and POU-homeo, are involved in DNA binding. At least six different autosomal recessive and two autosomal dominant Pit-1 mutations have been found in humans in a subtype of panhypopituitary dwarfism associated with GH, PrL and TSH deficiency (Table 2).

AUTOSOMAL RECESSIVE PIT-1 MUTATIONS

The first and second mutations were reported in two consanguineous Japanese families *(28,29)*. In one family, a C → T substitution in codon 172 converted a CGA(Arg) → TGA(Stop). Both parents were heterozygous and the affected child was homozygous for the mutation. In the second family, an G → A substitution in codon 143 changing a CGA(Arg) → CAA(Gln) was found. The patient was shown to be homozygous for this mutation whereas the parents and two unaffected siblings were shown to be heterozygous. Both mutations occur in the POU-specific domain and are believed to affect binding of the Pit-1 protein to the DNA.

The third and fourth Pit-1 mutations were found in two Dutch families who had postnatal growth failure with complete deficiencies of GH and PrL, whereas the T4 levels were low or normal prior to or following GH replacement *(30,31)*. Subjects having normal T4 levels were homozygous for a G → C substitution in codon 158 changing GCA(Ala) → CCA(Pro). This mutation interferes with formation of Pit-1 homodimers and dramatically reduces the altered Pit-1's ability to activate transcription. In the family with low T4 levels, the affected children were genetic compounds with one deleted and one Pit-1 gene with the previous mutation. These cases emphasize the importance of determining PrL levels and TSH responses to TRH in evaluating panhypopituitarism. Since GH and TSH deficiency often occur together, finding a low PrL level and absent TSH responses should raise the question of their having Pit-1 gene defects.

A fifth Pit-1 mutation was identified in a Thai patient with deficiency of GH, TSH, and PrL *(32)*. Both parents were healthy and found to be heterozygous for a G → T transversion in codon 250 which converted a GAA(Glu) → TAA(Stop) codon. The CPHD patient was found to be homozygous for the mutation. This mutation resulted in complete loss of the POU-homeodomain that is necessary for DNA binding.

A sixth Pit-1 mutation has been reported in a consanguineous family of Tunisian descent *(33)*. All four affected sibs were found to be homozygous for an T → G transversion in codon 135 converting a TTT(Phe) → TGT(Cys) in the POU-specific domain of Pit-1. The patients were found to have pituitary hypoplasia and deficiencies of GH, TSH, and PrL.

AUTOSOMAL DOMINANT PIT-1 MUTATIONS

The first dominant-negative mutation identified in the Pit-1 gene was a C → T substitution in codon 271 converting a CGG(Arg) → TGG(Trp) *(34,35)*. This mutation is located in the POU-homeodomain and does not affect binding of the mutant Pit-1 protein to DNA but functions as a dominant inhibitor of Pit-1 action by some, as of yet unknown mechanism. Three unrelated patients have been reported to be heterozygous for this mutation. Two of the patients were evaluated as adults and found to have pituitary hypoplasia and deficiencies of GH, PrL, and TSH. The third patient was identified at only 2 mo of age and found to have a normal pituitary and normal basal levels of TSH, but a delayed TSH response in a TRH stimulation test. The authors suggest that since Pit-1 may be necessary for anterior pituitary cell survival, the affected patient will develop hypoplasia and TSH deficiencies with age.

The second dominant-negative Pit-1 gene mutation was a C → T transition in the 24th codon converting a CCT(Pro) → CTT(Leu) *(29)*. This proline residue resides within the major transactivating domain of Pit-1 and is highly conserved in different species. The mechanism by which this mutation exerts its dominant-negative effect is also not known.

CURRENT PHARMACOLOGIC TREATMENT

Recombinant-derived GH is available worldwide and is administered by subcutaneous injection. To obtain an optimal outcome, children with GHD should be started on replacement therapy as soon as their diagnosis is established. The initial dosage of recombinant GH is based on body weight but the exact amount used and the frequency of administration may vary between different protocols. The dosage increases with increasing body weight to a maximum during puberty and is usually discontinued by ~17 yr of age (36,37).

Conditions that are treated with GH include those in which it has proven efficacy and a variety of others in which its use has been reported, but its use is not accepted as standard practice (38). Disorders in which GH treatment is of proven efficacy include GH deficiency, either isolated or in association with panhypopituitary dwarfism and Turner syndrome. The clinical responses of individuals with the first two disorders to GH replacement therapy varies depending on the severity and age at which treatment is begun, recognition and response to treatment of associated deficiencies, such as thyroid hormone deficiency, and if treatment is complicated by the development of anti-GH antibodies (39). The outcome of Turner syndrome subjects varies with the severity of their short stature, chromosomal complement, and age at which treatment was begun.

Additional disorders in which the use of GH has been reported but for which its efficacy is not accepted as standard practice include treatment of:

1. Selected skeletal dysplasias, such as achondroplasia;
2. Prader Willi syndrome;
3. Growth suppression secondary to exogenous steroids, such as chronic autoimmune diseases;
4. Chronic renal failure;
5. Extreme idiopathic short stature;
6. Russell–Silver syndrome; and
7. Intrauterine growth retardation.

There is, in general, insufficient data to establish the efficacy of GH replacement therapy in treating these disorders because of the limited number of subjects and lack of use of standardized protocols (40,41).

FUTURE DIRECTIONS

Several problems contribute to incomplete ascertainment of affected individuals, which in turn can result in less than optimal outcomes. These problems in ascertainment include the spectrum of severity, lack of a single provocative test that is both very sensitive and specific, and lack of an assay to test for qualitative changes in endogenous GH. Improvements in techniques that address these problems could facilitate the detection of and improve the outcome of treated patients in the future.

A number of genetic defects in GH biosynthesis (Tables 1 and 2) have been documented that prevent some affected individuals from secreting GH. These include those defects that result in the synthesis of truncated GH molecules, lack of GHRH receptor function, and mutant GH products that have dominant-negative effects on the normal GH products that are present. In the future, agonists of GH secretion, for example, those that complement the function of GHRH, may be found that can enhance release of the stored GH that is found in some of these cases. The efficacy of IGF-I in treating Laron dwarfism and IGHD patients who are resistant to exogenous GH because of anti-GH antibodies has been proven. Additional uses of IGF-1 or perhaps isoforms of IGF-1, which have prolonged half lives, may provide improved efficacy in the future.

Although potential applications of gene therapy to somatic cells are feasible, targeted and regulated expression that is pituitary specific remains impractical. Thus, potential applications of gene therapy to achieve appropriate hormonal regulation less dangerously than with exogenous GH replacement seem remote.

ACKNOWLEDGMENT

This work was supported in part by the NIH under Grant DK35592 (JAP), and by grants from the Genentech Foundation for Growth & Development (JDC and JAP).

REFERENCES

1. Carter-Su C, Schwartz J, Smit LS. Molecular mechanism of growth hormone action. Ann Rev Physiol 1996;58:187–207.
2. Argetsinger LS, Campbell GS, Yang X, Witthuhn BA, Silvennoinen O, et al. Identification of JAK2 as a growth hormone receptor-associated tyrosine kinase. Cell 1993;74:237–244.
3. Phillips JA III, Hjelle BL, Seeburg PH, Zachmann M. Molecular basis for familial isolated growth hormone deficiency. Proc Natl Acad Sci USA 1981;78:6372–6375.
4. Laron Z, Kelijman M, Pertzelan A, Keret R, Shoffner JM, Parks JS. Human growth hormone gene deletion without antibody formation or arrest during treatment—a new disease entity? Israel J Med Sci 1985;21:999–1006.
5. Matsuda I, Hata A, Jinno Y, Endo F, Akaboshi I, Nishi Y, et al. Heterogeneous phenotypes of Japanese cases with a growth hormone gene deletion. Jpn J Hum Genet 1987;32:227–235.
6. Vnencak-Jones CL, Phillips JA III, Chen EY, Seeburg PH. Molecular basis of human growth hormone gene deletions. Proc Natl Acad Sci USA 1988;85:5615–5619.
7. Vnencak-Jones CL, Phillips JA III, De-fen W. Use of polymerase chain reaction in detection of growth hormone gene deletions. J Clin Endo Metab 1990;70:1550–1553.
8. Mullis PE, Akinci A, Kanaka C, Eble A, Brook CGD. Prevalence of human growth hormone-1 gene deletions among patients with isolated growth hormone deficiency from different populations. Pediat Res 1992;31:532–534.
9. Duquesnoy P, Amselem S, Gourmelen M, LeBouc Y, Goossens M. A frameshift mutation causing isolated growth hormone deficiency type 1A. Am J Hum Genet 1990;47:A110.
10. Cogan JD, Phillips JA III, Sakati N, Frisch H, Schober E, Milner RDG. Heterogeneous growth hormone (GH) gene mutations in familial GH deficiency. J Clin Endo Metab 1993;76:1224–1228.
11. Cogan JD, Phillips JA III, Schenkman SS, Milner RDG, Sakati N. Familial growth hormone deficiency: a model of dominant and recessive mutations affecting a monomeric protein. J Clin Endo Metab 1994;79:1261–1265.
12. Miller-Davis S, Phillips JA III, Milner RDG, Al-Ashwal A, Sakati NA, Summar ML. Detection of mutations in GH genes and transcripts by analysis of DNA from dried blood spots and mRNA from lymphoblastoid cells. Endocr Soc Prog Abstr 1993;333.
13. Abdul-Latif HD, Brown MR, Parks JS, et al. Mutation of intron 4 of the GH-1 gene causes GH deficiency. Endocr Soc Prog Abstr 1995;470.
14. Igarashi Y, Ogawa M, Kamijo T, Iwatani N, Nishi Y, Kohno H, et al. A new mutation causing inherited growth hormone deficiency: a compound heterozygote of a 6.7 kb deletion and two base deletion in the third exon of the GH-1 gene. Hum Mol Genet 1993;2:1073,1074.
15. Cogan JD, Ramel B, Lehto M. A recurring dominant-negative mutation causes autosomal dominant growth hormone deficiency. J Clin Endo Metab 1995;80:3591–3595.
16. Phillips JA III, Cogan JD. Genetic basis of endocrine disease 6: molecular basis of familial human growth hormone deficiency. J Clin Endocr 1994;78:11–16.
17. Binder G, Ranke MB. Screening for growth hormone (GH) gene splice-site mutations in sporadic cases with severe isolated GH deficiency using ectopic transcript analysis. J Clin Endo Metab 1995;80:1247–1252.
18. Cogan JD, McCarthy EMS, Prince MA, Lekhakula S, Futrakul A, Bundey S, et al. A novel mechanism of aberrant pre-mRNA splicing in humans. Hum Mol Genet 1997;6:909–912.
19. Wajnrajch MP, Gertner JM, Moshang T, Saenger P, Leibel RL. Isolated growth hormone (GH) deficiency, type II (IGHD II) caused by substitution of arginine by histidine in c-terminal portion of the GH molecule. Endocr Soc Prog Abstr 1996;P2–313.

20. Kowarski AA, Schneider JJ, Ben-Galim E, Weldon VV, Daughaday WH. Growth failure with normal serum RIA-GH and low somatomedin activity: somatomedin restoration and growth acceleration after exogenous GH. J Clin Endocr 1978;47:461–464.
21. Valenta LJ, Sigel MB, Lesniak MA, Elias AN, Lewis UJ, Friesen HG, et al. Pituitary dwarfism in a patient with circulating abnormal growth hormone polymers. N Engl J Med 1985;312:214–217.
22. Takahashi Y, Kaji H, Okimura Y, Goji K, Abe H, Chihara K. Brief report: short stature caused by a mutant growth hormone. N Engl J Med 1996;334:432–436.
23. Woods KA, Fraser NC, Postel-Vinay MC, Savage MO, Clark AJL. A homozygous splice site mutation affecting the intracellular domain of the growth hormone (GH) receptor resulting in Laron syndrome with elevated GH-binding protein. J Clin Endo Metab 1996;81:1686–1690.
24. Berg MA, Argente J, Chernausek S, Gracia R, Guevara-Aguirre J, Hopp M, et al. Diverse growth hormone receptor gene mutations in Laron syndrome. Am J Hum Genet 1993;52:998–1005.
25. Lin SC, Lin CR, Gukovsky I, Lusis AJ, Sawchenko PE, Rosenfeld MG. Molecular basis of the little mouse phenotype and implications for cell type-specific growth. Nature 1993;364:208–213.
26. Wajnrajch MP, Gertner JM, Harbison MD, Chua SC Jr, Leibel RL. Nonsense mutation in the human growth hormone-releasing hormone receptor causes growth failure analogous to the little (lit) mouse. Nature Genet 1996;12:88–90.
27. Baumann G, Maheshwari H. The dwarfs of Sindh: severe growth hormone (GH) deficiency caused by a mutation in the GH-releasing hormone receptor gene. Acta Paediatr Sup 1997;423:33–38.
28. Tatsumi K, Miyai K, Notomi T, Kaibe K, Amino N, Mizuno Y, et al. Cretinism with combined pituitary hormone deficiency caused by a mutation in the PIT1 gene. Nature Genet 1992;1:56–58.
29. Ohta K, Nobukuni Y, Mitsubuchi H, et al. Mutations in the Pit-1 gene in children with combined pituitary hormone deficiency. Biochem Biophys Res Commun 1992;189:851–855.
30. Wit JM, Drayer NM, Jansen M, Walenkamp MJ, Hackeng WHL, Thijssen JHH, et al. Total deficiency of growth hormone and prolactin, and partial deficiency of thyroid stimulating hormone in two Dutch families: a new variant of hereditary pituitary deficiency. Hormone Res 1989;32:170–177.
31. Pfaffle RW, DiMattia GE, Parks JS, Brown MR, Wit JM, Jansen M, et al. Mutation of the POU-specific domain of Pit-1 and hypopituitarism without pituitary hypoplasia. Science 1992;257:1118–1121.
32. Irie Y, Tatsumi K, Ogawa M, Kamijo T, Preeyasombat C, Suprasongsin C, et al. A novel E250X mutation of the PIT1 gene in a patient with combined pituitary hormone deficiency. Endo J 1995;42:351–354.
33. Pelligrini-Bouiller I, Belicar P, Barlier A, Gunz G, Charvet JP, Jauet P, et al. A new mutation of the gene encoding the transcription factor Pit-1 is responsible for combined pituitary hormone deficiency. J Clin Endo Metab 1996;81:2790–2796.
34. Radovick S, Nation M, Du Y, Bergh LA, Weintraub BD, Wondisford FE. A mutation in the POU-homeodomain of Pit-1 responsible for combined pituitary hormone deficiency. Science 1992;257:1115–1118.
35. Cohen LE, Wondisford FE, Salvantoni A, et al. A hot spot in the Pit-1 gene responsible for combined pituitary hormone deficiency: clinical and molecular correlates. J Clin Endo Metab 1995;80:679–684.
36. Ranke MB. Growth hormone therapy in children: when to stop? Hormone Res 1995;43:122–125.
37. Rosen T, Johannsson G, Johansson JO, Bengtsson BA. Consequences of growth hormone deficiency in adults and the benefits and risks of recombinant human growth hormone treatment. Hormone Res 1995;43:93–99.
38. Strasburger CJ. Implications of investigating the structure-function relationship of human growth hormone in clinical diagnosis and therapy. Hormone Res 1994;41:113–120.
39. Illig R. Growth hormone antibodies in patients treated with different preparations of human growth hormone (HGH). J Clin Endo Metab 1970;31:679–688.
40. Neely EK, Rosenfeld RG. Use and abuse of human growth hormone. Ann Rev Med 1994;45:407–420.
41. Wyatt DT, Mark D, Slyper A. Survey of growth hormone treatment practices by 251 pediatric endocrinologists. J Clin Endo Metab 1995;80:3292–3297.

4

The Molecular Basis of Hypophosphatemic Rickets

Michael J. Econs, MD and Tim M. Strom, MD

CONTENTS

INTRODUCTION

Several hereditary disorders of isolated phosphate wasting have been described. These include X-linked hypophosphatemic rickets (HYP), autosomal dominant hypophosphatemic rickets (ADHR), hypophosphatemic bone disease (HBD), and hereditary hypophosphatemic rickets with hypercalciuria (HHRH). Phosphate wasting is also a prominent feature of the CLCN-5 disorders, including Dents disease, X-linked recessive nephrolithiasis (XRN) and X-linked recessive hypophosphatemic rickets (XLRH). The large number of hereditary renal phosphate wasting disorders indicates that control over renal phosphate homeostasis is a complex process. Investigators are starting to find genes that when mutated result in renal phosphate wasting. The discovery of these genes provides insights into phosphate homeostasis and helps to elucidate the pathophysiology of these disorders. Additionally, in some instances, the isolation of a disease gene allows clinicians to combine what were previously thought to be distinct disorders into one disorder.

X-LINKED HYPOPHOSPHATEMIC RICKETS

X-linked hypophosphatemic rickets (HYP) is the most common form of hereditary renal phosphate wasting with a prevalence of approx 1:20,000 *(1)*. The hallmark of this disease is isolated renal phosphate wasting with inappropriately normal calcitriol concentrations. An osteoblast defect has also been proposed to contribute to impaired

From: *Molecular and Cellular Pediatric Endocrinology*
Edited by: S. Handwerger © Humana Press Inc., Totowa, NJ

mineralization in the disorder *(see below)*. Classically, patients present with lower extremity deformities, rickets, growth retardation, bone pain, tooth abscesses, enthesopathy, and osteomalacia *(2)*. However, the severity of the disease is variable and affected members of the same family, who have the same genetic defect, may have markedly different phenotypes. HYP is an X-linked dominant disorder, and although controversy exists regarding whether there is a gene dosage effect, the available evidence suggests that males and females are affected equally *(3)*.

Much of our understanding of the pathophysiology of HYP has been derived from the two mouse models, the Hyp and Gy mice. In accord with the human disease, these mice have renal phosphate wasting, impaired mineralization and growth retardation. Linkage studies have mapped the two mutations to a region of the mouse X chromosome that is syntenic to the human HYP locus *(4,5)*. Both murine models have renal phosphate wasting, impaired mineralization, and growth retardation *(6,7)*. However, the Gy mouse also has inner ear abnormalities, deafness, hyperactivity, and circling behavior *(7)*. The Gy mouse is bred on the B6C3H background and the Hyp mouse is bred on the C57BL/6J background. Of note, the male Gy mouse does not survive on the C57BL/6J background *(8)*. As with the human disease there does not appear to be a marked difference in severity between male and female Hyp mice *(9)*, however, less data are available for the Gy.

The etiology of the phosphate wasting defect has been examined in the Hyp mouse. This defect has been directly demonstrated in the brush border membrane of the renal proximal tubule *(10)*. More recent studies demonstrate that the phosphate wasting in the proximal tubule is caused by a defect in the high-affinity/low-capacity sodium-dependent phosphate cotransport system *(11)*. This transporter (NPT-2) has recently been cloned *(12)* and the Hyp mutation results in an approx 50% decrease in NPT-2 mRNA and protein *(13,14)*. Tenenhouse et al. *(15)* report that the Gy mutations also results in an approx 50% decrease in NPT-2 mRNA and protein. However, Collins and Gishan *(16)* assert that HYP and Gy mice differ in this regard since they find normal levels of NPT-2 mRNA in the Gy, but decreased levels of NPT-2 protein in the Gy. Since human NPT-2 is located on chromosome 5q35 it is not a candidate gene for HYP *(17)*. However, the data suggest that the HYP gene is involved in regulation of NPT-2 expression and/or turnover.

Despite these results is was unclear as to whether the phosphate wasting results from a primary renal defect or whether the phosphate wasting is the result of elaboration of a humoral factor that alters phosphate transport in the renal proximal tubule. In this regard, Meyer et al. performed parabiosis experiments using Hyp and normal mice *(18)*. In these experiments mice are surgically joined together and vascular channels are allowed to develop between the animals resulting in crosscirculation between the two parabiosed animals. After performing these experiments they found that normal mice joined to Hyp mice had a progressive reduction in plasma phosphate over 3 wk and the normal mice joined to Hyp mice had a greater renal phosphate excretion index than normal mice joined to other normal mice. Furthermore, after separating the normal/Hyp pairs, plasma phosphate returned to normal in the normal mouse within 24 h and after 2 and 7 d these normal mice had "rebound hyperphosphatemia" as compared to mice separated from normal/normal pairs *(18)*.

Since parabiosis experiments have significant limitations, Nesbitt et al. *(19)* performed renal crosstransplantation between Hyp and normal mice. They found that when normal kidneys were transplanted into nephrectomized Hyp mice, the kidneys wasted phosphorus, but when Hyp kidneys were transplanted into nephrectomized normal mice, the kidneys retained phosphorus normally. Thus, the defect in the Hyp mouse is neither corrected nor transferred by renal crosstransplantation, indicating that the phosphate transport defect in the Hyp mouse is not caused by an intrinsic renal abnormality.

The above studies demonstrate that the defect in the Hyp mouse, and probably in the human disease, is not in the kidney. However, they do not establish which tissues are defective. Some investigators have focused on the osteoblast since there is a mineralization defect in the Hyp mouse. Ecarot et al. *(20,21)* transplanted periostea and osteoblasts from normal and Hyp mice into the gluteal muscles of normal and Hyp mice. As anticipated, when normal cells were transplanted into Hyp mice mineralization was impaired. However, when Hyp cells were transplanted into normal mice, reduction, but not normalization of the defect was observed leading these investigators to conclude that there is an intrinsic osteoblast defect in the Hyp mouse. Although these studies supported the hypothesis that there is a primary osteoblast defect in the Hyp mouse, they did not exclude the possibility that the putative circulating factor in the Hyp mouse could have led to an irreversible developmental defect in the Hyp osteoblast. Such a situation would be analogous to the permanent developmental defects that are produced in developing neural tissue by lack of sufficient thyroid hormone at a critical stage of development *(22)*.

An intrinsic osteoblast defect was also postulated by Lajeunesse et al. *(23)* who studied the effects of Hyp serum and Hyp osteoblast conditioned media on phosphate transport in primary mouse proximal tubule cultures (MPTC). They found that Hyp serum, when added to the culture media for at least 24 h, impaired phosphate transport in MPTC in a dose-dependent fashion. Furthermore, conditioned media from Hyp osteoblasts, but not normal osteoblasts, also inhibited phosphate transport in the MPTC. These data suggest that the Hyp osteoblast is responsible for the release and/or modification of a humoral factor(s) that inhibits phosphate reabsorption *(23)*. Whether the osteoblast is solely responsible for the production and/or modification of this factor or whether another cell type plays an important role in the pathogenesis of the phosphate wasting cannot be determined by these studies. However, these studies do implicate the osteoblast as a potentially important cell in maintenance of phosphate homeostasis.

The possibility that a hormonal factor plays a role in phosphate wasting is supported by existence of tumor induced osteomalacia. These tumors, which are frequently of mesenchymal origin, result in renal phosphate wasting and inappropriately low serum calcitriol concentrations. Both the phosphate wasting and low calcitriol concentrations resolve when the tumor is removed. Since tumors frequently secrete, in abnormal amounts and in an unregulated fashion, substances that have a role in normal physiology, it is plausible that the phosphate wasting observed in patients who have tumor induced osteomalacia is caused by overproduction of a factor(s) that normally controls renal phosphate reabsorption. We have referred to this factor as "phosphatonin" *(24)*. Unfortunately, this factor has only been partially purified *(25,26)* and its role in the phosphate wasting seen in HYP has yet to be determined.

Vitamin D Metabolism

In the setting of hypophosphatemia, increased calcitriol (1,25OH vitamin D) concentrations are anticipated since this is one of the homeostatic mechanisms that is present to return serum phosphate concentrations to normal. However, several investigators have found normal serum calcitriol concentrations in HYP patients (27–29). Thus, HYP patients have a relative insufficiency of calcitriol. Studies in the Hyp mouse confirm and expand the human observations. 25(OH)D-1α-hydroxylase, the enzyme that converts 25OH vitamin D into 1,25OH vitamin D, plays an important role in determining serum calcitriol concentrations. Lobaugh and Drezner (30) studied the activity of this enzyme in Hyp mice and compared it to normal mice on control and phosphate deplete diets. Normal mice on phosphate deplete diets profoundly increased 1α-hydroxylase activity compared to normal mice on the control diet whereas Hyp mice had a much lesser increment in 1α-hydroxylase despite having serum phosphorus concentrations that were similar to the phosphate deplete mice. Moreover, other investigators have found that the catabolism of 1,25(OH)$_2$D$_3$ is increased in Hyp mice as compared to controls (31,32).

Unfortunately, studies of 1α-hydroxylase activity in the Gy mouse are more controversial. Davidai et al. (33) found that activity of renal 25(OH)D-1α-hydroxylase in the Gy mouse was similar to that of normal mice on phosphate depleted diets, but much greater than that of normal mice on control diets. They concluded that, unlike the Hyp mouse, 1α-hydroxylase activity is appropriately regulated in the Gy mouse. Tenenhouse et al. (34) were unable to detect a statistically significant difference in calcitriol concentrations between Gy and normal mice on control diets, although there was a trend for Gy mice to have higher calcitriol concentrations. However, when Gy and normal mice were placed on phosphate restricted diets normal mice appropriately increased their calcitriol concentration, but the calcitriol concentration in phosphate deplete Gy mice paradoxically dropped substantially below that of Gy mice on the control diet. Meyer et al. (35) studied Gy and Hyp mice that were both bred on the B6C3H background (the background on which the Gy mice are usually bred). They did not find a difference in calcitriol concentrations between Hyp and Gy mice. However, both Hyp and Gy mice calcitriol concentrations were substantially effected by calcium concentrations in the diet. Thus, it is possible that much of the observed difference in vitamin D metabolism between Gy and Hyp mice was secondary to differences in background strain and diet. These findings are important since several investigators have asserted that the Hyp and Gy mice arose from mutations in two different genes, particularly in light of the occurrence of a recombination event between the two mutations (7). However, a definitive answer to this question required cloning the gene and characterizing the mutations.

Positional Cloning of the PEX Gene

Despite extensive study, as outlined above, the pathophysiology of HYP has not been fully elucidated. To gain a better understanding of the disorder we used the positional cloning approach to map and clone the HYP gene. (For a review of how this was accomplished see ref. 36.) The positional cloning approach has two major advantages: It does not require the investigator to make any assumptions about the gene's function and knowledge of tissue expression, although helpful, is not required. This approach is becoming more commonplace and it has been used to clone a wide variety of disease genes (37).

To locate a gene by the positional cloning approach investigators first use linkage analysis to determine the chromosomal location of the gene. Once a general location is known, they perform additional linkage analysis with multiple genetic markers from the region to find two markers that closely flank the disease gene. Subsequently, the investigators construct a "contig" map of human DNA between the flanking genetic markers.

They use this contig to identify genes contained within the contig and test these genes for mutation in affected individuals.

Early linkage studies by Machler et al. and Read et al. placed the HYP gene on Xp22 *(38,39)*. Subsequently, Thakker et al. *(40)* found that DXS41 and DXS43 are flanking markers for the HYP gene, but the distance between these markers was far to great to consider creating a contig map with the available technology. To refine the genetic map around the HYP locus we tested several restriction fragment length genetic markers in the Xp22 region for linkage to the HYP gene in five large kindreds *(41)*. We determined that HYP is located between DXS257 on the telomeric side and DXS41 on the centromeric side. The distance between these two flanking markers is approx 3.5 c*M*. Unfortunately, although the marker DXS365 was tightly linked to HYP [$Z_{(\theta)} = 13.98$ at $\theta = 0.0$] we were unable to locate DXS365 with respect to HYP since there were no recombination events between DXS365 and HYP. Indeed, the RFLP for DXS365 was not informative in the one mating that demonstrated a recombination event between DXS257 and HYP *(41)*. To be an informative mating the affected parent of the recombinant individual must be heterozygous for the marker. Additional linkage data obtained by Rowe et al. *(42)* determined that DXS274 was also linked to the HYP gene [$Z_{(\theta)} = 4.2$ at $\theta = 0.0$], but they were unable to locate it with respect to HYP since there were no recombination events between the RFLP DXS274 and HYP. Since tightly linked flanking markers are necessary prerequisites to obtain the HYP gene by positional cloning techniques, we extended our linkage studies to include an additional large HYP kindred to enable us to determine the positions of DXS365 and DXS274 relative to the HYP gene *(43)*.

Using the expanded family resources we demonstrated that DXS365 is telomeric to the HYP gene and DXS274 is centromeric to the gene *(43)*. Simultaneously, Rowe et al. *(44)* made a microsatellite repeat marker for DXS274. Microsatellite repeat markers are multiallele markers *(45)* that are generally more polymorphic than RFLPs. As a result they tend to have far fewer noninformative matings. Combining their results for the microsatellite repeat for DXS274 and the RFLP for DXS274 Rowe et al. determined that DXS274 lies centromeric to the HYP gene and telomeric to DXS41 *(44)*. Thus, the locus order supported by the above studies was Xtel-DXS43-(DXS257/DXS365)-HYP-DXS274-DXS41-Xcen, where a "/" between loci indicates that the order between them could not be determined. To determine the relative location of DXS257 and DXS365 we combined HYP kindreds from two groups of investigators *(43,44)* and analyzed recombination events in these families with a newly available microsatellite repeat for DXS365 *(46)*. Our data demonstrated that DXS365 was centromeric to DXS257 and was the closest telomeric marker to HYP *(47)*. The new order was now Xtel-DXS43-DXS257-DXS365-HYP-DXS274-DXS41-Xcen.

The flanking markers, DXS365 on the telomeric side and DXS274 on the centromeric side, were now close enough to try to bridge the distance between them with yeast artificial chromosomes (YAC). YACs are yeast vectors that contain large pieces of human DNA (up to 1 Mb) and can be propagated in yeast *(48)*. DXS365 and DXS274, and/or cosmids that contained these probes, were used to screen YAC libraries *(49)*. This screening identified four nonchimeric YACs on the centromeric side and two nonchimeric YACs on the telomeric side. To complete the contig we isolated a cosmid from the telomeric end of one of the centromeric YACs and used this cosmid to rescreen the YAC library. This "walking" technique allowed us to isolate several new YAC clones. One of these YAC clones overlapped with one of the YACs that was obtained by the initial library screen with DXS365, the telomeric marker. Thus, the distance between the two flanking markers DXS365, on the telomeric side, and DXS274, on the centromeric side, was spanned by a 3 YAC contig that covered approx 1.5 Mb of genomic DNA *(49)*.

To further define the region we developed new microsatellite markers, DXS1683 and DXS7474, from two of the YACs *(50,51)*. Both of these markers were physically mapped to lie on opposite ends of the YAC in the center of the contig *(49)*. We tested these markers in 20 large HYP kindreds. Two recombinants were seen between DXS1683 and HYP. Both of these matings placed DXS1683 on the centromeric side of the HYP gene *(47)*. Similarly, there were two recombination events between DXS7474 and HYP which placed DXS7474 telomeric to HYP *(52)*. These results allowed us to place the HYP gene on one YAC between DXS1683 and DXS7474 in a physical distance of approx 350 kb *(52)*.

Since the distance between the new flanking markers is relatively short and since cosmids have several advantages over YACs, we constructed a cosmid contig *(53)* across the region. The cosmid contig allowed us to change our approach to mutation detection. In addition to trying to isolate cDNAs from the HYP region and test them for mutation in our 20 large kindreds, we used the cosmids to screen large numbers of affected individuals for deletions. These affected individuals were either members of small kindreds that were not suitable for linkage studies or were isolated cases. Through the collaborative efforts of the five laboratories that make up the HYP consortium *(53)*, we obtained DNA samples from approx 150 unrelated affected individuals. We looked for deletions by hybridizing whole cosmids to Southern blots of restriction enzyme digested genomic DNA from these individuals. Although we did not think that deletions would be common in this disease, the detection of even one deletion with a cosmid would be a strong indication that the cosmid contained the HYP gene.

We found three affected individuals who demonstrated deletions in DNA contained within cosmid 611 and we found a fourth affected individual who demonstrated a small (approx 1 kb) deletion within cosmid 1005, which lies immediately centromeric to cosmid 611 *(53)*. This latter deletion does not overlap with the other three deletions. Thus, we focused our efforts on these cosmids.

Cloning the PEX Gene

To clone the gene the members of the HYP consortium employed three complementary approaches. We used the cosmids that were identified by patient deletions to screen cDNA libraries made from fetal brain, fetal liver, and adult muscle. We also performed exon trapping *(54)* to detect exons from genes that were contained within the contig. Additionally, we performed automated sequencing of the cosmids and used standard computer programs to search for exons within the genomic sequence. All three lines of investigation revealed the presence of a candidate gene in the region. Sequence analysis of this gene indicated that it contains significant homology at the peptide level to the M13 family of endopeptidase genes, which includes neutral endopeptidase, endothelin-converting enzyme-1 and 2 (ECE-1 and 2) and the Kell antigen. Further analysis revealed that in all four patients who had deletions, the deletions involved at least one exon from this gene *(53)*. We labeled this gene "PEX" for *p*hosphate regulating gene with homologies to *e*ndopeptidases on the *X* chromosome.

As is typical for the M13 endopeptidases, PEX has the 10 conserved cysteines that are seen in other members of this class and it has a short N-terminal cytoplasmic domain and a single transmembrane domain. Thus, most of the molecule is in the extracellular space. There are two conserved zinc binding motifs, one of which is conserved in most of the metalloendopepdiases (exon17) and one of which is conserved in the M13 (exon19) family *(53,55)*. Cloning the human PEX gene has led to relatively rapid cloning of the mouse Pex gene, which has high homology to human PEX *(56,57)*. Of interest, neither the human nor murine PEX/Pex genes have "classic" Kozak sequences *(58)*. PEX is one of only 3% of known genes that does not have a purine at the −3 position before the ATG initiation sequence *(55–57)*. This finding may be significant since, in general, genes that do not have good Kozak sequences tend to be posttranscriptionally regulated *(59)*.

Although little is known about the Kell blood group protein, endothelin converting enzyme 1 and 2 and neutral endopeptidase function as ectoenzymes. Neutral endopeptidase degrades/inactivates several small peptides including substance P, bradykinin, and enkephalins *(60)*. Endothelin converting enzyme 1 and 2, on the other hand, serve to convert Big endothelin to endothelin, the active form *(61,62)*. Thus, it is likely that PEX functions to either activate or degrade a peptide hormone.

EXPRESSION PATTERN

Although RT-PCR can be used to amplify PEX from lymphocyte and fetal brain RNA *(53)*, it is not likely that these are the physiologically relevant tissues of expression. PEX is probably expressed in teeth since database searches *(55)* identified a highly significant match between the 5' end of PEX and an expressed sequence tag containing the 5' end of a rat incisor cDNA clone, which is likely to be the 5' UTR of the rat homolog of PEX (Genebank accession number R47026). Indeed, defective PEX functioning in teeth may predispose HYP patients to dental abscesses, which occur in 55% of HYP patients *(63)*. Du et al. *(56)* detected a 6.6 kb transcript in mouse bone and mouse osteoblasts with Northern blots using a mouse Pex cDNA. In light of the experiments that demonstrate an osteoblast defect in Hyp mice, it is not surprising that PEX is expressed in the osteoblast. However, it is too early to conclude that the osteoblast plays a central role in the phosphate wasting that is seen in this disease. In a more recent study, Beck et al. *(64)* detected Pex message from mouse calvaria, long bone, and lung and, to a lesser extent, brain, testis, and muscle by RT-PCR. They did not find Pex message in mouse kidney, heart, or liver. These findings in bone and lung were confirmed by RNase protection assay, a method that requires greater expression levels than RT-PCR. Of note, levels of expression of Pex are two orders of magnitude less than that of B actin *(64)*. They also detected Pex expression on northern blots of poly A RNA from mouse bone and lung. These authors also looked for PEX expression in human fetal tissues. They found expression by RT-PCR in calvaria, long bone, lung, ovary, and skeletal muscle *(64)*. RNase protection confirmed expression in calvaria, ovary, lung, and muscle. Of note, PEX expression was approximately seven times more abundant in calvaria than in lung, ovary, or muscle *(64)*. Additional data is provided by Grieff et al. *(65)* who found PEX expression in adult ovary and lung as well as fetal lung and liver. In light of these findings there are several tissues that could play a role in phosphate homeostasis and PEX may have roles in processes unrelated to phosphate homeostasis.

PEX MUTATIONS

Although the PEX deletions that we found in four patients were consistent with PEX being the HYP gene, it was possible, although unlikely, that these deletions also involved another gene, which was the "real" HYP gene. To establish with certainty that PEX was the HYP gene, we looked for point mutations in our HYP patients. In our initial efforts, we detected a frameshift mutation caused by the loss of a TC dinucleotide in exon 6. We also found two point mutations in the splice acceptor site of exon 7. These two mutations led to exon skipping (53). More recent efforts (55,66) have demonstrated mutations in almost every exon and PEX mutations have been found by other investigators (67–69). Although mutation detection is still ongoing, there does not appear to be a single common mutation that results in the HYP phenotype. Additionally, the mutations described so far, appear to be loss of function mutations.

Recent success in cloning the mouse Pex gene (56,57) provides an opportunity to interpret previous studies of Gy and Hyp mice in a new light. Since there are phenotypic differences and an alleged biochemical difference between Hyp and Gy mice several investigators have proposed that there were two separate genes that when mutated resulted in phosphate wasting (8,33,70). The occurrence of a single recombinant event (7) between these two mutations further misled investigators to assume that two closely linked genes that regulated phosphate transport existed on the X chromosome. Strom et al. (57) have determined that the Hyp mouse has a deletion of the last 7 Pex exons and the Gy mouse has a deletion at the 5' end of the gene that involves the first 3 exons and an undetermined amount of upstream sequence. The human PEX gene covers a distance of over 220 kb of genomic DNA (55) and it is likely that the mouse Pex gene covers a similar distance. Since the Hyp and Gy mutation occur at opposite ends of the gene it is not surprising that a recombination event occurred between the two deletions.

Despite the fact that the Hyp and Gy both have mutations in Pex, there are still phenotypic differences between the two mutants. One enticing possibility is that the location of the mutations affects the phenotype. However, both mutations appear to lead to loss of gene function. Alternatively, one or both of the deletions may involve another gene in the region that may influence the overall phenotype. Indeed it is quite likely that the Gy mutation may involve another gene since the Gy male does not survive on the C57BL/6J background (8). Part of the phenotypic differences observed between the two murine mutants may be secondary to background strain differences. Of note, when Hyp mice are bred on to the B6C3H background (the background on which the Gy mouse is bred) some of the mice circle (8). Additionally, as noted above, differences in the biochemical manifestations of the mutations may be related to background strain and dietary differences. In any event, the identification of the Hyp and Gy mutations provides strong evidence that Pex is the only phosphate regulating gene on this portion of the X chromosome.

Possible Roles for PEX in Normal Phosphate Homeostasis

Despite that fact that mutations in the PEX gene are responsible for X-linked hypophosphatemic rickets, its role in pathophysiology of HYP is not immediately obvious. Several observations should be taken into account when considering possible mechanisms. First, HYP is an X-linked dominant disorder with little, if any, gene dosage effect. In this regard, it is possible that mutations in the PEX gene result in a dominant negative effect. Alternatively, HYP could be a haploinsufficiency disorder in which having half the normal amount of PEX gene could result in the disease phenotype. This later possibility is supported by the murine Gy mutation, which involves the 5' end of the Pex gene and should result in lack of message production. Second, as noted above, the Hyp and Gy mouse mutations result in decreased levels of NPT-2, the high-affinity/low-capacity sodium-dependent phosphate cotransporter. Thus, it is likely that one PEX function is to directly or indirectly regulate the expression of this transporter. Third, studies demonstrating PEX expression in osteoblasts and those studies that demonstrate an osteoblast defect in the Hyp mouse indicate that the osteoblast defect is responsible for at least part of the mineralization abnormalities that are seen in the disease. These studies also indicate that osteoblast could play a role in regulating phosphate homeostasis, although there is currently insufficient data to fully support this contention. Fourth, the existence of tumors that secrete "phosphatonin" as well as parabiosis data in the Hyp mouse support the notion that the pathophysiology of the disease involves the elaboration of a humoral phosphate wasting factor. Since PEX mutations, which result in the disease phenotype, are loss of function mutations and not activating mutations, it is clear that PEX is not "phosphatonin." However, the PEX gene product may play a role in regulating the concentration of phosphatonin.

In this regard, there are several possible roles for the normal PEX protein in phosphate homeostasis. Since PEX is a member of the neutral endopeptidase family, it is possible that PEX serves to degrade/inactivate phosphatonin. Thus, mutations in PEX could interfere with this process and result in excessive concentrations of phosphatonin. However, if this is the case, one might predict that parabiosis between a Hyp and normal mouse would rescue the Hyp phenotype (i.e., the normal Pex protein should be able to degrade excessive phosphatonin from the mutant animal). However, parabiosis did not rescue the Hyp phenotype. Instead, normal mice, when parabiosed to Hyp mice, waste phosphate *(18)*. Although resolution of this apparent discrepancy awaits additional data, it is possible that the kidney is exposed to the high phosphatonin level before the PEX protein has a chance to degrade the phosphatonin. Alternatively, the normal animal may not be able to adequately upregulate PEX to metabolize the excessive quantities of phosphatonin that are generated by the mutant animal. Another potential mechanism of action that is keeping with an enzymatic role for PEX is that, under normal circumstances, PEX could function to activate a phosphate conserving hormone. This possibility has become more plausible in light of recent data that human staniocalcin stimulates phosphate reabsorption when administered to rats *(71)*. However, this model would also predict that parabiosis of normal mouse to Hyp mouse would rescue the Hyp phenotype. An additional possibility that fits in with the currently available data is that the PEX gene indirectly functions to inhibit the expression of phosphatonin. Thus, mutations of the PEX gene would result in over expression of phosphatonin and lead to renal phosphate wasting. Although this model does not conflict with available data, there is currently very little data that addresses this question.

Adult Onset Vitamin D Resistant Hypophosphatemic Osteomalacia

Despite recognition that there is variability in the clinical spectrum of HYP, one group of investigators has proposed that there are two forms of X-linked hypophosphatemic rickets. Frymoyer and Hodgkin *(72)* described a 133-person kindred with what they referred to as "adult onset vitamin D resistant hypophosphatemic osteomalacia." The inheritance pattern was consistent with X-linked dominant transmission. Hypophosphatemic young adults had minimal femoral bowing and older adults (defined as over age 40) were "progressively disabled by severe bowing" *(72)*. In several instances, radiographs from adults demonstrated bone overgrowth at tendonous insertions (enthesopathy) as is seen in HYP. There were 14 hypophosphatemic children in the kindred. Moderate bowing was observed in one 17-yr-old who had closed epiphyses.

Although "mild femoral bowing" was observed in some of the other 13 children, none of these affected children had radiographic evidence of rickets. Based largely on this lack of radiographically evident rickets, these authors concluded that there are two forms of X-linked hypophosphatemic rickets.

Since the absence of radiographic evidence of rickets was used to define this new disease, we tested the hypothesis that radiographic evidence of rickets is an invariant feature of HYP. To perform these studies we obtained radiographs from affected children who were from several well established HYP families. We found rachitic abnormalities in 5 of 11 wrist radiographs and 13 of 15 knee radiographs. Indeed, two children aged 3.8 and 5.2 yr displayed no radiographic evidence of rickets at either the wrist or knee, although their relatives exhibited rickets (73).

In light of our findings that radiographic evidence of rickets is not an invariant feature of HYP, we felt that it was premature to define new disease entities based largely on the lack of rickets in affected children. However, since none of the 13 affected children described by Frymoyer and Hodgkin had radiographic evidence of rickets, the possibility still exists that their kindred does have a distinct disorder. The identification of PEX provides us with an opportunity to examine this question further. We have been able to examine and obtain DNA samples from many members of this kindred. Linkage analysis indicates that the disease is linked to the HYP (Xp22.1) region (Econs unpublished observations). We are currently analyzing DNA from this kindred to search for a PEX mutation. The identification of a PEX mutation in affected members of this kindred, coupled with the observation that some members of the kindred have classic HYP would rule out the contention that there are two forms of X-linked dominant hypophosphatemic rickets. Thus, identification of the PEX gene may provide additional clinical insights.

AUTOSOMAL-DOMINANT FORMS OF RENAL PHOSPHATE WASTING

In addition to HYP there are two proposed autosomal-dominant forms of isolated renal phosphate wasting: autosomal-dominant hypophosphatemic rickets (ADHR) and hypophosphatemic bone disease (HBD). Both of these disorders are less common than HYP and have been less well studied, although ongoing studies may provide an opportunity to understand the pathogenesis of these disorders.

Autosomal-Dominant Hypophosphatemic Rickets (ADHR)

Bianchine et al. described a small family with an autosomal-dominant form of renal phosphate wasting (74,75). The father was a markedly affected man who had isolated renal phosphate wasting, short stature and an impressive windswept deformity (valgus on one side and varus on the other). He had two affected daughters and one affected son. These investigators reported that the father had a marked tendency towards fracture with or without trauma. Otherwise, the clinical course in these individuals appeared to be similar to that of HYP patients.

We have recently had the opportunity to evaluate a large ADHR kindred with over twenty affected individuals (76). This kindred provided us with an opportunity to explore the phenotypic variability of this disease in a large number of individuals who all have the same mutation. Affected kindred members have isolated renal phosphate wasting with inappropriately normal serum calcitriol concentrations. In contrast to HYP, ADHR displays variable penetrance. The family contains two subgroups of affected individuals. One subgroup consists of patients who presented with phosphate wasting as adults or adolescents. These individuals complained of bone pain, weakness and insufficiency fractures, but did not have lower extremity deformities. The second group consists of individuals who presented during childhood with phosphate wasting, rickets and lower extremity deformity in a pattern similar to the classic presentation of HYP. Surprisingly, some of the children in this group presented with phosphate wasting and rickets, but later lost the phosphate-wasting defect after puberty *(76)*. In addition to these two groups there appear to be at least two unaffected individuals who are carriers for the ADHR mutation *(76)*. Thus, the clinical manifestations of ADHR are even more variable than those observed in HYP.

Hypophosphatemic Bone Disease (HBD)

Hypophosphatemic bone disease (HBD) was originally described by Scriver et al. *(77)* who studied five small families in which affected members had isolated renal phosphate wasting, short stature, and lower extremity deformity. In one family (family 4), there was a male to male transmission, indicating an autosomal dominant pattern of inheritance in this family. These investigators stated that HBD differed from ADHR since affected children in their kindreds did not display radiographic evidence of rickets. In other respects, the patients appeared to be similar to other patients with phosphate wasting. As noted above, radiographic evidence of rickets is not always present in HYP *(73)*. By analogy, it is possible that radiographic evidence of rickets may not be universal in children with ADHR. Of note, in the original description of HBD family 4, which was the only family that demonstrated a father to son transmission, contained two members who were said to have a clinical picture consistent with HYP (including rickets in at least one of these individuals) in addition to the two individuals who had HBD *(77)*. The paternal grandmother of the propositus, who was also the aunt of the two individuals who reportedly had HYP, had a serum phosphorus of 3.1 mg/dL. In light of the incomplete penetrance that is observed in ADHR and the fact that the occurrence of two different uncommon renal phosphate wasting disorders in the same family is unlikely, this family may have had ADHR. Thus, HBD may not be a distinct clinical entity. However, definitive evidence as to whether ADHR and HBD are distinct entities or forme fruste of one another awaits identification of the gene(s) that cause these disorders. Indeed, even if these diseases result from mutations in the same gene, it will be important to characterize the mutations that cause ADHR and HBD since different mutations in the same gene can give rise to different phenotypes. One example of this phenomenon is the dystrophin gene in which missense mutations give rise to Beckers muscular dystrophy and nonsense mutations result in Duchenne muscular dystrophy *(78)*. In any case, the weight of the evidence currently favors the hypothesis that ADHR and HBD are the same disorders.

Positional Cloning Efforts
in Autosomal-Dominant Phosphate-Wasting Disorders

We have recently initiated studies aimed at identifying the gene(s) responsible for ADHR. In this regard we are performing linkage studies in the large ADHR kindred described above. Since the high-affinity/low-capacity sodium-dependent phosphate cotransporter plays an important role in the maintenance of phosphate homeostasis we considered it a strong candidate gene. Kos et al. *(17)* located this transporter to the long arm of chromosome 5 (5q35) so in our initial studies we used markers from this region to look for linkage with ADHR. Our results excluded linkage of the ADHR gene to markers on 5q35 ruling out mutations in NPT-2 as a cause of ADHR in this family (Econs et al., unpublished observations). Since another phosphate cotransporter has been identified on the short arm of chromosome 6 *(79)*, we extended our study to include markers from this region in the linkage analysis. Our results also excluded linkage to this region (Econs et al., unpublished observations). In absence of further candidate genes, we undertook a genome wide linkage search with markers spaced every 20 c*M* across the genome. Results from these studies should facilitate the eventual identification of the ADHR gene as has been done for HYP. The use of several large ADHR families may provide us with information about whether ADHR results from mutation in one gene or whether mutations in several different genes can give rise to the ADHR phenotype.

Hereditary Hypophosphatemic Rickets with Hypercalciuria

Hereditary hypophosphatemic rickets with hypercalciuria (HHRH) was first described in a Bedouin tribe *(80)*. In concert with other disorders of phosphate wasting, HHRH results in decreased serum phosphate levels and reduced tubular phosphate reabsorption, and normal serum calcium concentrations. However, in contrast to other phosphate-wasting disorders, serum levels of 1,25-dihydroxyvitamin D are elevated despite suppressed parathyroid function and there is a marked increase in urinary calcium excretion. Oral calcium and phosphate loading tests show that there is intestinal hyperabsorption of calcium and phosphate. It has been suggested that the pivotal defect consists of renal phosphate depletion, which stimulates renal 25-hydroxyvitamin D 1-α hydroxylase, followed by an increase of 1,25-dihydroxyvitamin D. This, in turn, will enhance intestinal calcium and phosphate absorption, increase the renal calcium filtered load and suppress parathyroid gland function, both events leading to hypercalciuria *(80)*.

The accurate diagnosis of HHRH has important therapeutic implications. In contrast to HYP, phosphate supplemetion alone can cause a complete remission of the disease whereas the addition of active vitamin D can be harmful and create complications, such as hypercalcemia, kidney stones, and renal damage *(81)*.

Since the original report *(80)* of HHRH Tieder et al. *(82)* have further characterized this family. Of the 59 family members that they studied there were nine individuals with HHRH and an additional 21 members who had idiopathic hypercalciuria, slightly reduced serum phosphate levels and elevated serum 1,25-dihydroxyvitamin D concentrations *(82)*. It has been suggested, that HHRH is inherited in an autosomal recessive mode and heterozygotes can be affected by idiopathic hypercalciuria. The data of the bedouin tribe are compatible to an autosomal recessive mode of inheritance assuming incomplete penetrance of the recessive phenotype, however, the mode of inheritance has not been unequivocally established. Of note, an autosomal dominant form of HHRH has been described, where the clinical and biochemical abnormalities are less pronounced *(83)*.

Since these first reports, only one other kindred *(84)* and a few sporadic cases *(81,85,86)* have been reported. Linkage analysis has not been reported for HHRH. There are a few candidate genes, such as NPT1, NPT2, and stanniocalcin which have been mapped by FISH analysis and somatic cell hybrid panels to chromosome 6p21.3-p23 *(79)*, chromosome 5q35 *(17)* and chromosome 8p21 *(71)*, respectively. In two German families, we could exclude cosegregation of the disease with the markers D5S408 and D5S498, which are localized on the distal part of the long arm of chromosome 5. However, testing of cosegregation of the disease with one of these genes in small families is difficult when the exact map position is not known. In light of the uncertain mode of inheritance, it will be imperative to perform nonparametric analysis *(87)* to locate the HHRH gene(s).

HYPOPHOSPHATEMIA RESULTING FROM MUTATIONS IN THE CLCN-5 GENE

Enia et al. *(88)* described a kindred with X-linked recessive hypophosphatemic rickets (XLRH), however, the abnormalities that are seen in the disease are not confined to renal phosphate wasting. Recently Lloyd et al. *(89)* have demonstrated that XLRH, Dent's disease, and X-linked recessive nephrolithiasis (XRN) all result from inactivating mutations in the CLCN-5 gene, which codes for a putative voltage-gated chloride channel. Although Lloyd et al. asserted that mutations in the CLCN-5 gene give rise to three phenotypically distinct disorders, the similarities observed between patients with the three diseases indicate that all of the patients have the same disease. In addition to phosphate wasting all three diseases result in proteinuria, hypercalciuria, nephrolithiasis, nephrocalcinosis, and eventual renal failure *(90–93)*. Patients with Dent's disease and XLRH both manifest rickets and osteomalacia. Although rickets was not observed in the one XRN family, there was only one child in this kindred *(90)* and the clinical description fails to include the radiographs necessary to determine the presence of rickets. Even if this patient did not have rickets, rickets does not appear to be an invariant feature in this disease. Indeed in the most recent description of Dent's disease *(92)*, there were two affected male children who did not have rickets.

Overall, when one examines the available clinical data, the phenotypic differences observed between affected individuals from the same family exceed those differences observed between the different diseases. It is likely that the observed phenotypic differences between the different families resulted from the small numbers of affected individuals within each kindred and that each group of investigators chose to emphasize a particular aspect of the disease. Considering the phenotypic similarities between the diseases and the fact that mutations responsible for all the disorders result in total loss of chloride channel function *(89)*, there is no basis with which to consider these as separate disease entities. In light of the fact that mutations in the CLCN-5 gene result in generalized tubular dysfunction, it is likely that this gene does not play a specific role in phosphate homeostasis, but mutations in this gene lead to proximal tubular dysfunction which results in phosphate wasting as a secondary event.

CONCLUSION

Phosphate homeostasis is a complex process, but new methods of analysis are shedding light on phosphate homeostasis and the hereditary disorders of phosphate wasting. In several instances, advances in molecular genetics not only help investigators gain a better understanding of the pathogenesis of these diseases, but allow clinicians to understand the variability in the clinical presentation of these disorders.

ACKNOWLEDGMENTS

This work was supported by the NIH under Grants AR42228, AR27032, MO1-RR-30, and NIA 5 P60 AG11268 (National Institute on Aging, Claude Pepper Older Americans Independence Center) and by grants from the Deutsche Forschungsgemeinschaft and the Commission of the European Communities (CT930027).

REFERENCES

1. Davies M, Stanbury SW. The rheumatic manifestations of metabolic bone disease. Clin Rheumatic Dis 1981;7:595–646.
2. Econs MJ, Drezner MK. Bone disease resulting from inherited disorders of renal tubule transport and vitamin D metabolism. In: Favus MJ, Coe FL, eds. Disorders of Bone and Mineral Metabolism. Raven, New York, 1992; pp. 935–950.
3. Whyte MP, Schranck FW, Armamento-Villareal R. X-linked hypophosphatemia: A search for gender, race, anticipation, or parent of origin effects on disease expression in children. J Clin Endo Metab 1996;81:4075–4080.
4. Kay G, Thakker RV, Rastan S. Determination of a molecular map position for *Hyp* using a new inter-specific backcross produced by in vitro fertilization. Genomics 1991;11:651–657.
5. Sonin NV, Taggart RT, Meyer MH, Meyer RA, Jr. Placement of the Gyro *(Gy)* mutation on the molecular map of chromosome X of the mouse. J Bone Min Res 1995;10:S300 (abst).
6. Eicher EM, Southard JL, Scriver CR, Glorieux FH. Hypophosphatemia: Mouse model for human familial hypophosphatemic (vitamin D resistent) rickets. Proc Natl Acad Sci USA 1976;73:4667–4671.
7. Lyon MF, Scriver CR, Baker LRI, Tenenhouse HS, Kronick J, Mandla S. The *Gy* mutation: Another cause of X-linked hypophosphatemia in mouse. Proc Natl Acad Sci USA 1986;83:4899–4903.
8. Meyer RA, Jr., Meyer MH, Gray RW, Bruns ME. Femoral abnormalities and vitamin D metabolism in X-linked hypophosphatemic (*Hyp* and *Gy*) mice. J Ortho R 1995;13:30–40.
9. Qiu ZQ, Tenenhouse HS, Scriver CR. Parental origin of mutant allele does not explain absence of gene dose in X-linked *Hyp* mice. Genet Res 1993;62:39–43.
10. Tenenhouse HS, Scriver CR, McInnes RR, Glorieux FH. Renal handling of phosphate in vivo and in vitro by the X-linked hypophosphatemic male mouse: Evidence for a defect in the brush border membrane. Kidney Intern 1978;14:235–244.
11. Tenenhouse HS, Klugerman AH, Neal J. Effect of phosphonoformic acid, dietary phosphate and the *Hyp* mutation on kinetically distinct phosphate transport processes in mouse kidney. Biochim Biophys Acta 1989;984:207–213.
12. Werner A, Moore ML, Mantei N, Biber J, Slemenza G, Murer H. Cloning and expression of cDNA for a Na/Pi cotransport system of kidney cortex. Proc Natl Acad Sci USA 1991;88:9608–9612.
13. Tenenhouse HS, Werner A, Biber J, Ma S, Martel J, Roy S, et al. Renal Na$^+$-phosphate cotransport in murine X-linked hypophosphatemic rickets. J Clin Invest 1994;93:671–676.
14. Collins JF, Scheving AL, Ghishan FK. Decreased transcription of the sodium-phosphate transporter gene in the hypophosphatemic mouse. Am J Physiol 1995;F:439–448.
15. Tenenhouse HS, Beck L. Renal Na$^+$-phosphate cotransporter gene expression in X-linked *Hyp* and *Gy* mice. Kidney Intern 1996;49:1027–1032.
16. Collins JF, Ghishan FK. The molecular defect in the renal sodium-phosphate transporter expression pathway of Gyro *(Gy)* mice is distinct from that of hypophosphatemic *(Hyp)* mice. FASEB J 1996;10:751–759.
17. Kos CH, Tihy F, Econs MJ, Murer H, Lemieux N, Tenenhouse HS. Localization of a renal sodium phosphate cotransporter gene to human chromosome 5q35. Genomics 1994;19:176,177.
18. Meyer RA, Jr., Meyer MH, Gray RW. Parabiosis suggests a humoral factor is involved in X-linked hypophosphatemia in mice. J Bone Min Res 1989;4:493–500.
19. Nesbitt T, Coffman TM, Griffiths R, Drezner MK. Cross-transplantation of kidneys in normal and *Hyp* mice: Evidence that the *Hyp* phenotype is unrelated to an intrinsic renal defect. J Clin Invest 1992;89:1453–1459.
20. Ecarot-Charrier B, Glorieux FH, Travers R, Desbarats M, Bouchard F, Hinek A. Defective bone formation by transplanted hyp-mouse bone cells into normal mice. Endocrinology 1988;123:768–773.
21. Ecarot B, Glorieux FH, Desbarats M, Travers R, Labelle L. Effect of 1,25 dihydroxyvitamin D3 treatment on bone formation by transplanted cells from normal and X-linked hypophosphatemic mice. J Bone Min Res 1995;10:424–431.
22. Cao XY, Jiang XM, Dou ZH, Rakeman MA, Zhang ML, O'Donnell K, et al. Timing of vulnerability of the brain to iodine deficiency in endemic cretinism. N Engl J Med 1994;331:1739–1744.
23. Lajeunesse D, Meyer RA, Jr., Hamel L. Direct demonstration of a humorally-mediated inhibition of renal phosphate transport in the Hyp mouse. Kidney Intern 1996;50:1531–1538.
24. Econs MJ, Drezner MK. Tumor-induced osteomalacia: Unveiling a new hormone. N Engl J Med 1994;330:1679–1681.

25. Cai Q, Hodgson SF, Kao PC, Lennon VA, Klee GG, Zinsmiester AR, et al. Inhibition of renal phosphate transport by a tumor product in a patient with oncogenic osteomalacia. N Engl J Med 1994;330:1645–1649.

26. Rowe PS, Ong AC, Cockerill FJ, Goulding JN, Hewison M. Candidate 56 and 58 kDa protein(s) responsible for mediating the renal defects in oncogenic hypophosphatemic osteomalacia. Bone 1996;18:159–169.

27. Scriver CR, Reade TM, DeLuca HF, Hamstra AJ. Serum 1,25-dihydroxyvitamin D levels in normal subjects and in patients with hereditary rickets or bone disease. N Engl J Med 1978;299:976–979.

28. Drezner MK, Haussler MR. Correspondence. N Engl J Med 1979;300:435.

29. Lyles KW, Clark AG, Drezner MK. Serum 1,25-dihydroxyvitamin D levels in subjects with X-linked hypophosphatemic rickets and osteomalacia. Calcif Tissue Int 1982;34:125–130.

30. Lobaugh B, Drezner MK. Abnormal regulation of renal 25-hydroxyvitamin D-1a-hydroxylase activity in the X-linked hypophosphatemic mouse. J Clin Invest 1983;71:400–403.

31. Cunningham J, Gomes H, Seino Y, Chase LR. Abnormal 24-hydroxylation of 25-hydroxyvitamin D in the X-linked hypophosphatemic mouse. Endocrinology 1983;112:633–637.

32. Tenenhouse HS, Yip A, Jones G. Increased renal catabolism of 1,25-Dihydroxyvitamin D_3 in murine X-linked hypophosphatemic rickets. J Clin Invest 1988;81:461–465.

33. Davidai GA, Nesbitt T, Drezner MK. Normal regulation of calcitriol production in *Gy* mice: Evidence for biochemical heterogeneity in the X-linked hypophosphatemic diseases. J Clin Invest 1990;85:334–339.

34. Tenenhouse HS, Meyer RA, Jr., Mandla S, Meyer MH, Gray RW. Renal phosphate transport and vitamin D metabolism in X-linked hypophosphatemic *Gy* mice: Responses to phosphate deprivation. Endocrinology 1992;131:51–56.

35. Meyer RA, Jr., Meyer MH, Morgan PL. Effects of altered diet on serum levels of 1,25-dihydroxyvitamin D and parathyroid hormone in X-linked hypophosphatemic (*Hyp* and *Gy*) mice. Bone 1996;18:23–28.

36. Econs MJ. Positional cloning of the HYP gene: A review. Kidney Int 1996;49:1033–1037.

37. Collins F. Positional cloning moves from perditional to traditional. Nature Gen 1995;9:347–350.

38. Machler M, Frey D, Gai A, Orth U, Wienker TF, Fanconi A, et al. X-linked dominant hypophosphatemia is closely linked to DNA markers DXS41 and DXS43 at Xp22. Hum Genet 1986;73:271–275.

39. Read AP, Thakker RV, Davies KE, Mountford RC, Brenton DP, Davies M, et al. Mapping of human X-linked hypophosphatemic rickets by multilocus linkage analysis. Hum Genet 1986;73:267–270.

40. Thakker RV, Read AP, Davies KE, Whyte MP, Weksberg R, Glorieux F, et al. Bridging markers defining the map position of X-linked hypophosphatemic rickets. J Med Genet 1987;24:756–760.

41. Econs MJ, Barker DF, Speer MC, Pericak-Vance MA, Fain PR, Drezner MK. Multilocus mapping of the X-linked hypophosphatemic rickets gene. J Clin Endo Metab 1992;75:201–206.

42. Rowe PSN, Read AP, Mountford R, Benham F, Kruse TA, Camerino G, et al. Three DNA markers for hypophosphatemic rickets. Hum Genet 1992;89:539–542.

43. Econs MJ, Fain PR, Norman M, Speer MC, Pericak-Vance MA, Becker PA, et al. Flanking markers define the X-linked hypophosphatemic rickets gene locus. J Bone Min Res 1993;8:1149–1152.

44. Rowe PSN, Goulding J, Read A, Mountford R, Hanauer A, Oudet C, et al. New markers for linkage analysis of hypophosphatemic rickets. Hum Genet 1993;91:571–575.

45. Weber JL, May PE. Abundant class of human DNA polymorphisms which can be typed using the polymerase chain reaction. Am J Hum Genet 1989;44:388–396.

46. Browne D, Barker D, Litt M. Dinucleotide repeat polymorphisms at the DXS365, DXS443 and DXS451 loci. Hum Mol Genet 1992;1:213.

47. Econs MJ, Rowe PSN, Francis F, Barker DF, Speer MC, Norman M, et al. Fine structure mapping of the human X-linked hypophosphatemic rickets gene locus. J Clin Endo Metab 1994;79:1351–1354.

48. Burke DT, Carle GF, Olson MF. Cloning of large segments of exogenous DNA into yeast by means of artificial chromosome vectors. Science 1987;236:806–812.

49. Francis F, Rowe PSN, Econs MJ, See CG, Benham F, O'Riordan JLH, et al. A YAC contig spanning the hypophosphatemic rickets gene candidate region. Genomics 1994;21:229–237.

50. Econs MJ, Francis F, Rowe PSN, Speer MC, O'Riordan J, Lehrach H, et al. Dinucleotide repeat polymorphism at the DXS1683 locus. Hum Mol Genet 1994;3:680.

51. Rowe PSN, Francis F, Goulding J. Rapid isolation of DNA sequences flanking microsatellite repeats. Nucleic Acid Res 22, 1994;5135,5136.

52. Rowe PSN, Goulding JN, Francis F, Oudet C, Econs MJ, Hanauer A, et al. The gene for X-linked hypophosphatemic rickets maps to a 200–300 kb region in Xp22.1-Xp22.2, and is located on a single YAC containing a putative vitamin D response element (VDRE). Hum Genet 1996;97:345–352.

53. HYP Consortium. Lab 1: Francis F, Hennig S, Korn B, Reinhardt R, de Jong P, Poustka A, Lehrach H. Lab 2: Rowe PSN, Goulding JN, Summerfield T, Mountford R, Read AP, Popowska E, Pronicka E, Davies KE, O'Riordan JLH. Lab 3: Econs MJ, Nesbitt T, Drezner MK. Lab 4: Oudet C, Hanauer A. Lab 5: Strom T, Meindl A, Lorenz B, Cagnoli M, Mohnike KL, Murken J, Meitinger T. Positional cloning of PEX: A gene with homologies to endopeptidases is mutated in patients with X-linked hypophosphatemic rickets. Nature Genet 1995;11:130–136.

54. Buckler AJ, Chang DD, Graw SL, Brook JD, Haber DA, Sharp PA, et al. Exon amplification—a strategy to isolate mammalian genes based on RNA splicing. Proc Natl Acad Sci USA 1991;88:4005–4009.

55. Francis F, Strom TM, Hennig S, Boeddrich A, Lorenz B, Brandau O, et al. Genomic organization of the human PEX gene mutated in X-linked dominant hypophosphatemic rickets. Genome Res 1997;7:573–585.

56. Du L, Desbarats M, Viel J, Glorieux FH, Cawthorn C, Ecarot B. cDNA cloning of the murine Pex gene implicated in X-linked hypophosphatemia and evidence for expression in bone. Genomics 1996;36:22–28.

57. Strom TM, F. Francis, B. Lorenz, A. Boeddrich, MJ Econs, H. Lehrach, et al. Pex gene deletions in *Gy* and *Hyp* mice provide mouse models for X-linked hypophosphatemia. Hum Mol Genet 1997;6:165–171.

58. Kozak M. An analysis of 5' noncoding sequences from 699 vertebrate messenger RNAs. Nucleic Acid Res 1987;15:8125–8148.

59. Kozak M. An analysis of vertebrate mRNA sequences: intimations of translational control. J Cell Biol 1991;115:887–903.

60. Welches WR, Brosnihan KB, Ferrario CM. A comparison of the properties and enzymatic activities of the three angiotensin processing enzymes: angiotensin converting enzyme, prolyl endopeptidase and neutral endopeptidase 24.11. Life Sci 1993;52:1461–1480.

61. Xu D, Emoto N, Giaid A, Slaughter C, Kaw S, de Wit D, et al. ECE-1: A membrane-bound metalloprotease that catalyzes the proteolytic activation of big endothelin-1. Cell 1994;78:473–485.

62. Emoto N, Yanagisawa M. Endothelin-converting enzyme-2 is a membrane bound, phosphoramidon-sensitive metalloprotease with acidic pH optimum. J Biol Chem 1995;270:15,262–15,268.

63. Econs MJ, Samsa GP, Monger M, Drezner MK, Feussner JR. X-linked hypophosphatemic rickets: A disease often unknown to affected patients. Bone Min 1994;24:17–24.

64. Beck L, Soumounou Y, Martel J, Krishnamurthy G, Gauthier C, Goodyear CG, et al. Pex/PEX tissue distribution and evidence for a deletion in the 3' region of the Pex gene in X-linked hypophosphatemic mice. J Clin Invest 1997;99:1200–1209.

65. Grieff M, Mumm S, Waeltz P, Mazzarella R, Whyte MP, Thakker RV, et al. Expression and cloning of the Human X-linked hypophosphatemia gene cDNA. Biochem Biophys Res Commun 1997;231: 635–639.

66. Rowe PSN, Oudet C, Francis F, Hanauer A, Econs MJ, Strom TM, et al. The PEX gene is mutated in families with X-linked hypophosphatemic rickets (HYP): Evidence for PEX function (Zn^{+2} metalloprotease). Hum Mol Genet 1997;6:539–549.

67. Holm IA, Huang X, Zacconi NM, Kunkel LM. Mutations in the PEX gene in X-linked hypophosphatemic rickets (HYP). Am J Hum Genet 1996;59S:A43 (abst).

68. Dixon PH, Wooding C, Trump D, Schlessinger D, Whyte MP, Thakker RV. Seven novel mutations in the PEX gene indicate molecular heterogeneity for X-linked hypophosphatemic rickets. J Bone Min Res 1996;11:S136 (abst).

69. Mokrzycki AK, Tassabehji M, Davies M, Rowe P, Mawer EB, Read AP. PEX mutations in families with X-linked hypophosphatemic rickets. Am J Hum Genet 1996;59S:A273 (abst).

70. Scriver CR, Tenenhouse HS. X-linked hypophosphatemia: A homologous phenotype in humans and mice with unusual organ-specific gene dosage. J Inher Metab Dis 1992;15:610–624.

71. Olsen HS, Cepeda MA, Zhang QQ, Rosen CA, Vozzolo BL, Wagner GF. Human stanniocalcin: A possible hormonal regulator of mineral metabolism. Proc Natl Acad Sci USA 1996;93: 1792–1796.

72. Frymoyer JW, Hodgkin W. Adult-onset vitamin D-resistant hypophosphatemic osteomalacia. J Bone Joint Surg 1977;59:101–106.

73. Econs MJ, Feussner JR, Samsa GP, Effman EL, Vogler JB, Martinez S, et al. X-linked hypophosphatemic rickets without "rickets". Skeletal Radiol 1991;20:109–114.

74. Bianchine JW, Stambler AA, Harrison HE. Familial hypophosphatemic rickets showing autosomal dominant inheritance. Birth Defects Org Art Ser 1971;VII(6):287–294.

75. Harrison HE, Harrison HC. Rickets and osteomalacia. In: Major Problems in Clinical Pediatrics, Vol. 20: Disorders of Calcium and Phosphate Metabolism in Childhood and Adolescence. WB Saunders, Philadelphia, PA, 1979; pp. 230–249.

76. Econs MJ, McEnery PT. Autosomal dominant hypophosphatemic rickets/osteomalacia: Clinical characterization of a novel renal phosphate wasting disorder. J Clin Endo Metab 1997;82:674–681.

77. Scriver CR, MacDonald W, Reade T, Glorieux FH, Nogrady B. Hypophosphatemic norachitic bone disease: an entity distinct from X-linked hypophosphatemia in the renal defect, bone involvement, and inheritance. Am J Med Gen 1977;1:101–117.

78. Koenig M, Beggs AH, Moyer M, Scherpf S, Heindrich K, Bettecken T, et al. The molecular basis for Duchenne versus Becker muscular dystrophy: correlation of severity with type of deletion. Am J Hum Genet 1989;45:498–506.

79. Chong SS, Kozak CA, Liu L, Kristjansson K, Dunn ST, Bourdeau JE, et al. Cloning, genetic mapping, and expression analysis of a mouse renal sodium-dependent phosphate cotransporter. Am J Physiol 1995;268:F1038–F1045.

80. Tieder M, Modai D, Samuel R, Arie R, Halabe A, Bab I, et al. Hereditary hypophosphatemic rickets with hypercalciuria. N Engl J Med 1985;312:611–617.

81. Chen C, Carpenter T, Steg N, Baron R, Anast C. Hypercalciuric hypophosphatemic rickets, mineral balance, bone histomorphometry, and therapeutic implications of hypercalciuria. Pediatrics 1989;84: 276–280.

82. Tieder M, Modai D, Shaked U, Samuel R, Arie R, Halabe A, et al. "Idiopathic" hypercalciuria and hereditary hypophosphatemic rickets. Two phenotypical expressions of a common genetic defect. N Engl J Med 1987;316:125–129.

83. Proesmans WC, Fabry G, Marchal GJ, Gillis PL, Bouillon R. Autosomal dominant hypophosphataemia with elevated serum 1,25 dihydroxyvitamin D and hypercalciuria. Pediatr Nephrol 1987;1:479–484.

84. Tieder M, Arie R, Bab I, Maor J, Liberman UA. A new kindred with hereditary hypophosphatemic rickets with hypercalciuria: implications for correct diagnosis and treatment. Nephron 1992;62: 176–181.

85. Nishiyama S, Inoue F, Makuda I. A single case of hypophosphatemic rickets with hypercalciuria. J Pediatr Gastroenterol Nutr 1986;5:826–829.

86. Schnabel D, von Mühlendahl KE, Morlot M, Wassmann A, Grüters A, Kruse, K. The hereditary syndrome of hypophosphatemic rickets and hypercalciuria (HHRH): possible diagnostic pitfalls and clinical follow-up (abstract). Horm Res 1996;46(suppl 2):84.

87. Lander ES, Schork NJ. Genetic dissection of complex traits. Science 1994;265:2037–2048.

88. Enia G, Zoccali C, Bolino A, Romeo G. New X-linked hypophosphatemic rickets with hypercalciuria leading to progressive renal failure. Nephrol Dial Transplant 1992;7:757,758 (abst).

89. Lloyd SE, Pearce SHS, Fisher SE, Steinmeyer K, Schwappach B, Scheinman SJ, et al. A common molecular basis for three inherited kidney stone diseases. Nature 1996;379:445–449.

90. Frymoyer PA, Scheinman SJ, Duham PB, Jones DB, Hueber, P, Schroeder ET. X-linked recessive nephrolithiasis with renal failure. N Engl J Med 1991;325:681–686.

91. Bolino A, Devoto M, Enia G, Zoccali C, Weissenbach J, Romeo G. Genetic mapping in the Xp11. 2 region of a new form of X-linked hypophosphatemic rickets. Eur J Hum Genet 1993;1:269–279.

92. Wrong OM, Norden AGW, Feest TG. Dent's disease; a familial proximal renal tubular syndrome with low-molecular-weight-proteinuria, hypercalciuria, nephrocalcinosis, metabolic bone disease, progressive renal failure and marked male predominance. Q J Med 1994;87:473–493.

93. Reinhart SC, Norden AGW, Lapsley M, Thakker RV, Frymoyer PA, Scheinman SJ. Phenotypes of males and carrier females in X-linked recessive nephrolithiasis (XRN) J Am Soc Nephrol 1993; 4:265 (abst).

5

The Roles of Growth Hormone, Prolactin, and Placental Lactogen in Human Fetal Development

Critical Analysis of Molecular, Cellular, and Clinical Investigations

Michael Freemark, MD

CONTENTS

BACKGROUND

Human growth hormone (hGH), human prolactin and human placental lactogen (hPL, also called human chorionic somatomammotropin or hCS) constitute a family of somatogenic and lactogenic polypeptide hormones that have similarities in structure and biological function. With diverse effects on growth factor production, nutrient metabolism, hormone secretion, and mammary function, the somatogens and lactogens play central roles in growth and sexual development, reproduction, immune function, and intermediary metabolism. In the pregnant mother, hGH, human prolactin, and hPL exert effects on insulin production and carbohydrate and lipid metabolism that ensure the delivery of

From: *Molecular and Cellular Pediatric Endocrinology*
Edited by: S. Handwerger © Humana Press Inc., Totowa, NJ

nutrients to the fetus for normal growth and development *(1–3)*. Through induction of maternal IGF-I *(4)* and other growth factors, hGH may stimulate the growth of maternal tissues, such as the uterus and placenta *(5,6)*. And through actions on the maternal breast and hypothalamus *(7–9)*, prolactin and hPL may prepare the mother for feeding and caring for her newborn young after birth.

Initial investigations suggested that the effects of the somatogens and lactogens on fetal growth and development were mediated only indirectly through effects on maternal metabolism. However, hGH, human prolactin, and hPL are secreted directly into the fetal as well as the maternal circulations, and PL and prolactin are detected in abundance in the extraembryonic coelomic and amniotic fluids. In addition, recent studies demonstrate widespread expression of somatogenic and lactogenic receptors in the human fetus and direct biological actions of hGH, human prolactin, and hPL in fetal tissues. Together with studies of patients with GH resistance associated with mutations of the GH receptor and of transgenic mice with deletions of the prolactin receptor, these recent findings suggest novel roles for the somatogens and lactogens in fetal development.

EXPRESSION AND REGULATION OF SOMATOGENIC AND LACTOGENIC HORMONES IN THE HUMAN FETUS

As reviewed in recent manuscripts *(10)* and in other chapters in this compendium, the genes encoding hGH and hPL reside on chromosome 17, band q22–24, within a 66-kb cluster of five genes including the hGH-N gene, which is expressed in the anterior pituitary gland and in lymphoid and hematopoietic cells *(11)*, and four genes expressed in the placental syncytiotrophoblasts: the hGH-V gene *(12)*, which encodes a 22-kDa protein that differs from pituitary GH by 13 amino acids; the hPL-A and hPL-B genes, which encode identical mature 22.2-kDa proteins that differ by a single amino acid in their signal peptides *(13)*; and the hPL-L gene. Initially thought to be a pseudogene, the hPL-L gene appears to be expressed in minute amounts during normal pregnancy *(14)*. The protein encoded by the gene has not yet been identified. Alternative splicing of the primary pituitary hGH-N transcript results in the production of a 22-kDa hGH (191 amino acids) and a 20-kDa hGH that lacks amino acids 32–46. The 20-kDa hGH molecule has somatogenic potency equivalent to that of 22 kDa hGH, but binds with sevenfold lower affinity to prolactin receptors *(15)*. The 22-kDa hGH can be cleaved within the somatotrope to yield a 17.5-kDa hGH lacking the N-terminal amino acids 1–43. The 17.5-kDa hGH (hGH 44–191) binds with high affinity to prolactin receptors, but not GH receptors; it has potent diabetogenic activity but lacks the growth-promoting and insulin-like activities of 22-kDa hGH *(16)*.

The gene encoding human prolactin resides on chromosome 6 and is expressed in the anterior pituitary, in decidualized endometrium and myometrium, in thymocytes, splenocytes, and peripheral lymphocytes, and monocytes *(18)*. The prolactin molecule produced by the decidua is identical in structure and biological activity to the 23-kDa prolactin produced by the pituitary gland. The decidua likely provides the source of prolactin found in amniotic fluid but does not appear to secrete prolactin into the fetal or maternal circulations during pregnancy.

The concentrations of hGH, prolactin, and hPL in fetal serum and in amniotic fluid vary independently of maternal concentrations, owing to the failure of the somatogenic and lactogenic hormones to traverse the placental/decidual barrier and to differential secretion and regulation within the fetal and maternal compartments.

Human Growth Hormone

During early gestation, circulating GH in the pregnant mother originates in the anterior pituitary, encoded by the hGH-N gene. Beginning at 19–22 wk of gestation the synthesis and secretion of maternal pituitary GH decline. Concomitantly, the placenta initiates production and secretion of the GH variant, encoded by the hGH-V gene *(19)*. The GH variant has somatogenic potency equivalent to that of pituitary GH but its potency in lactogenic bioassays is 20-fold less than that of pituitary GH *(20)*. The levels of GH variant increase slowly throughout the latter half of pregnancy, reaching a peak concentration of 15–20 ng/mL in maternal serum at term. Maternal plasma concentrations of GH variant correlate positively with maternal IGF-I concentrations *(4)*, suggesting that the GH variant may regulate maternal IGF-I production after midgestation.

In the human fetus, immunoreactive hGH is first detected in the anterior pituitary between 7 and 9 wk of gestation *(21)*. Fetal pituitary GH mRNA and GH content increase markedly to peak between 25 and 29 wk, remaining relatively constant thereafter. GH is detected in human fetal plasma as early as 70 d of gestation. Initial studies in human abortuses *(22)* demonstrated that fetal plasma GH levels increase from 15 to 50 ng/mL at 10–14 wk of gestation to a maximum of 60–320 ng/mL (mean 150 ng/mL) at 20–24 wk; subsequently fetal GH levels decline to a mean of 30–40 ng/mL in umbilical cord blood. Direct measures of hormone levels in normal human fetuses using periumbilical cord sampling *(23)* reveal a decline in GH concentrations from a mean of 33.6 ± 2.1 ng/mL at 18–29 wk of gestation to a mean of 21.9 ± 1.4 ng/mL at 30–40 wk. The higher levels of GH measured in aborted fetuses may reflect the stress of the operative procedure. In amniotic fluid, the concentration of GH rises to a peak (10–20 ng/mL) at midgestation and declines slightly towards term *(24)*. The GH in the fetal circulation and in amniotic fluid appears to originate in the fetal pituitary because the GH variant (GH-V) is not detected in fetal serum or in amniotic fluid either at midgestation or at term *(19)*. It is unclear whether the pituitary GH detected in fetal serum represents the 22 or 20 kDa isoform or the cleaved 17.5 kDa hGH.

The exaggerated production of GH in the fetus has been examined in studies in the chronically catheterized fetal lamb (reviewed in ref. *21*). In the fetal lamb, pituitary GH is secreted in high amplitude pulses. Heightened production of GH in the fetus results from an exaggerated pituitary response to growth hormone releasing hormone and diminished responses to somatostatin and to insulin-like growth factor-I (IGF-I). The inhibitory responses to somatostatin and IGF-I mature late in gestation, possibly a consequence of the rise in fetal plasma glucocorticoids.

Immaturity of the human fetal GH secretory axis is reflected in the paradoxical secretory response to thyrotropin releasing hormone in late gestation, the poor suppressibility of GH secretion by glucose prior to a month of age, and the lack of a sleep-associated rise in plasma GH until the third month of postnatal life. HGH levels in human umbilical cord blood correlate negatively with birth weight and with fetal plasma IGF-I concentrations and are elevated in growth-retarded neonates *(25–27)*. Conversely, GH secretion is diminished in congenital hypothyroidism, reflecting the effects of thyroid hormone on pituitary GH synthesis *(28,29)*. The levels of GH in amniotic fluid vary independently of those in fetal serum and are normal in anencephaly *(30,31)*.

Human Prolactin

In the pregnant mother prolactin levels rise progressively after 8 wk of gestation, reaching a peak of 200–400 ng/mL at term. The increase in maternal prolactin parallels the rise in maternal levels of estrogen, which stimulates pituitary prolactin gene transcription.

Immunoreactive prolactin is detected in the fetal pituitary *(21)* and in the extraembryonic coelomic fluid *(32)* at 9–10 wk of gestation. The fetal pituitary content of prolactin increases markedly between 15 and 23 wk and rises more slowly thereafter. In fetal plasma, prolactin can be detected as early as 11–12 wk of gestation *(33)*. Prolactin levels are low (10–20 ng/mL) until 25–27 wk of pregnancy; subsequently, fetal serum concentrations rise sharply to a peak of 150–170 ng/mL in umbilical cord blood. The prenatal rise in fetal serum prolactin is thought to be driven by a striking increase in fetal serum estrogens (especially 17 β estradiol) beginning at 20 wk of gestation *(21,33)*. The role of thyrotropin releasing hormone (TRH), which stimulates prolactin production in the postnatal period, is less clear: TRH levels in the fetus are high during mid-late gestation, reflecting production from hypothalamic as well as extrahypothalamic sources (pancreas, stomach, and placenta); nevertheless, several studies failed to detect an effect of TRH on human fetal prolactin production *(33a)*. The dramatic increase in fetal (as well as maternal) serum prolactin levels in late gestation can be prevented by the administration of bromocryptine, a dopamine agonist, to the pregnant mother *(34)*. In anencephaly, fetal prolactin levels are normal *(33)*.

Prolactin is detected in amniotic fluid as early as 8 wk of gestation *(24,35,36)*. Concentrations of the hormone in amniotic fluid are low prior to 14 wk and then rise to a peak (1000–4000 ng/mL) at 18–26 wk of pregnancy. Subsequently, levels decline to a mean of 450 ng/mL at term. As noted previously the prolactin in amniotic fluid appears to originate in the decidua. Decidual synthesis of prolactin is induced by growth factors such as IGF-I, insulin, and relaxin, inhibited by lipocortin I, and modulated by peptide releasing and inhibitory factors that remain poorly characterized (reviewed in ref. *37*). In contrast to pituitary prolactin, the synthesis and release of decidual prolactin are not regulated by dopamine agonists or thyrotropin releasing hormone. Consequently, the administration of bromocryptine to pregnant mothers has no effects on the levels of prolactin in amniotic fluid *(34,38)*.

Human Placental Lactogen

HPL can be detected in the syncytiotrophoblast within 5–10 d after implantation of the fertilized ovum *(39)*. In the pregnant mother, serum hPL levels rise progressively beginning at 3–4 wk of gestation, reaching a peak of 5000–15,000 ng/mL several weeks prior to term. A modest reduction in maternal plasma hPL concentrations precedes the onset of labor. In amniotic fluid, the levels of hPL range from 300 to 400 ng/mL in early–midgestation *(40,41)*. Concentrations in amniotic fluid rise to maximal levels (750–850 ng/mL) at 34–36 wk and decline prior to term. HPL appears to be secreted directly into the amniotic fluid because there is no transfer of the hormone from the maternal or fetal blood.

HPL is found in extraembryonic coelomic fluid *(42)* and is detected in fetal blood as early as 7–8 wk of gestation *(22,43)*. Studies in human abortuses *(22,43)* suggest a striking rise in fetal serum hPL concentrations between 12 and 20 wk of pregnancy, with peak levels approximating 50–500 ng/mL, followed by a progressive decline in fetal PL levels to a mean of 15–30 ng/mL in term cord blood. However, direct fetal periumbilical cord blood sampling at various times during pregnancy *(44)* reveals a different pattern of hormone expression. In the intact human fetus, hPL levels rise from a mean of 5 ng/mL at 20 wk of gestation to a mean of 20–30 ng/mL at birth. Differences between the levels of hPL measured in abortuses and those measured in intact fetuses may reflect the stress of the abortion and/or the disruption of the normal fetal/placental circulation.

For reasons related to the dangers of human, and particularly fetal, experimentation, it has been difficult to study the factors that regulate PL concentrations in the mother or fetus. In vitro studies by Handwerger et al. suggest roles for numerous hormones, cytokines, and growth factors in the regulation of hPL gene expression (see Chapter 15). In vivo, the major factor controlling maternal plasma PL concentrations appears to be the relative mass of the placenta. In addition, a number of studies suggest that PL concentrations in the pregnant mother are regulated by nutrient availability; for example, prolonged (48–60 h) fasting stimulates a rise in maternal hPL concentrations (45). However, short-term changes in plasma glucose, insulin, triglycerides, fatty acids, or amino acids have inconsistent or no effects on maternal plasma hPL concentrations. Similarly, sex steroids, glucocorticoids, and various hypothalamic and pituitary hormones exert little or no effect on maternal plasma hPL levels. Parallel studies of the effects of these nutrients and hormones on fetal hPL concentrations have never been conducted. Studies in intact and aborted fetuses at mid- and late gestation and in newborn infants at term have demonstrated positive correlations between fetal plasma hPL concentrations and fetal weight and fetal plasma IGF-I and IGF-II concentrations (44,46). However studies of cord blood hPL levels in growth retarded neonates and in infants of diabetic mothers have yielded inconsistent results, possibly reflecting the heterogeneity of the underlying diseases (47–49).

In the ovine fetus, plasma concentrations of PL rise during prolonged maternal fasting, but not during the acute induction of fetal hypoglycemia or hyperglycemia (50). Hypoxic stress and surgery produce dramatic though transient elevations in fetal oPL levels (51). The significance of these observations for the human fetus remains unclear, though findings in the ovine fetus are consistent with those in pregnant women.

SOMATOGENIC AND LACTOGENIC RECEPTORS IN FETAL TISSUES

The hGH and Human Prolactin Receptor Family

The biological actions of hGH, prolactin and hPL are mediated through binding to specific, high-affinity receptors located on the plasma membranes of target tissues. Two receptors for the human somatogenic and lactogenic hormones have been characterized: the hGH receptor (hGHR) and the human prolactin receptor (hPRLR) (52–55). The GH and PRL receptors are encoded by genes located on chromosome 5 (5p13–p14). Each receptor is a single chain polypeptide comprising extracellular, transmembrane and cytoplasmic domains (Fig. 1). The extracellular domain functions as a hormone binding unit. Two pairs of cysteine residues situated near the amino terminus of each receptor, are critical for protein folding. In the PRLR, but not the GHR, a tryptophan-serine-residue-tryptophan-serine (WSXWS) motif lying just proximal to the transmembrane region appears essential for protein–protein interactions, homodimerization of the receptor, and cellular trafficking. Within the proximal cytoplasmic domain of the PRL and GH receptors lies a proline-rich motif (Box 1) that interacts with a receptor-associated tyrosine kinase termed Janus kinase 2 (JAK 2). The proline-rich motif is critical for receptor-mediated signaling. Binding of ligand to the full-length hGH or hPRL receptors is

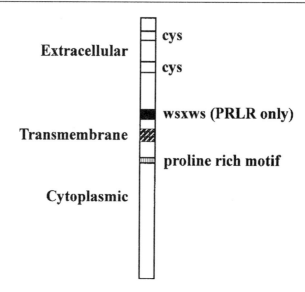

Fig. 1. Schematic drawing of shared features of the GH and PRL receptors. cys, pair of cysteine residues; wsxws, tryptophan-serine motif. The wsxws motif is characteristic of PRL receptors but not GH receptors. The corresponding sequence in the hGH receptor is ygefs.

accompanied by activation of JAK2 and tyrosine phosphorylation of the receptor, activation of other cellular kinases including the Fyn, Raf-1, and mitogen-activator protein (MAP) kinases, and tyrosine phosphorylation of various cytosolic proteins including insulin receptor substrate-1 and signal transducers and activators of transcription (STATs) 1, 3, and 5. The phosphorylated STAT dissociated from the receptor dimerizes and is translocated to the nucleus, where it activates DNA elements in the promoter regions of target genes.

Efficient signaling through the hGH and human prolactin receptors appears to require receptor dimerization. In the two-site model of GH receptor activation initially proposed by Wells and his colleagues (56,57), hGH first binds to a single GH receptor molecule. At low hormone concentrations this hormone-receptor complex then binds an additional molecule of receptor, effectively dimerizing the receptor and facilitating signal transduction. Very high concentrations of hormone (1–10 μM) favor the formation of 1:1 hormone-receptor complexes, preventing receptor homodimerization and signal transduction (55–57). Like the interaction between GH and the GHR, the interaction between lactogenic hormones such as human prolactin and hPL and the human prolactin receptor is thought to conform to the two-site model of receptor activation (55,58).

Alternative splicing of the GH and PRL receptor transcripts plays an important role in receptor physiology. The hGH receptor is expressed as distinct isoforms that contain or lack the extracellular exon 3. Structure-function studies have not yet compared the relative signal-transducing capacities of the two GHR isoforms. Isoforms of the PRL receptor which differ by lengths of the cytoplasmic domains are expressed in rodent (52–55) and human (58a) tissues. The PRLR isoforms have differential capacities for transducing signals of lactogenic hormones (58b); the full-length ("long") and intermediate isoforms are fully active, whereas the short isoform may function as a dominant negative inhibitor of long isoform bioactivity (58c).

Table 1
Affinity of Binding (Kd, nM) of Human Somatogens
and Lactogens to the hGH and hPRL Receptors

	Human GHR	Human PRLR
hGH-N	0.34	0.033
hGH-V	0.35	0.24–1.0[a]
hPRL	NB	2.6
hPL	770	0.046

NB, no binding to the GHR.
[a]Estimate based on the relative binding of hGH-N and hGH-V
to rat prolactin receptors and Nb2 lymphoma cells.

Posttranslational processing of the GH and PRL receptors also subserves important functions in the physiology of the somatogenic and lactogenic hormones. In the serum of human adults, approx 40–50% of circulating GH is bound to high- and low-affinity GH binding proteins (59). The high affinity hGH binding protein represents the extracellular domain of the hGHR cleaved from the membrane-bound protein and as such binds both hGH-N and hGH-V. Binding of hGH to the high affinity GH binding protein increases the circulating half-life of the hormone and may enhance its growth-promoting activity in vivo (60). The levels of the high affinity GH binding protein in umbilical cord blood are only one-eighth to one-tenth those in adult serum (61), possibly reflecting a relative deficiency of hGH receptors in fetal tissues. A prolactin binding protein has not yet been identified in human serum. However, human milk contains a protein that binds hGH and hPRL with high affinity (62), and a high-affinity prolactin binding protein is detected in rabbit milk (63).

Recent studies have characterized the interactions between hGH, human prolactin and hPL and the recombinant hGH and human prolactin receptors (Table 1). The hGHR binds hGH-N and hGH-V with high affinity (Kd 0.34 nM) and hPL with low affinity (Kd 770 nM); it does not interact with human prolactin (55,57,64,65). Thus, at the physiological concentrations measured in human fetal serum, the only hormone likely to bind to, and transmit a signal through, the hGHR is pituitary hGH (fetal serum does not contain detectable levels of hGH-V). The hPRLR (55,58,64) binds hGH-N (Kd 33 pM) and hPL (Kd 46 pM) with very high affinity and human prolactin with lesser high affinity (Kd 2.6 nM). Interestingly, the binding of hGH and hPL to the hPRLR requires zinc (55,66), whereas the binding of hPRL to the PRLR does not. The concentrations of zinc required for optimal binding of hGH or hPL (10–50 μM) are comparable to the concentrations of zinc in human fetal and maternal serum (9–12 μM), suggesting that zinc availability during pregnancy may modulate the fetal tissue response to the various lactogenic hormones (67,68).

Receptor Expression in Human Fetal Tissues

hGH Receptors

The expression of hGHR mRNA in human fetal tissues has been examined (69) using the technique of reverse transcription-polymerase chain reaction (RT-PCR). Messenger RNA encoding the membrane-bound hGHR is expressed in the liver, kidney, skin, muscle, lung, adrenal, brain, spleen, intestine, and pancreas of the human fetus at 7–20 wk of gestation. Two isoforms of hGHR mRNA are expressed in fetal tissues: the full-length

GHR mRNA and an isoform lacking exon 3. The expression of the two isoforms varies on a person-to-person basis rather than in a tissue-specific manner, but the expression of the exon-3 deleted isoform may predominate in the fetus. The significance of this finding is unclear because the two isoforms bind hGH and hPL with similar affinities *(70)*.

The cellular distribution of GHR protein in the human fetus at 8.5–20 wk of gestation has been analyzed using immunohistochemical techniques. Initial studies by Hill et al. *(71)* in human abortuses at 14–16 wk of gestation demonstrated weak GHR immunoreactivity in human fetal hepatocytes, pancreatic duct epithelial cells, renal tubular epithelial cells, cerebral cortical neuronal cell bodies, and germinal cells of the epidermis. No immunoreactive staining was observed in skeletal or cardiac muscle, epiphyseal growth plate, lung, intestine, or adrenal gland. Subsequent studies of human abortuses *(72,73)* demonstrated low levels of GHR immunoreactivity in fetal hepatocytes, bile duct epithelial cells, and renal tubular and glomerular epithelial cells at 8.5 wk of gestation. Faint staining was noted in fetal adrenal cortical cells beginning at 13–14 wk of gestation; undifferentiated definitive zone cells were immunonegative. Maturing chondrocytes and perichondrial cells were immunopositive at 16 wk of gestation, while GHR immunoreactivity was first detected in small intestinal villous epithelial cells and crypts at 19–20 wk of gestation. Despite evidence of expression of pulmonary GHR mRNA in early gestation, the lung was immunonegative throughout fetal development. In contrast, vascular smooth muscle cells and endothelial cells and dermal fibroblasts were immunopositive as early as 8 wk postconception. In the liver, adrenal cortex, small intestine, and epidermis, the intensity of GHR immunostaining increased markedly between early gestation and the neonatal and adult periods. Ontogenetic studies of hormone binding are consistent with the results of immunohistochemical studies: the binding of radiolabeled hGH to hepatic membranes of children and human adults exceeds greatly the binding of radiolabeled hGH to human fetal liver membranes *(74)*.

These observations suggest a relative paucity of hGH receptors in the human fetus in early and midgestation with progressive maturation of the GHR in late gestation or in the perinatal period. Findings in subprimate species are consistent with studies in human fetal and postnatal tissues. Low levels of GHR mRNA and GH binding activity are detected in diverse tissues of the fetal sheep, rabbit, rat, and mouse in mid–late gestation *(75–81)*. In skeletal muscle of the fetal sheep, the levels of GHR mRNA increase between early (d 51) and mid (d 95) gestation *(77)*. In the liver, GHR mRNA levels and GH binding activity increase dramatically soon after birth in the sheep and rabbit *(75–77,80)* and rise precipitously after postnatal d 10 in the rat *(78,82)*, coincident with the induction of hepatic IGF-I mRNA and GH-dependent serine protease inhibitors (Spi 2.1 and 2.3). And in the rat hypothalamus *(83)*, the levels of GHR mRNA increase 8- to 10-fold between embryonic d 15 and postnatal d 7. The emergence of the GH receptor in late gestation suggests a mechanism by which GH may assume control of growth and metabolism during the perinatal and postnatal periods.

Prolactin Receptors

Recent studies *(84–88)* demonstrate widespread expression of prolactin receptor mRNA, immunoreactive protein, and lactogenic binding activity in the human fetus and fetal rat in early and midgestation and reveal striking changes in the cellular distribution of prolactin receptors during fetal and perinatal development. Messenger RNA encoding the membrane-bound PRLR is expressed in diverse human and rat fetal tissues including

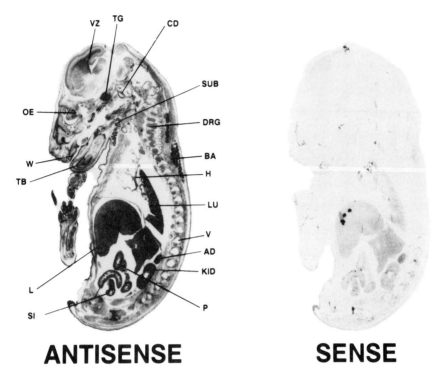

ANTISENSE   **SENSE**

Fig. 2. Tissue distribution of PRLR mRNA in the fetal rat (E18.5). Sections were hybridized with antisense and sense strand RNA probes encoding the rat PRLR. VZ, ventricular zone neuroepithelium; TG, trigeminal ganglion; CD, cochlear duct; SUB, submandibular gland; DRG, dorsal root ganglion; BA, brown adipocytes; H, heart; LU, lung; V, vertebrae; AD, adrenal gland; KID, kidney; P, pancreas; SI, small intestine; L, liver; TB, tooth bud; W, whisker primordia; OE, olfactory epithelium. From Royster et al. *(86)* with permission.

the liver, small intestine, stomach, adrenal, heart, lung, pancreas, thymus, kidney, brain, choroid plexus, the trigeminal and dorsal root ganglia, the cochlear duct, the cartilage of endochondral bones, the enamel epithelium of the tooth bud, and the submandibular gland, brown adipose tissue, and testis (Fig. 2). Expression of PRLR mRNA is demonstrable as early as 52 d of gestation in the human fetus and 11.5 d of gestation in the fetal rat.

Histochemical analysis *(86,88)* of PRLR expression in the early gestational human fetus (7.5–10 wk) and fetal rat (E12.5–E16.5) reveals intense PRLR immunoreactivity in tissues derived from embryonic mesoderm, including the periadrenal and perinephric mesenchyme, the pulmonary and duodenal mesenchyme, the skeletal and cardiac myocytes, and the mesenchymal precartilage and maturing chondrocytes of the endochondral craniofacial and long bones, vertebrae, and ribs. Subsequently, there are striking changes in the cellular distribution and magnitude of expression of PRLRs in a number of tissues. In the fetal adrenal the initial mesenchymal PRLR expression is succeeded by the emergence of PRLR immunoreactivity in deeper fetal cortical cell layers; the latter is apparent by 14 wk of gestation in the human fetus and by embryonic d E18.5–E20.5 in the fetal rat. In the fetal kidney and lung, the invagination of cortical mesenchyme is accompanied by progressive PRLR immunoreactivity in renal tubular and bronchial airway epithelial cells. In the renal tubules and collecting ducts, the PRLR is expressed

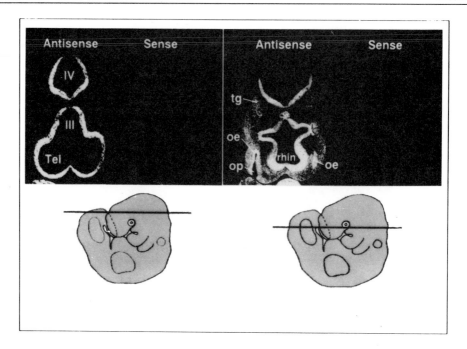

Fig. 3. Expression of PRLR mRNA in the brain of the rat embryo. Transverse sections of rat embryos on d E12.5 were hybridized with antisense and sense strand RNA probes encoding the rat PRLR. Specific staining is shown in white. oe, olfactory epithelium; op, olfactory pit; rhin, rhinencephalic neuroepithelium; tel, telencephalic vesicle; tg, trigeminal ganglion; III, third ventricle; IV, fourth ventricle. Note the staining in the cranial mesenchyme interposed between the surface ectoderm and the ventricular neuroepithelium. From Freemark et al. *(87)* with permission.

primarily on luminal surfaces, consistent with the effects of lactogenic hormones on tubular fluid and electrolyte transport in postnatal animals. In the pulmonary airways, the PRLR is expressed initially in basal epithelial cells and subsequently in surface epithelial cells lining the bronchiolar lumen. In the pancreas, the PRLR is detected in acinar cells and ducts in early gestation; in late gestation and in the postnatal period, the PRLR is expressed predominantly in pancreatic islets, colocalizing with insulin and glucagon. Finally, in fetal hepatocytes, PRLR immunoreactivity increases markedly between embryonic d E52 and E96 in the human fetus and between d E16.5 and E18.5 in the fetal rat. The widespread expression of the PRLR in the human fetus in early and midgestation, and the changing distribution of PRLRs in fetal tissues during ontogeny, suggest roles for the lactogenic hormones in tissue differentiation and development.

Further evidence supporting a role for lactogens in tissue differentiation is provided by studies of the ontogenesis of PRLR expression in the rat olfactory system *(87)*. At midgestation (E12.5), messenger RNAs encoding the long and short isoforms of the rat PRLR are detected in the medial and lateral nasal processes, the epithelial lining of the olfactory pit, and the neuroepithelium lining the cerebral ventricles in the region of the rhinencephalon (Fig. 3). With advancing gestation the PRLR is expressed intensely, though discontinuously, in the olfactory epithelium as well as in the mesenchymal prechondrocytes of the developing craniofacial bones (Fig. 4). PRLRs are first detected in the olfactory bulb on embryonic d 18.5, localizing initially to the periventricular

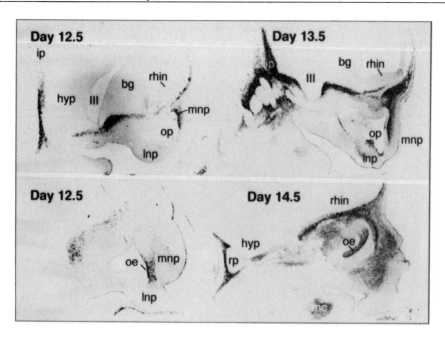

Fig. 4. PRLR immunoreactivity in the fetal olfactory system and craniofacial tissues. Numbers in the upper left corners represent days of gestation. oe, olfactory epithelium; op, olfactory pit; hyp, hypothalamus; mnp, medial nasal process; lnp, lateral nasal process; rp, Rathke's pouch; bg, basal ganglia; ip, interpeduncular fossa. Note the striking immunoreactivity in the nasal processes, oe, and frontonasal mesenchyme and in the mesenchyme of Meckel's cartilage (mc, lower right figure). From Freemark et al. *(87)* with permission.

neuroepithelium. Subsequently, there is robust staining of the bulbar mitral and tufted cell neurons, accompanied by intense expression in the sensory neuronal cell bodies of the olfactory epithelium. On postnatal d 5, the PRLR is expressed in abundance in mitral and tufted cells of the olfactory bulb and in neuronal cell bodies of the anterior olfactory nucleus and the piriform cortex (Fig. 5). Interestingly, the levels of PRLR mRNA in the olfactory bulb of the fetal and neonatal rat exceed greatly the levels of PRLR mRNA in the olfactory bulb of the lactating rat. These observations implicate novel roles for the lactogenic hormones in olfactory development and suggest new mechanisms by which the lactogens may regulate neonatal behavior and maternal–infant interactions.

The roles of lactogenic hormones in fetal development may be clarified by studies of "knockout" mice with deletions of the mouse prolactin receptor. Initial *(52,89,90)* studies reveal striking reproductive abnormalities in PRLR-deficient mice: homozygous females are sterile owing to defects in implantation and ovarian function; heterozygous females have delayed mammary development and lactate poorly after the first pregnancy, and maternal behavior is aberrant. Twenty percent of the homozygous males show delayed fertility, for reasons unknown. Finally, PRLR-deficient mice have reduced bone mineral density and mineral content and delayed bone formation, even as early as embryonic d 18.5. Other effects of the PRLR knockout on the mouse embryos have not been examined, but critical organ dysfunction is unlikely given that the homozygous mutants survive to adulthood.

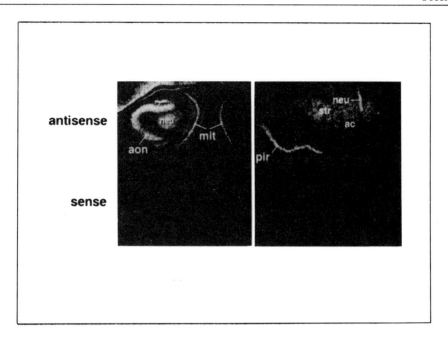

Fig. 5. PRLR expression in the neonatal olfactory cortex. Coronal sections of rat brain (postnatal d 5) were hybridized with antisense and sense RNA probes encoding the rat PRLR. aon, anterior olfactory nucleus; pir, piriform cortex; mit, mitral cells of olfactory bulb; str, striatum; neu, neuroepithelium. No staining of the anterior commissure (ac) was observed. From Freemark et al. *(87)* with permission.

PLACENTAL LACTOGEN BINDING SITES

In a study of human abortuses at 12–20 wk of gestation *(43)*, specific binding of radiolabeled hPL was detected in diverse tissues including the liver, adrenal, kidney, lung, skin, heart, intestine, brain, and skeletal muscle. The binding of radiolabeled hPL to human fetal liver and lung *(43* and MF, unpublished observations) was inhibited by unlabeled hGH and human prolactin as well as hPL, consistent with binding of hPL to the human PRLR. In microsomal membranes of human fetal skeletal muscle, however, the binding of hPL was not inhibited by either hGH or human prolactin (Fig. 6). This observation, together with studies of the biological actions of hPL, hGH and human prolactin in human fetal myoblasts and fibroblasts *(see below)*, suggest a distinct signaling mechanism by which hPL may exert biological effects in the human fetus.

The possible existence of a distinct PL receptor is suggested by studies in the sheep and cow. In microsomal membranes of fetal sheep liver *(75,91,92)*, the specific binding of radiolabeled ovine PL (oPL) exceeds greatly that of ovine GH (oGH) and ovine prolactin. The affinity of binding of oPL is 20–50 times higher than that of oGH and 1000–2000 times higher than that of ovine prolactin, and the apparent Mr of the oPL binding site in ovine fetal liver (38–44 kDa), as determined by affinity crosslinking *(93,94)*, differs from that of the oGH binding site in postnatal sheep liver (53/108 kDa). In bovine endometrium *(95,96)*, as in fetal sheep liver, the affinity of binding of PL is 100–1000 times greater than that of GH and prolactin. The significance of these observations remains unclear because fetal sheep liver and bovine endometrium contain distinct GH and prolactin receptors. Certain findings might be explained by differences in the mechanisms by which the

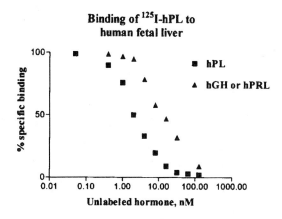

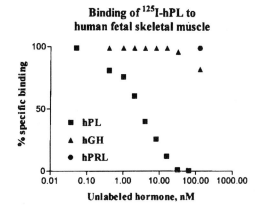

Fig. 6. Binding of hPL, hGH and hPRL to microsomal membranes of human fetal liver and skeletal muscle. Redrawn from Hill et al. *(43)* with permission.

ungulate PLs and the ungulate GHs interact with ungulate GH receptors. Whereas bovine GH forms a 1:2 hormone:receptor complex with the bovine GH receptor, bovine PL forms only 1:1 hormone:receptor complexes with the bovine GH receptor *(97)*. The failure of the ungulate PLs to dimerize the ungulate GH receptor may explain their weak or apparent lack of somatotropic activity in the cow and sheep *(98–101)*. On the other hand, the binding of hPL in the human fetus is likely to be accompanied by receptor dimerization because hPL exerts direct metabolic and somatotropic effects in human fetal tissues *(see below)*. The possible existence of a distinct PL receptor remains a major unresolved puzzle in clarifying the roles of the somatogenic and lactogenic hormones in fetal development.

REGULATION OF SOMATOGENIC
AND LACTOGENIC RECEPTORS IN FETAL TISSUES

The roles of hormonal and nutritional factors in the regulation of fetal somatogenic and lactogenic receptors have been examined only in the sheep. Fasting of the pregnant ewe for 72 h in mid–late gestation causes a 50–70% reduction in the number of oPL binding sites in fetal and maternal liver *(102,103)*. The binding of oPL to fetal liver is restored by refeeding or by the administration of intravenous glucose to the pregnant ewe. The changes in oPL binding in the sheep fetus during fasting suggest a novel hormonal adaptation to nutritional deprivation during pregnancy. Nutrition-dependent changes in PL binding in the ovine fetus correlate positively with changes in fetal plasma glucose, insulin and IGF-I concentrations and negatively with fetal plasma oPL concentrations *(102,103)*. Nevertheless, glucose and insulin have no effect on the binding of oPL to cultured fibroblasts from fetal sheep. However, the binding of oPL to fetal sheep fibroblasts is increased 1.5–fivefold by the glucocorticoid dexamethasone *(103,104)*.

Glucocorticoids appear to play a major role in the induction of the GH receptor in the late-gestational fetal lamb. The induction of GH receptor mRNA and IGF-I mRNA in ovine fetal liver during the week prior to parturition *(75–77)* is prevented by fetal adrenalectomy *(105)*; GH receptor and IGF-I mRNA levels in adrenalectomized animals are restored by the direct administration of cortisol to the fetus *(105)*. These observations suggest that the fetal cortisol surge in late gestation is critical for maturation of the GH receptor and the somatotropic axis during the perinatal period.

GH AND PROLACTIN RECEPTORS IN UTEROPLACENTAL TISSUES

During pregnancy, the GH and prolactin receptors are expressed in the human amnion, chorion, decidua, and placental trophoblast *(106–108)*. The full-length GHR predominates in the chorion and decidua, whereas the amnion and placental villi express primarily the exon-3 deleted isoform. The roles of the GH and PRL receptors in uteroplacental tissues are unknown. Previous investigations suggested that lactogenic activity in the human amnion may serve to regulate the composition of fluids and electrolytes in amniotic fluid *(109–111)*. Recent findings indicate that prolactin and hPL stimulate the production of parathyroid hormone related peptide (PTH-RP) in isolated amnion cells *(112)*, suggesting that lactogens may regulate calcium transport in uteroplacental tissues. Additional evidence for a role for the lactogens in mineral and/or nutrient transport is provided by recent studies demonstrating the expression of PRLR mRNA and immunoreactive protein in the rat visceral yolk sac *(87)*.

BIOLOGICAL ACTIONS OF THE SOMATOGENIC AND LACTOGENIC HORMONES IN THE HUMAN FETUS AND THEIR ROLES IN FETAL GROWTH

Metabolic Actions

Metabolic effects of the somatogenic and lactogenic hormones have been examined in a number of fetal tissues including the adrenal, lung, liver, pancreas, thymus, and skeletal muscle.

A role for lactogenic hormones in the production of fetal adrenocortical steroid hormones is suggested by studies in the chronically catheterized baboon fetus. The iv administration of prolactin to the baboon fetus at midgestation stimulates a two- to threefold increase in fetal plasma dehydroepiandrosterone concentrations but no increase in fetal plasma cortisol concentrations *(113)*. Similar effects of lactogenic hormones have been recorded in human fetal adrenal slices, baboon fetal adrenocortical cells, and isolated adrenocortical cells from human adults *(114–117)*. Limited evidence suggests that the effects of lactogens on fetal dehydroepiandrosterone production in vivo may predominate at midgestation *(118,119)*. The demonstration of prolactin receptors in the human fetal adrenal cortex *(88)* at 14–20 wk is consistent with these observations. However, no

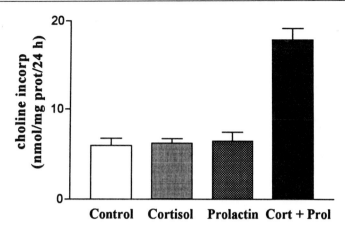

Fig. 7. Data adapted and redrawn from Mendelson et al. *(121)* with permission.

effects of prolactin were noted in other studies of dehydroepiandrosterone or cortisol production in isolated human fetal adrenocortical cells (reviewed in refs. *119,120*). The interpretation of in vitro studies is complicated by the fact that human fetal adrenal cells in culture undergo morphologic and maturational changes that may alter cellular function and prolactin receptor expression (*120* and M. F., unpublished observations).

A role for lactogenic hormones in the development of the human fetal lung is suggested by studies in pulmonary explants from human abortuses at midgestation. In concert with glucocorticoids, prolactin stimulated a two- to threefold increase in pulmonary surfactant production and lamellar body secretion (*121,122*, Fig. 7). On the other hand, cortisol, prolactin, and hPL reduced the production of IGF-I in lung explant cultures *(123)*. These observations suggest a role for lactogens in pulmonary maturation, a hypothesis supported by some *(124,125)*, but not all *(126,127)*, clinical studies in premature infants demonstrating a negative correlation between umbilical cord prolactin levels and the incidence of respiratory distress syndrome.

Clinical experience substantiates a role for lactogenic and somatogenic hormones in perinatal carbohydrate metabolism. Newborn infants with GH deficiency or with GH insensitivity resulting from defects in the hGH receptor are predisposed to severe hypoglycemia in the neonatal period *(128)*. Increased sensitivity to insulin likely plays a role; but the neonatal hypoglycemia may also result in part from deficient storage of glycogen in fetal liver because ovine PL, GH and prolactin *(91,129)*, in concert with insulin *(130)*, stimulate glycogen synthesis and inhibit glycogenolysis *(131)* in isolated hepatocytes from fetal sheep and fetal rats. The glycogenic effects of somatogens and lactogens in human fetal liver have not yet been examined. However, both hPL and hGH stimulate DNA synthesis and IGF-I production in isolated human fetal hepatocytes *(132)*.

The somatogens and lactogens also regulate the production of IGF-I as well as insulin in the fetal pancreas. In cultured explants of human pancreas at 12–21 wk of gestation, both hPL and hGH stimulated a 50% increase in insulin content and release and a twofold increase in pancreatic IGF-I content and release *(133)*. The effect of hPL on insulin production exceeded that of hGH, and the actions of both hormones were observed only when media glucose concentrations exceeded 5.5 m*M*. Similar findings have been recorded in studies of human adults and fetal and neonatal rats and mice *(134–136)*. These observations implicate a role for the lactogenic and somatogenic hormones in the induc-

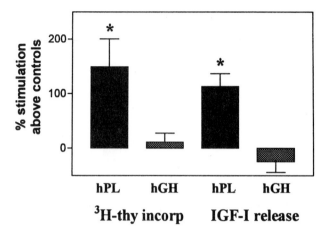

Fig. 8. Data adapted and redrawn from Hill et al. *(143)* with permission.

tion of glucose-sensitive insulin release in late gestation. HGH, prolactin and hPL also stimulate also stimulate DNA synthesis in isolated islets from neonatal rats and mice *(134–136)* and promote the formation of islet-like cell clusters in cultures of human fetal pancreas *(137)*. These findings suggest roles for the somatogens and lactogens in the regulation of islet development and growth.

GH and PRL receptors are expressed in the human fetal thymus and in the thymus of the fetal rat and cow *(85,86,88,137a)*. In the fetal rat, the expression of PRLRs increases markedly between d 17 and 20 of fetal life *(86)*. That the GHRs and PRLRs play roles in thymic development is suggested by a recent study that demonstrated that GH, PRL and PL stimulate increases in the mRNA levels of interleukin-1α, interleukin-1β, and interleukin-6 in fetal bovine thymic stromal cells *(137b)*.

The high prevalence of micropenis in newborn males with GH deficiency or GH resistance *(138,139)* implicates a role for somatogenic hormones in the regulation of human phallic growth *in utero*. The mechanisms by which GH regulates phallic growth are unclear, but recent studies *(140)* in the fetal mouse suggest a role for the somatogens in the differentiation of the male reproductive tract.

The results of the various studies cited above can be explained by the interactions of hGH, human prolactin, and hPL with the hGH and human prolactin receptors. However, studies in fetal skeletal muscle and in isolated human fetal myoblasts and fetal skin fibroblasts are more difficult to interpret. In postnatal skeletal muscle, hGH stimulates amino acid uptake, protein synthesis, and the production of IGF-I. In isolated fetal rat diaphragm *(141,142)*, and in cultured human fetal myoblasts and fibroblasts *(143)*, on the other hand, neither GH nor prolactin stimulate amino acid uptake nor IGF-I production. These findings might be explained by the relatively low level of expression of hGHRs and hPRLRs in fetal muscle. However, ovine PL stimulated a 50% increase in amino acid uptake in fetal rat diaphragm *(142)*, and hPL stimulated 1.5- to 3-fold increases in amino acid uptake, DNA synthesis and IGF-I production in human fetal myoblasts and fibroblasts in culture *(143,144*; Fig. 8). The effects of hPL on ^{3}H-thymidine incorporation and amino acid transport were blunted though not abolished by an antiserum to IGF-I, suggesting that the action of hPL is mediated in part through the paracrine release of IGF-I *(143,144)*. Together with studies demonstrating a positive correlation between cord blood hPL levels and IGF concentrations *(44,46)*, these observations suggest a possible role for hPL in the control of fetal growth. The mechanisms by which PL exerts anabolic effects in fetal skeletal muscle are unclear, but the absence of effects of GH and prolactin suggests that the biological activity of hPL may be mediated through binding to a distinct hPL receptor or to a modified or variant GH or prolactin receptor.

Roles in Fetal Growth

Although GH, prolactin and PL bind with high affinity to fetal receptors and exert direct metabolic effects in fetal tissues, a role for these hormones in fetal development and growth has been challenged by clinical and experimental studies conducted during the past 25 yr. Much of this evidence has been reviewed previously *(145)* and can be summarized as follows.

First, a deficiency of somatogenic or lactogenic hormones in the human fetus is not associated with fetal growth failure. There are minimal or modest (and inconsistent) reductions (0.8 ± 1.4 SD below the mean) in birth length in patients with isolated GH deficiency, pituitary aplasia or anencephaly *(145,146)*. Moreover, birth weight and length are normal in prolactin-deficient newborns whose mothers received bromocryptine during pregnancy *(34)*. Finally, patients with deletions of the human growth hormone V gene and the hPL A and B genes *(147–150)* are generally, but not always *(150a)*, of normal birth length and weight and have no apparent metabolic, immunologic or reproductive abnormalities. In striking contrast, mutations or deletions of the IGF-I or IGF-II genes are accompanied by severe intrauterine growth retardation *(151,152)*.

Second, a deficiency or excess of GH in experimental animals has little or no effect on fetal growth. For example, dwarf mice deficient in pituitary GH have normal tail lengths at birth and modest (14%) reductions in birth weight, though serum IGF-I and IGF-II concentrations are reduced significantly *(153)*. Decapitation, encephalectomy or hypophysectomy of fetal rabbits, rhesus monkeys, rats, mice, or pigs is not accompanied by fetal growth failure or reductions in serum IGF I concentrations, and electrolytic destruction of the ovine fetal medial-basal hypothalamus with concomitant GH deficiency has no effects on fetal plasma IGF-I or IGF-II concentrations *(145)*. Conversely, an excess of fetal GH is not accompanied by fetal overgrowth. For example, transgenic mice expressing high levels of pituitary GH *(154)* or GH releasing hormone *(155)* are normally sized at birth and do not grow excessively until 14–21 d of age.

Third, a deficiency or functional abnormality of the GH receptor in the human fetus is not accompanied by fetal growth failure. Birth length is reduced modestly and variably (1.6 ± 2.0 SD below the mean) in states of GH insensitivity *(138,139)* resulting from mutations of the GH receptor gene ("Laron dwarfism"). The near-normal growth in utero is thought to reflect the low level of expression, and relative unimportance, of GH receptors in normal fetal tissues. The induction of GH receptors in the perinatal period explains the severe growth failure that is demonstrable soon after birth.

Although persuasive, the evidence cited above has important limitations. For example, see the following.

1. Whereas circulating hPL is derived exclusively from the placenta during normal pregnancy, hGH and human prolactin are produced by extrapituitary tissues including decidual cells and lymphocytes *(11,18)*. Controlled by mechanisms distinct from those that regulate pituitary GH and prolactin, the production of GH and PRL by decidual cells persists in the absence of normal fetal pituitary function; for example, the levels of GH in amniotic

fluid are normal in anencephaly despite deficient pituitary GH production *(30,31)*, and the levels of prolactin in amniotic fluid are normal in pregnant women treated with bromocryptine *(34,38)*. Amniotic fluid containing prolactin (as well as hPL and hGH) is inhaled and swallowed by the fetus and may exert direct trophic or maturational effects on fetal tissues such as the lung and gastrointestinal tract *(156–159)*. Such actions, as yet poorly defined, may theoretically mitigate the effects of reductions in fetal serum pituitary GH and prolactin associated with hypopituitarism or with the administration of bromocryptine to the mother.

2. Overlapping biological actions of various somatogenic and lactogenic hormones may provide a redundancy of function that may protect the fetus against the loss of a single hormone. In a number of experimental systems, for instance, the biological actions of PL are similar to those of GH and/or prolactin. Thus, expression of PL may theoretically compensate for the absence of GH and/or PRL in states associated with hypopituitarism. Conversely, the expression of prolactin or hGH may compensate for reductions in fetal expression of PL in patients with deletions of one or more of the hPL genes. There is currently no experimental evidence to confirm or refute such speculation. However, preliminary studies suggest that variant genes that are normally expressed at negligible levels (for example, the hPL-L gene) may be expressed in pregnant patients bearing deletions of the hPL-A and B genes *(160)*.

3. The relatively low levels of binding of radiolabeled GH, prolactin, and PL in fetal tissues must be interpreted in light of changes in tissue composition during development. The liver provides a useful example. The somatogenic and lactogenic hormones bind to fetal and postnatal hepatocytes rather than to hepatic hematopoietic cells or Kupfer cells *(73,86)*. In early and midgestation the fetal liver is comprised by relatively equal numbers of hematopoietic cells and hepatocytes. In late gestation and in postnatal life, the number of hematopoietic cells wanes whereas the relative hepatocyte content of the liver increases. Changes in the binding of GH, prolactin, and PL to the liver during development may therefore reflect, at least in part, the structural changes in the organ itself. Nevertheless, recent studies from our laboratory *(88)* indicate that changes in the magnitude of expression of somatogenic and lactogenic receptors in specific cell types (e.g., hepatocytes) accounts for some of the ontogenetic changes in hormone binding that have been observed in previous studies.

4. Investigators have tended to combine the results of studies of animals with relatively short gestational periods, such as rats, mice, and rabbits, with studies of humans and other animals with far longer gestational periods. This may complicate the interpretation of results, since the rat or mouse fetus in late gestation has achieved a state of tissue and organ maturation that resembles in many ways the state of maturation of the human fetus at midgestation. If the growth-promoting actions of somatogens or lactogens in the fetus are exerted only late in gestation, then the consequences of hormone deficiency or resistance on linear growth may become apparent (and demonstrable experimentally) only after birth in rats and mice.

5. Finally, previous studies of patients with clinical states of hormone deficiency and hormone resistance may have overlooked subtle but significant effects of the somatogenic and lactogenic hormones on fetal development and growth. For example, newborn infants ("Laron dwarfs") with mutational defects in the GH receptor may have small hands and feet, frontal bossing and depressed nasal bridge, blue sclerae, hypoplastic nails, and sparse hair *(138,139)*. These observations suggest that hGH exerts important effects on skeletal and craniofacial development and on the maturation and function of the fetal integument. It is unclear whether these clinical complications result directly from the

absence of GH action in fetal tissues or from a deficiency in GH-dependent growth factors, such as IGF-I.

CONCLUSIONS AND AVENUES FOR FUTURE RESEARCH

Fetal metabolism and growth are complex processes subject to regulation by a multitude of genetic, nutritional, environmental and hormonal factors. Whereas none of the somatogenic or lactogenic hormones appears to play an indispensable role in fetal metabolism, GH, prolactin and PL likely serve important functions in embryonic and fetal development. Clinical observations establish a role for GH in perinatal carbohydrate metabolism and in the regulation of phallic growth and strongly suggest roles for somatogenic hormones in development of the craniofacial bones and the human integument. Studies of the ontogeny of GH receptors in fetal tissues, together with clinical studies demonstrating modest reductions in birth length in GH-deficient and GH-resistant patients, suggest that the effects of GH on fetal linear growth are exerted relatively late in gestation.

The effects of prolactin and hPL on human fetal development are more difficult to assess because of the lack of a clinical model of tissue resistance to lactogenic hormones. In this regard, studies of the effects of prolactin receptor deficiency in transgenic mice should provide important information regarding the roles of the lactogens in fetal metabolism and growth. Studies of the ontogenesis of prolactin receptors and the biological actions of lactogenic hormones in fetal tissues suggest roles for lactogens in adrenocortical function, pulmonary maturation, hepatic growth factor production, and pancreatic hormone secretion. The effects of the lactogens on fetal skeletal growth remain speculative, though the expression of prolactin receptors in human fetal chondrocytes and skeletal myocytes and the direct anabolic effects of hPL in fetal myoblasts suggest roles for lactogenic hormones in cartilage and muscle growth and development.

Unresolved issues continue to bedevil the field. For example, why does the human fetus express three different hormones that have lactogenic activity? Do the differences in the mechanisms by which hGH, human prolactin, and hPL interact with the GHR and the PRLR forge differences in biological activity that are important for fetal development? Does hPL exert biological effects through binding to a receptor distinct from the GH and prolactin receptors? What roles do the somatogens and lactogens play in tissue differentiation in early development? How are such effects mediated? Do the lactogenic hormones in amniotic fluid exert direct effects on the human fetus in utero? And how do nutritional factors and trace mineral (e.g., zinc) availability in the pregnant mother modulate the fetal tissue response to somatogenic and lactogenic hormones? These and other important questions clearly warrant further investigation by Pediatric endocrinologists and developmental and reproductive biologists.

ACKNOWLEDGMENTS

The author would like to thank Dr. Stuart Handwerger and various collaborators, former fellows, and technical assistants in the United States, Canada, and France. This work was supported in part by grants from the NICHD (HD24192 and HD00901), March of Dimes (1-7488-1104), and the Juvenile Diabetes Foundation (196029). Dr. Freemark is the recipient of a Research Career Development Award from the National Institute of Child Health and Development.

REFERENCES

1. Nicoll CS, Bern HA. On the actions of PRL among the vertebrates: is there a common denominator? In: Wolstenholme GEW, Knight J, eds. Lactogenic Hormones. Churchill Livingstone, London, 1972, pp. 299–337.
2. Meites J. Biological functions of PRL. In: Hoshino K, ed. PRL Gene Family and Its Receptors. Elsevier, Amsterdam, 1988, pp. 123–130.
3. Ogren L, Talamantes F. Prolactins of pregnancy and their cellular source. Int Rev Cytol 1988; 112:1–65.
4. Caufriez A, Frankenne F, Hennen G, Copinschi G. Regulation of maternal IGF-I by placental GH in normal and abnormal human pregnancies. Am J Physiol 1993;265:E572–577.
5. Fant M, Munro H, Moses AC. An autocrine/paracrine role for insulin-like growth factors in the regulation of human placental growth. J Clin Endo Metab 1986;63:499–505.
6. Sterle JA, Cantley TC, Lamberson WR, Lucy MC, Gerrard DE, Matteri RL, et al. Effects of recombinant porcine somatotropin on placental size, fetal growth, and IGF-I and IGF-II concentrations in pigs. J Anim Sci 1995;73:2980–2985.
7. Pihoker C, Robertson MC, Freemark M. Rat placental lactogen I binds to the choroid plexus and hypothalamus of the pregnant rat. J Endocrinol 1993;139:235–242.
8. Bridges R, Freemark M. Human placental lactogen infusions into the medial preoptic area stimulate maternal behavior in steroid-primed, nulliparous female rats. Horm Behav 1995;29:216–226.
9. Bridges RS, Robertson MC, Shiu RPC, Friesen HG, Stuer AM, Mann PE. Endocrine communication between conceptus and mother: placental lactogen stimulation of maternal behavior. Neuroendocrinol 1996;64:57–64.
10. Chen EY, Liao Y-C, Smith DH, Barrera-Saldana HA, Gelinas RE, Seeburg PH. The human growth hormone locus: nucleotide sequence, biology and evolution. Genomics 1989;4:479–497.
11. Weigent DA, Blalock JE. The production of growth hormone by subpopulations of rat mononuclear leukocytes. Cellular Immunol 1991;135:55–65.
12. Frankenne F, Scippo ML, Van Beeumen J, Igout A, Hennen G. Identification of placental human growth hormone as the growth hormone-V gene expression product. J Clin Endo Metab 1990;71:15–18.
13. Walker WH, Fitzpatrick SL, Barrera-Saldana HA, Resendez-Perez D, Saunders GF. The human placental lactogen genes: structure, function, evolution and transcriptional regulation. Endocr Rev 1991;12:316–328.
14. MacLeod JN, Lee AK, Liebhaber SA, Cooke NE. Developmental control and alternative splicing of the placentally expressed transcripts from the human growth hormone gene cluster. J Biol Chem 1992;267:14,219–14,226.
15. Stewart TA, Clift S, Pitts-Meek S, Martin L, Terrell TG, Liggitt D, et al. Evaluation and functions of the 22 kilodalton (kDa), the 20 kDa, and the N-terminal polypeptide forms of human growth hormone using transgenic mice. Endocrinology 1992;130:405–414.
16. Haro L, Singh RN, Lewis UJ, Martinez AO, Galosy SS, Staten NR, et al. Human growth hormone deletion mutant (hGH 44-191) binds with high affinity to lactogenic receptors but not to somatogenic receptors. Biochem Biophys Res Commun 1996;222:421–426.
17. Handwerger S, Richards RG, Markoff E. The physiology of decidual prolactin and other decidual protein hormones. Trends Endo Metab 1992;3:91–95.
18. Pellegrini I, Lebrun J-J, Ali S, Kelly PA. Expression of prolactin and its receptor in human lymphoid cells. Mol Endo 1992;6:1023–1031.
19. Frankenne F, Closset J, Gomez F, Scippo ML, Smal J, Hennen G. The physiology of growth hormones in pregnant women and partial characterization of the placental GH variant. J Clin Endo Metab 1988;66:1171–1180.
20. MacLeod JN, Worsley I, Ray J, Friesen HG, Liebhaber SA, Cooke NE. Human growth hormone-variant is a biologically active somatogen and lactogen. Endocrinology 1991;128:1289–1302.
21. Grumbach MM, Gluckman PD. The human fetal hypothalamus and pituitary gland: The maturation of neuroendocrine mechanisms controlling the secretion of fetal pituitary growth hormone, prolactin, gonadotropins, adrenocorticotropic-related peptides and thyrotropin. In: Tulchinsky D, Little AB, eds. Maternal-Fetal Endocrinology. Saunders, Philadelphia, 1994, pp. 193–262.
22. Kaplan SL, Grumbach MM, Shepard TH. The ontogenesis of human fetal hormones. I. Growth hormone and insulin. J Clin Invest 1972;51:3080–3093.
23. Leger J, Oury JF, Noel M, Baron S, Benali K, Blot P, et al. Growth factors and intrauterine growth retardation. I. Serum growth hormone, insulin-like growth factor I, IGF II, and IGF binding protein

3 levels in normally grown and growth-retarded human fetuses during the second half of gestation. Pediatr Res 1996;40:94–100.

24. Kletzky OA, Rossman F, Bertolli SI, Platt LD, Mishell DR, Jr. Dynamics of human chorionic gonadotropin, prolactin and growth hormone in serum and amniotic fluid throughout normal human pregnancy. Am J Obstet Gynecol 1985;151:878–884.

25. Varvarigou A, Vagenakis AG, Makri M, Beratis NG. Growth hormone, insulin-like growth factor I and prolactin in small for gestational age neonates. Biol Neonate 1994;65:94–102.

26. Leger J, Noel M, Limal JM, Czernichow P. Growth factors and intrauterine growth retardation. II. Serum growth hormone, IGF I, and IGF binding protein 3 levels in children with intrauterine growth retardation compared with normal control subjects: prospective study from birth to two years of age. Pediatr Res 1996;40:101–107.

27. Nieto-Diaz A, Villar J, Matorras-Weinig R, Valenzuela-Ruiz P. Intrauterine growth retardation at term: association between anthropometric and endocrine parameters. Acta Obstet Gynecol Scand 1996;75:127–131.

28. Nogami H, Yokose T, Tachibana T. Regulation of growth hormone expression in fetal rat pituitary gland by thyroid or glucocorticoid hormone. Am J Physiol 1995;268:E262–267.

29. Rodriguez-Garcia M, Jolin T, Santos A, Perez-Castillo A. Effect of perinatal hypothyroidism on the developmental regulation of rat pituitary growth hormone and thyrotropin genes. Endocrinology 1995;136:4339–4350.

30. Wisniewski L, Jezuita J, Bogoniowska Z, Grzes A. Insulin and human growth hormone in the amniotic fluid in normal pregnancy and in cases of fetal central nervous system anomalies. Zeitschrift fur Geburtshilfe und Perinatologie 1983;187:151,152.

31. Kubota T, Tsuzuki T, Saito M. Determination of prolactin, growth hormone, beta-endorphin, and cortisol in both maternal plasma and amniotic fluid during human gestation. Acta Endocrinol 1989;121:297–303.

32. Wathen NC, Campbell DJ, Patel B, Touzel R, Chard T. Dynamics of prolactin in amniotic fluid and extraembryonic coelomic fluid in early human pregnancy. Early Hum Devel 1993;35:167–172.

33. Aubert MJ, Grumbach MM, Kaplan SL. The ontogenesis of human fetal hormones. III. Prolactin. J Clin Invest 1975;56:155–164.

33a. Roti E, Gardini E, Minelli R, Bianconi L, Alboni A, Braverman LE. Thyrotropin releasing hormone does not stimulate prolactin release in the preterm human fetus. Acta Endocrinol 1990;122:462–466.

34. Bigazzi M, Ronga R, Lancranjan I, Ferraro S, Branconi F, Buzzoni P, et al. A pregnancy in an acromegalic woman during bromocryptine treatment: effects on growth hormone and prolactin in the maternal, fetal and amniotic compartments. J Clin Endo Metab 1979;48:9–12.

35. Clements JA, Reyes FI, Winter JSD, Faiman C. Studies on human sexual development IV. Fetal pituitary and serum and amniotic fluid concentrations of prolactin. J Clin Endo Metab 1977;44:408–413.

36. Kubota T, Tsuzuki H, Saito M. Determination of prolactin, growth hormone, beta-endorphin, and cortisol in both maternal plasma and amniotic fluid during human gestation. Acta Endocrinol 1989;121:297–303.

37. Handwerger S, Markoff E, Richards RG. Regulation of the synthesis and release of decidual prolactin by placental and autocrine/paracrine factors. Placenta 1991;12:121–130.

38. Lehtovirta P, Ranta T. Effect of short-term bromocryptine treatment on amniotic fluid prolactin concentration in the first half of pregnancy. Acta Endocrinol 1981;97:559–561.

39. Braunstein GD, Rasor JL, Engvall E, Wade ME. Interrelationships of human chorionic gonadotropin, human placental lactogen and pregnancy-specific beta1 glycoprotein throughout normal human gestation. Am J Obstet Gynecol 1980;138:1205–1213.

40. Berle P. Pattern of the human chorionic somatomammotrophic (HCS) concentration ratio in maternal serum and amniotic fluid during normal pregnancy. Acta Endocrinol 1974;76:364–368.

41. Lolis D, Kaskarelis D. Human placental lactogen levels in amniotic fluid in normal and toxemic pregnancies. Acta Obstet Gynecol Scand 1978;57:367–369.

42. Wathen NC, Cass PL, Campbell DJ, Kitau MJ, Chard T. Levels of placental protein 14, human placental lactogen and unconjugated oestriol in extraembryonic coelomic fluid. Placenta 1992;13:195–197.

43. Hill DJ, Freemark M, Strain AJ, Handwerger S, Milner RDG. Placental lactogen and growth hormone receptors in human fetal tissues: relationship to fetal plasma human placental lactogen concentrations and fetal growth. J Clin Endo Metab 1988;66:1283–1290.

44. Lassarre C, Hardouin S, Daffos F, Forestier F, Frankenne F, Binoux M. Serum insulin-like growth factors and insulin-like growth factor binding proteins in the human fetus. Relationships with growth in normal subjects and in subjects with intrauterine growth retardation. Pediatr Res 1991;29:219–225.

45. Talamantes F, Ogren L. Human placental lactogen. In: Adashi E, Rock JA, Rosenwaks Z, eds. Reproductive Endocrinology, Surgery and Technology. Lippincott-Raven, Philadelphia, 1996, pp. 769–781.

46. Kastrup KW, Andersen HJ, Lebech P. Somatomedin in newborns and the relationship to human chorionic somatotropin and fetal growth. Acta Pediatr Scand 1978;67:757–762.

47. Botta RM, Donatelli M, Bucalo ML, Bellomonte ML, Bompani GD. Placental lactogen, progesterone, total estriol and prolactin plasma levels in pregnant women with insulin-dependent diabetes mellitus. Eur J Obstet Gynecol 1984;16:393–401.

48. Espinoza-Lopez I, Smith RF, Gillmer M, Schidlmeir A, Hockaday TDR. High levels of growth hormone and placental lactogen in pregnancy complicated by diabetes. Diabetes Res 1986;3:119–125.

49. Braunstein GD, Mills JL, Reed GF, Jovanovic LG, Holmes LB, Aarons J, et al. Comparison of serum placental protein hormone levels in diabetic and normal pregnancy. J Clin Endo Metab 1989;68:3–8.

50. Brinsmead MW, Bancroft BJ, Thorburn GD, Waters MJ. Fetal and maternal ovine placental lactogen during hyperglycemia, hypoglycemia and fasting. J Endocr 1981;90:337–343.

51. Gluckman PD, Kaplan SL, Rudolph AM, Grumbach MM. Hormone ontogeny in the ovine fetus. II. Ovine chorionic somatomammotropin in mid- and late gestation in the fetal and maternal circulations. Endocrinology 1979;104:1828–1834.

52. Bole-Feysot C, Goffin V, Edery M, Binart N, Kelly P. Prolactin and its receptor: actions, signal transduction pathways and phenotypes observed in prolactin receptor knockout mice. Endocr Rev 1998;19:225–268.

53. Horseman N, Yu-Lee L-Y. Transcriptional regulation by the helix bundle peptide hormones: growth hormone, prolactin and hematopoietic cytokines. Endocr Rev 1994;15:627–649.

54. Gao J, Hughes JP, Auperin B, Buteau H, Edery M, Zhuang H, et al. Interactions among JANUS kinases and the prolactin receptor in the regulation of a PRL response element. Mol Endocrinol 1996;10: 847–856.

55. Goffin V, Shiverick KT, Kelly PA, Martial JA. Sequence-function relationships within the expanding family of prolactin, growth hormone, placental lactogen, and related proteins in mammals. Endocr Rev 1996;17:385–410.

56. Cunningham BC, Ultsch M, DeVos AM, Mulkerrin MG, Clauser KR, Wells JA. Dimerization of the extracellular domain of the human growth hormone receptor by a single hormone molecule. Science 1991;254:821–825.

57. Fuh G, Cunningham BC, Fukunaga R, Nagata S, Goeddel DV, Wells JA. Rational design of potent antagonists to the human growth hormone receptor. Science 1992;256:1677–1680.

58. Fuh G, Colosi P, Wood WI, Wells JA. Mechanism-based design of prolactin receptor antagonists. J Biol Chem 1993;268:5376–5381.

58a. Nagano M, Chastre E, Choquet A, Bara J, Gespach C, Kelly PA. Expression of prolactin and growth hormone receptor genes and their isoforms in the gastrointestinal tract. Am J Physiol 1995;268: G431–G442.

58b. O'Neal KD, Yu-Lee LY. Differential signal transduction of the short, Nb2, and long prolactin receptors. Activation of interferon regulatory factor-1 and cell proliferation. J Biol Chem 1994;269:26,076–26,082.

58c. Perrot-Applanat M, Gualillo O, Pezet A, Vincent V, Edery M, Kelly PA. Dominant negative and cooperative effects of mutant forms of prolactin receptor. Mol Endocrinol 1997;11:1020–1032.

59. Baumann G. Growth hormone binding to a circulating receptor fragment—the concept of receptor shedding and receptor splicing. Exp Clin Endo Diab 1995;103:2–6.

60. Clark RG, Mortensen DL, Carlsson LMS, Spencer SA, McKay P, Mulkerrin M, et al. Recombinant human growth hormone binding protein enhances the growth-promoting activity of human GH in the rat. Endocrinology 1996;137:4308–4315.

61. Merimee TJ, Russell B, Quinn S. Growth hormone binding proteins of human serum: developmental patterns in normal man. J Clin Endo Metab 1992;75:852–854.

62. Mercado M, Baumann G. A growth hormone/prolactin binding protein in human milk. J Clin Endo Metab 1994;79:1637–1641.

63. Postel-Vinay MC, Belair L, Kayser C, Kelly PA, Djiane J. Identification of prolactin and growth hormone binding proteins in rabbit milk. Proc Natl Acad Sci USA 1991;88:6687–6690.

64. Lowman HB, Cunningham BC, Wells JA. Mutational analysis and protein engineering of receptor-binding determinants in human placental lactogen. J Biol Chem 1991;266:10,982–10,988.
65. Baumann G, Davila N, Shaw MA, Ray J, Liebhaber SA, Cooke NE. Binding of human growth hormone variant (placental GH) to GH binding proteins in human plasma. J Clin Endo Metab 1991;73:1175–1179.
66. Cunningham BC, Bass S, Fuh G, Wells JA. Zinc mediation of the binding of human growth hormone to the human prolactin receptor. Science 1990;250:1709–1712.
67. Veena R, Narang AP, Banday AW, Bhan VK. Copper and zinc levels in maternal and fetal cord blood. Int J Gynecol Obstet 1991;35:47–49.
68. Goldenberg RL, Tamura T, Neggers Y, Copper RL, Johnston KE, DuBard MB, et al. The effect of zinc supplementation on pregnancy outcome. JAMA 1995;274:463–468.
69. Zogopoulos G, Figueiredo R, Jenab A, Ali Z, Lefebvre Y, Goodyer CG. Expression of exon 3-retaining and-deleted human growth hormone receptor messenger RNA isoforms during development. J Clin Endo Metab 1996;81:775–782.
70. Sobrier ML, Duquesnoy P, Duriez B, Anselem S, Goosens M. Expression and binding properties of two isoforms of the human growth hormone receptor. FEBS Lett 1993;319:16–20.
71. Hill DJ, Riley SC, Bassett NS, Waters MJ. Localization of the growth hormone receptor, identified by immunocytochemistry, in second trimester human fetal tissues and in placenta throughout gestation. J Clin Endo Metab 1992;75:646–650.
72. Werther GA, Haynes K, Waters MJ. Growth hormone receptors are expressed on human fetal mesenchymal tissues-identification of messenger ribonucleic acid and GH-binding protein. J Clin Endo Metab 1993;76:1638–1646.
73. Simard M, Manthos H, Lefebvre Y, Goodyer CG. Ontogeny of growth hormone receptors in human tissues: an immunohistochemical study. J Clin Endo Metab 1996;81:3097–3102.
74. Freemark M. Unpublished observations.
75. Freemark M, Comer M, Handwerger S. Placental lactogen and growth hormone binding sites in sheep liver: striking differences in ontogeny and function. Am J Physiol 1986;251:E328–E333.
76. Adams TE, Baker L, Fiddes RJ, Brandon MR. The sheep growth hormone receptor: molecular cloning and ontogeny of mRNA in the liver. Mol Cell Endocrinol 1990;73:135–145.
77. Klempt M, Bingham B, Breier BH, Baumbach WR, Gluckman PD. Tissue distribution and ontogeny of growth hormone receptor messenger ribonucleic acid and ligand binding to hepatic tissue in the midgestation sheep fetus. Endocrinology 1993;132:1071–1077.
78. Tiong TS, Herington AC. Ontogeny of messenger RNA for the rat growth hormone receptor and serum binding protein. Mol Cell Endocrinol 1992;83:133–141.
79. Edmondson SR, Werther GA, Russell A, LeRoith D, Roberts CT, Jr, Beck F. Localization of growth hormone receptor/binding protein messenger ribonucleic acid (mRNA) during rat fetal development: relationship to insulin-like growth factor-I mRNA. Endocrinology 1995;136:4602–4609.
80. Ymer SI, Herington AC. Developmental expression of the growth hormone receptor gene in rabbit tissues. Mol Cell Endocrinol 1992;83:39–49.
81. Ilkbahar YN, Wu K, Thordarson G, Talamantes F. Expression and distribution of messenger ribonucleic acids for growth hormone receptor and GH-binding protein in mice during pregnancy. Endocrinology 1995;136:386–392.
82. Berry SA, Bergad PL, Bundy MV. Expression of growth hormone-responsive serpin mRNAs in perinatal rat liver. Am J Physiol 1993;264:E973–980.
83. Hasegawa O, Minami S, Sugihara H, Wakabayashi I. Developmental expression of the growth hormone receptor gene in the rat hypothalamus. Dev Brain Res 1993;74:287–290.
84. Freemark M, Kirk K, Pihoker C, Robertson MC, Shiu RPC, Driscoll P. Pregnancy lactogens in the rat conceptus and fetus: circulating levels, distribution of binding, and expression of receptor messenger ribonucleic acid. Endocrinology 1993;133:1830–1842.
85. Freemark M, Nagano M, Edery M, Kelly PA. Prolactin receptor gene expression in the fetal rat. J Endocrinol 1995;144:285–292.
86. Royster M, Driscoll P, Andrews J, Kelly PA, Freemark M. The prolactin receptor in the fetal rat: cellular localization of messenger RNA, immunoreactive protein and ligand binding activity and induction of expression in late gestation. Endocrinology 1995;136:3892–3900.
87. Freemark M, Driscoll P, Andrews J, Kelly PA, Freemark M. Ontogenesis of prolactin receptor gene expression in the rat olfactory system: potential roles for lactogenic hormones in olfactory development. Endocrinology 1996;137:934–942.

88. Freemark M, Driscoll P, Maaskant R, Petryk A, Kelly PA. Ontogenesis of prolactin receptors in the human fetus in early gestation: implications for tissue differentiation and development. J Clin Invest 1997;99:1107–1117.

89. Ormandy CJ, Binart N, Camus A, Lucas B, Buteau H, Barra J, et al. Structure and targeted mutation of the mouse prolactin receptor gene. Annual Meeting of the Endocrine Society, 1995; Washington, DC (abst # P1–541).

90. Ormandy CJ, Camus A, Barra J, Damotte D, Lucas B, Buteau H, et al. Null mutation of the prolactin receptor gene produces multiple reproductive defects in the mouse. Genes Dev 1997;11:167–178.

91. Freemark M, Handwerger S. The glycogenic effects of placental lactogen and growth hormone in ovine fetal liver are mediated through binding to specific fetal oPL receptors. Endocrinology 1986;118:613–618.

92. Pratt SL, Kappes SM, Anthony RV. Ontogeny of a specific high affinity binding site for ovine placental lactogen in fetal and postnatal liver. Domestic Anim Endocrinol 1995;12:337–347.

93. Freemark M, Comer M, Korner G, Handwerger S. A unique placental lactogen receptor: Implications for fetal growth. Endocrinology 1987;120:1865–1872.

94. Freemark M, Comer M. Purification of a distinct placental lactogen receptor, a new member of the GH/prolactin receptor family. J Clin Invest 1989;83:883–889.

95. Galosy SS, Gertler A, Elberg G, Laird DM. Distinct placental lactogen and prolactin receptors in bovine endometrium. Mol Cell Endo 1991;78:229–236.

96. Kessler MA, Duello TM, Schuler LA. Expression of prolactin related hormones in the early bovine conceptus, and potential for paracrine effects on the endometrium. Endocrinology 1991;129: 1885–1895.

97. Staten NR, Byatt JC, Krivi GG. Ligand-specific dimerization of the extracellular domain of the bovine growth hormone receptor. J Biol Chem 1993;268:18,467–18,473.

98. Oliver MH, Harding JE, Breier BH, Evans PC, Gallaher BW, Gluckman PD. The effects of ovine placental lactogen infusion on metabolites, insulin-like growth factors and binding proteins in the fetal sheep. J Endocrinol 1995;144:333–338.

99. Ogawa E, Breier BH, Bauer MK, Gluckman PD. Ovine placental lactogen lacks direct somatogenic and anticatabolic actions in the postnatal lamb. J Endocrinol 1995;145:87–95.

100. Klempt M, Breier BH, Min SH, MacKenzie DD, McCutcheon SN, Gluckman PD. IGFBP-2 expression in liver and mammary tissue in lactating and pregnant ewes. Acta Endocrinol 1993;129:453–457.

101. Byatt JC, Eppard PJ, Veenhuizen JJ, Sorbet RH, Buonomo FC, Curran DF, et al. Serum half-life and in vivo actions of recombinant bovine placental lactogen in the dairy cow. J Endocrinol 1992;132: 185–193.

102. Freemark M, Comer M, Mularoni T, D'Ercole AJ, Grandis AJ, Kodack L. Nutritional regulation of the placental lactogen receptor in fetal liver: implications for fetal metabolism and growth. Endocrinology 1989;125:1504–1512.

103. Freemark M, Keen A, Fowlkes J, Mularoni T, Comer M, Grandis A, et al. The placental lactogen receptor in maternal and fetal sheep liver: regulation by glucose and role in the pathogenesis of fasting during pregnancy. Endocrinology 1992;130:1063–1070.

104. Fowlkes J, Freemark M. Placental lactogen binding sites in isolated fetal fibroblasts: characterization, processing and regulation. Endocrinology 1993;132:2477–2483.

105. Li J, Owens JA, Saunders JC, Fowden AL, Gilmour RS. The ontogeny of hepatic growth hormone receptor and insulin-like growth factor I gene expression in the sheep fetus during late gestation: developmental regulation by cortisol. Endocrinology 1996;137:1650–1657.

106. Urbanek M, MacLeod JN, Cooke NE, Liebhaber SA. Expression of a human growth hormone receptor isoform is predicted by tissue-specific alternative splicing of exon 3 of the hGH receptor gene transcript. Mol Endo 1992;6:279–287.

107. Frankenne F, Alsat E, Scippo ML, Igout A, Hennen G, Evain-Brion D. Evidence for the expression of growth hormone receptors in human placenta. Biochem Biophys Res Commun 1992;182:481–486.

108. Maaskant R, Bogic LV, Gilger S, Kelly PA, Bryant-Greenwood GD. The human prolactin receptor in the fetal membranes, decidua and placenta. J Clin Endo Metab 1996;81:396–405.

109. Page KR, Abramovich DR, Smith MR. Water transport across isolated term human amnion. J Mem Biol 1974;18:49–60.

110. Josimovich JB, Merisco K, Boccella L. Amniotic prolactin control over amniotic and fetal extracellular fluid water and electrolytes in the rhesus monkey. Endocrinology 1977;100:564–570.

111. Tyson JE, Mowat GS, McCoshen JA. Simulation of a probable biologic effect of decidual prolactin on fetal membranes. Am J Obstet Gynecol 1984;148:296–300.

112. Dvir R, Golander A, Jaccard N, Yedwab G, Otremski I, Spirer Z, et al. Amniotic fluid and plasma levels of parathyroid hormone-related protein and hormonal modulation of its secretion by amniotic fluid cells. Eur J Endocrinol 1995;133:277–282.
113. Pepe GJ, Albrecht ED. Regulation of baboon fetal adrenal androgen production by adrenocorticotropin, prolactin, and growth hormone. Biol Reprod 1985;33:545–550.
114. Brown TB, Ginz B, Milne CM, Oakey RE. Stimulation by polypeptides of dehydroepiandrosterone sulphate synthesis in human foetal adrenal slices. J Endocrinol 1981;91:111–122.
115. Taga M, Tanaka K, Liu T, Minaguchi H, Sakamoto S. Effect of prolactin on the secretion of dehydroepiandrosterone and its sulfate and cortisol by the human fetal adrenal in vitro. Endocrinol Jpn 1981;28:321–327.
116. Pepe GJ, Waddell BJ, Albrecht ED. The effects of adrenocorticotropin and prolactin on adrenal dehydroepiandrosterone secretion in the baboon fetus. Endocrinology 1988;122:646–650.
117. Glasow A, Breidert M, Haidan A, Anderegg U, Kelly PA, Bornstein SR. Functional aspects of the effect of prolactin on adrenal steroidogenesis and distribution of the PRL receptor in the human adrenal gland. J Clin Endo Metab 1996;81:3103–3111.
118. Walker ML, Pepe GJ, Albrecht ED. Regulation of baboon fetal adrenal androgen formation by pituitary peptides at mid- and late-gestation. Endocrinology 1988;122:546–551.
119. Pepe GJ, Albrecht ED. Regulation of the primate fetal adrenal cortex. Endocr Rev 1990;11:151–176.
120. DiBlasio AM, Fujii DK, Yamamoto M, Martin MC, Jaffe RB. Maintenance of cell proliferation and steroidogenesis in cultured human fetal adrenal cells chronically exposed to adrenocorticotropic hormones: rationalization of in vitro and in vivo findings. Biol Reprod 1990;42:683–691.
121. Mendelson CR, Johnston JM, MacDonald PC, Snyder JM. Multihormonal regulation of surfactant synthesis by human fetal lung in vitro. J Clin Endo Metab 1981;53:307–317.
122. Snyder JM, Longmuir KJ, Johnston JM, Mendelson CR. Hormonal regulation of the synthesis of lamellar body phosphatidylglycerol and phosphatidylinositol in fetal lung tissue. Endocrinology 1983;112:1012–1018.
123. Snyder JM, D'Ercole AJ. Somatomedin C/insulin-like growth factor I production by human fetal lung tissue maintained in vitro. Exp Lung Res 1987;13:449–458.
124. Gluckman PD, Ballard PL, Kaplan SL, Liggins GC, Grumbach MM. Prolactin in umbilical cord blood and the respiratory distress syndrome. J Pediatr 1978;93:1011–1014.
125. Hauth JC, Parker CR, MacDonald PC, Porter JC, Johnston JM. A role of fetal prolactin in lung maturation. Obstet Gynecol 1978;51:81–88.
126. Schober E, Simbruner G, Salzer H, Husslein P, Spona J. The relationship of prolactin in cord blood, gestational age, and respiratory compliance after birth in newborn infants. J Perinat Med 1982;10:23–26.
127. Yuei BH, Phillips WDP, Cannon W, Sy L, Redford D, Burch P. Prolactin, estradiol, and thyroid hormones in umbilical cord blood of neonates with and without hyaline membrane disease: A study of 405 neonates from mid-pregnancy to term. Am J Obstet Gynecol 1982;142:698–703.
128. Lovinger RD, Kaplan SL, Grumbach MM. Congenital hypopituitarism associated with neonatal hypoglycemia and microphallus: four cases secondary to hypothalamic hormone deficiencies. J Pediatr 1975;87:1171–1181.
129. Freemark MF, Handwerger S. Ovine placental lactogen stimulates glycogen synthesis in fetal rat hepatocytes. Am J Physiol 1984;246:E121–E124.
129a. Schoknecht PA, McGuire MA, Cohick WS, Currie WB, Bell AW. Effect of chronic infusion of placental lactogen on ovine fetal growth in late gestation. Domest Anim Endocrin 1996;13:519–528.
130. Freemark M, Handwerger S. Synergistic effects of oPL and insulin on glycogen metabolism in fetal rat hepatocytes. Am J Physiol 1984;247:E714–718.
131. Freemark M, Handwerger S. Ovine placental lactogen inhibits glucagon-induced glycogenolysis in fetal rat hepatocytes. Endocrinology 1985;116:1275–1280.
132. Strain AJ, Hill DJ, Swenne I, Milner RDG. Regulation of DNA synthesis in human fetal hepatocytes by placental lactogen, growth hormone and insulin-like growth factor I/somatomedin C. J Cell Physiol 1987;132:33–40.
133. Swenne I, Hill DJ, Strain AJ, Milner RDG. Effects of human placental lactogen and growth hormone on production of insulin and somatomedin c/ IGF-I by human fetal pancreas in tissue culture. J Endocrinol 1987;113, 297–303.
134. Brelje TC, Scharp DW, Lacy PE, Ogren L, Talamantes F, Robertson M, et al. Effect of homologous placental lactogen, prolactins, and growth hormones on islet beta-cell division and insulin secretion in rat, mouse, and human islets: implication for placental lactogen regulation of islet function during pregnancy. Endocrinology 1993;132:879–887.

135. Brelje TC, Sorenson RL. Role of prolactin versus growth hormone on islet beta cell proliferation in vitro: implications for pregnancy. Endocrinology 1991;128:45–57.
136. Swenne I, Hill DJ, Strain AJ, Milner RD. Growth hormone regulation of insulin-like growth factor I production and DNA replication in fetal rat islets in tissue culture. Diabetes 1987;36:288–294.
137. Sandler S, Andersson A, Korsgren O, Tollemar J, Petersson B, Groth C-G, et al. Tissue culture of human fetal pancreas: growth hormone stimulates the formation and insulin production of islet-like cell cultures. J Clin Endo Metab 1987;65:1154–1158.
137a. Scott P, Kessler MA, Schuler LA. Molecular cloning of the bovine prolactin receptor and distribution of prolactin and growth hormone receptor transcripts in fetal and utero-placental tissues. Mol Cell Endocrinol 1992;89:47–58.
137b. Tseng Y-H, Kessler MA, Schuler LA. Regulation of interleukin (IL)-1 alpha, IL-1beta, and IL-6 expression by growth hormone and prolactin in bovine thymic stromal cells. Mol Cell Endocrinol 1997;128:117–127.
138. Savage MO, Blum WF, Ranke MB, Postel-Vinay MC, Cotterill AM, Hall K, et al. Clinical features and endocrine status in patients with growth hormone insensitivity (Laron syndrome). J Clin Endo Metab 1993;77:1465–1471.
139. Rosenfeld RG, Rosenbloom AL, Guevara-Aguirre J. Growth hormone insensitivity due to primary GH receptor deficiency. Endocr Rev 1994;15:369–390.
140. Nguyen AP, Chandorkar A, Gupta C. The role of growth hormone in fetal mouse reproductive tract differentiation. Endocrinology 1996;137:3659–3666.
141. Nutting DF. Ontogeny of sensitivity to growth hormone in rat diaphragm muscle. Endocrinology 1976;98:1273–1283.
142. Freemark M, Handwerger S. Ovine placental lactogen, but not growth hormone, stimulates amino acid transport in fetal rat diaphragm. Endocrinology 1982;112:402–404.
143. Hill DJ, Crace CJ, Milner RDG. Incorporation of 3H-thymidine by isolated human fetal myoblasts and fibroblasts in response to human placental lactogen: possible mediation of hPL action by release of immunoreactive SM-C. J Cell Physiol 1985;125:337–344.
144. Hill DJ, Crace CJ, Strain AJ, Milner RDG. Regulation of amino acid uptake and deoxyribonucleic acid synthesis in isolated human fetal fibroblasts and myoblasts: effect of human placental lactogen, somatomedin-C, multiplication stimulating activity and insulin. J Clin Endo Metab 1986;62:753–760.
145. Gluckman PD. The role of pituitary hormones, growth factors and insulin in the regulation of fetal growth. Oxford Rev Reprod 1986;8:1–60.
146. Gluckman PD, Gunn AJ, Wray A, Cutfield WS, Chatelain PG, Guilbaud O, et al. Congenital idiopathic growth hormone deficiency associated with prenatal and early postnatal growth failure. J Pediatr 1992;121:920–923.
147. Wurzel J, Parks JS, Herd HE, Nielson PV. A gene deletion is responsible for absence of human chorionic somatomammotropin. DNA 1982;1:251–257.
148. Goosens M, Brauner R, Czernichow P, Duquesnoy P, Rappaport R. Isolated growth hormone deficiency thype IA associated with a double deletion in the human GH gene cluster. J Clin Endo Metab 1986;62:712–716.
149. Simon P, Decoster C, Brocas H, Schwers J, Vassart G. Absence of human chorionic somatomammotropin during pregnancy associated with two types of gene deletion. Hum Genet 1986;74:235–238.
150. Akinci A, Kanaka C, Eble A, Akar N, Vidinlisan S, Mullis PE. Isolated growth hormone deficiency type IA associated with a 45 kilobase gene deletion within the human GH gene cluster. J Clin Endo Metab 1992;75:437–441.
150a. Rygaard K, Revol A, Esquivel-Escobedo D, Beck BL, Barrera-Saldana JC. Absence of human placental lactogen and placental growth hormone (HGH-V) during pregnancy: PCR analysis of the deletion. Hum Genet 1998;102:87–92.
151. Baker J, Liu J-P, Robertson EJ, Efstratiadis A. Role of insulin-like growth factors in embryonic and postnatal growth. Cell 1993;75:73–82.
152. Woods KA, Camacho-Hubner C, Savage MO, Clark AJL. Intrauterine growth retardation and postnatal growth failure associated with deletion of the insulin-like growth factor I gene. N Engl J Med 1996;335:1363–1367.
153. Kim JD, Nanto-Salonen K, Szczepankiewicz J, Rosenfeld RG, Glasscock GF. Evidence for pituitary regulation of somatic growth, insulin-like growth factors I and II and their binding proteins in the fetal rat. Pediatr Res 1993;33:144–151.

154. Palmiter RD, Norstedt G, Gelinas RE, Hammer RE, Brinster RL. Metallothionein-human GH fusion genes stimulate growth of mice. Science 1983;222:809–814.
155. Hammer RE, Brinster RL, Rosenfeld MG, Evans RM, Mayo KE. Expression of human growth hormone-releasing factor in transgenic mice results in increased somatic growth. Nature 1985; 315:413–416.
156. Johnson JW, Tyson JE, Mitzner W, Beck JC, Andreassen B, London WT, Villar J. Amniotic fluid prolactin and fetal lung maturation. Am J Obstet Gynecol 1985;153:372–380.
157. Peters CA, Reed LM, Docimo S, Luetic T, Carr M, Retik AB, et al. The role of the kidney in lung growth and maturation in the setting of obstructive uropathy and oligohydramnios. J Urol 1991;146:597–600.
158. Mulvihill SJ, Stone MM, Fonkalsrud EW, Debas HT. Trophic effect of amniotic fluid on fetal gastrointestinal development. J Surg Res 1986;40:291–296.
159. Avial CG, Harding R. The development of the gastrointestinal system in fetal sheep in the absence of ingested fluid. J Pediatr Gastroenterol 1991;12:96–104.
160. Frankenne F, Hennen G, Parks JS, Nielsen PV. A gene deletion in the hGH/hCS gene cluster could be responsible for the placental expression of hGH and/or hCS like molecule absent in normal subjects. 68th Ann Meet Endocrine Soc, Anaheim, CA, 1986, abst # 388.

6

Growth Hormone Releasing Hormone
Biological and Molecular Aspects

Paul L. Hofman, MBChB, FRACP
and O. H. Pescovitz, MD

CONTENTS

INTRODUCTION

Growth hormone (GH) synthesis and release is regulated by two hypothalamic peptides: somatostatin, which inhibits GH secretion, and growth hormone-releasing hormone (GHRH), which stimulates its release. Although somatostatin was the first to be identified in 1973 *(1)*, the presence of a hypothalamic GH stimulating substance had been predicted in 1960 from rodent studies in which hypothalamic lesions induced growth impairment *(2)*. However, because of methodological problems, particularly the loss of biological activity during purification, GHRH proved difficult to isolate. It was not until 1982 that GHRH was isolated from two separate pancreatic tumors obtained from individuals who presented with the clinical features of acromegaly *(3,4)*. The finding that GHRH mRNA and peptides isolated from pancreas were identical to those produced endogenously by the hypothalamus *(5,6)*, opened the door to a wealth of new discoveries. These have led to advances in understanding the transcriptional and translational regulation of the GHRH gene, characterization of the GHRH gene products, understanding

From: *Molecular and Cellular Pediatric Endocrinology*
Edited by: S. Handwerger © Humana Press Inc., Totowa, NJ

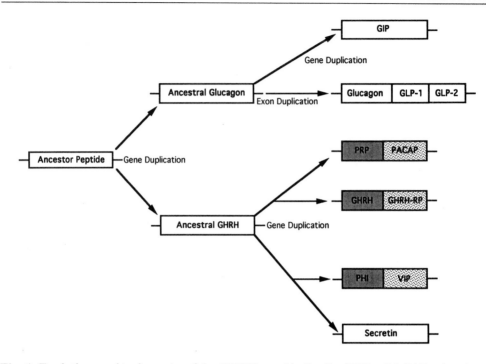

Fig. 1. Evolutionary development of the GHRH peptide family. PRP = PACAP related peptide; PACAP = pituitary adenylyl cyclase activating protein; VIP = vasoactive intestinal polypeptide; PHI = peptide histidine isoleucine; GIP = gastric inhibitory factor; GLP = glucagon-like
peptide.

the role of GHRH in regulating GH secretion, identification of the GHRH receptor and
the discovery of GHRH receptor mutations in mice, and humans. In this chapter, these
advances will be reviewed.

GHRH GENE STRUCTURE

The GHRH gene is a member of a large family of gut-brain factors that includes
glucagon, secretin, vasoactive intestinal polypeptide (VIP), peptide histidine isoleucine
(PHI), gastric inhibitory polypeptide (GIP), pituitary adenylyl cyclase activating polypeptide (PACAP), and PACAP related peptide (PRP). From an evolutionary perspective,
GHRH belongs to a branch of this family including the PHI, VIP, PRP, PACAP and
secretin polypeptides. It has greatest homology with PHI (37–63%) and PRP (35–55%)
followed by VIP (25–37%), PACAP (24–32%) and GIP (5–19%) (7). GHRH appears to
have evolved from the ancestral gene encoding PRP and PACAP approx 750 million yr
ago by gene duplication (Fig. 1) (7).

Humans and rodents have a single copy of the GHRH gene (8). Using FISH and
microsatellite markers this gene has been localized to chromosome 20q12- (9) in humans
and chromosome 2 in mice (10).

Most studies to date have focused on hypothalamic GHRH. However, in humans
GHRH mRNA transcripts and immunoreactive GHRH peptides have also been identified
in placenta (11), testis (11), and leukocytes (12). Similarly in rodents, GHRH mRNA and
GHRH-like peptides have been found in many other tissues including placenta (13–16),

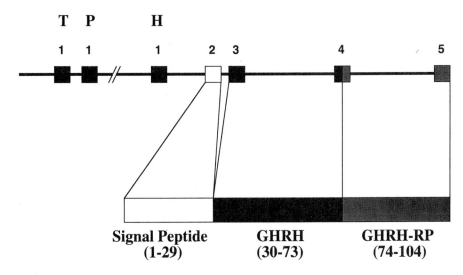

Fig. 2. Schematic representation of the GHRH gene and its relationship to the preproGHRH polypeptide. There are three first exons which appear tissue specific (T = testicular; P = placental, H = hypothalamus) and are not translated. All known GHRH mRNA transcripts contain exons 2–5 and encodes the GHRH precursor peptide. The mature GHRH is encoded in exons 3 and 4. As the biological activity of GHRH is dependent on the amino terminus, exon 4 is not necessary for a functional peptide. Exons 4 and 5 encode the 31 amino acid GHRH-RP peptide.

testis *(17)*, stomach *(18)*, small intestine *(19,20)* spleen *(20)*, pancreas *(18)*, adrenal gland *(20)*, kidney *(20)*, ovary *(20,21)*, and skeletal muscle *(20)*.

Hypothalamic, testicular and placental GHRH mRNAs share four common exons that encode the GHRH precursor peptide (Fig. 2) *(8,15,16,22)*. Interestingly, the GHRH cDNAs from each of these tissues have unique untranslated first exons that are spliced to the common exons 2–5 *(23)*. The testis and placental first exons are located 700 basepairs apart and are separated by more than 10 kb from the hypothalamic GHRH first exon *(22)*.

Analysis of the 5'-flanking regions from these first exons suggests unique promotor sequences. The 5'-flanking region from the hypothalamic-specific first exon includes TATA and CCAAT-like elements and are well conserved in human, rat and mouse genes *(8,14–16)*. The rat placental 5'-flanking region lacks both TATA box motifs and G+C rich sequences, but contains the sequence 5'-CGTCCTGCT-3' (position-153) and a putative inverse CCAAT box *(16)*. Analysis of the 5'-flanking region of the testicular GHRH gene for potential promoter sequences has shown both a TATA-like motif and sequences homologous to spermatogenic-specific *cis*-acting elements *(22)*.

It has been recently shown that the homeobox gene *Gsh-1* has consensus binding sites within both the testicular and hypothalamic promotor regions of the GHRH gene *(24)*. Homeobox genes encode a family of DNA binding proteins and the *Gsh-1* gene encodes a product necessary for GHRH gene transcription and translation. Interestingly *Gsh-1* knockout mice demonstrate biochemical evidence of GHRH deficiency and a phenotype that includes extreme postnatal dwarfism, sexual infantilism, leukopenia, marked peri-natal mortality, and a significantly shortened lifespan in the survivors. The extent of the *Gsh-1* knockout phenotype suggests that either *Gsh-1* regulates other developmentally important peptides, or that GHRH gene expression results in diverse tissue-specific functions.

The demonstration of unique promotor regions, transcription initiation sites and RNA processing in hypothalamus, placenta and testis provides a mechanism for tissue-specific gene expression and raises the possibility that GHRH may have important functions at extrahypothalamic sites *(22,23)*.

PROTEIN STRUCTURE, PROCESSING, AND METABOLISM

Hypothalamic GHRH mRNA comprises approx 750 base pairs including a poly-adenylation signal *(8)*. In humans, it is translated into a 108-amino acid precursor peptide *(25)*. This preproGHRH includes a signal peptide, the 44 amino acid GHRH (GHRH$_{1-44}$-NH$_2$), and a 31-amino acid carboxyl terminal peptide we have designated as GHRH related peptide (GHRH-RP; Fig. 3) *(26)*. Proteolytic processing of this precursor peptide involves cleavage of the signal peptide and the carboxyl terminal peptide to form a 45-amino acid peptide (GHRH$_{1-45}$) *(8)*. In humans, proteolytic cleavage of GHRH$_{1-45}$ occurs at a dibasic arg–arg amino terminal bond and at a gly–arg carboxyl terminal bond *(8,25)*. An amidation reaction subsequently occurs with the loss of the terminal glycine residue which acts as an amide donor to amino acid 44 (leucine) *(26)*.

The final amidated product (GHRH$_{1-44}$-NH$_2$) is the major GHRH form produced by the human hypothalamus. Two other nonamidated GHRH peptides have been identified in human tissues, a 40-amino acid GHRH (GHRH$_{1-40}$-OH) and a 37-amino acid GHRH (GHRH$_{1-37}$-OH) *(25,27)*. Although in general, processed peptides are flanked by paired basic amino acids *(28)*, cleavage has been reported at sites containing a single arginine, such as in the processing of arginine vasopressin-neurophysin *(29)* and ACTH from proopiomelanocortin *(30)*. The alternative GHRH products, GHRH$_{1-37}$-OH and GHRH$_{1-40}$-OH represent cleavage at other single arginine sites and are most likely natural variants. The forms GHRH$_{1-44}$-OH and GHRH$_{1-40}$-OH have been identified in the hypothalamus and placenta whereas GHRH$_{1-37}$-OH has only been identified in a GHRH secreting pancreatic tumor *(3,4,31)*. All three GHRH forms have similar bioactivity.

GHRH has been characterized in many species *(31)*. The amino terminal end of the GHRH peptide is most conserved across species, with the greatest similarity to human GHRH seen in the larger mammals (e.g., porcine, ovine, caprine, and bovine). The biological activity of GHRH is influenced predominantly by the more conserved amino terminal residues, with loss of the first two amino acids rendering the peptide inactive *(6,31)*. Although loss of carboxyl terminal amino acids results in some loss of function, synthetic GHRH$_{1-29}$ retains most of the biological potency of the natural 1–44 form *(6,31)*.

Unlike larger mammals, rodent and human GHRH gene products demonstrate greater differences *(31–33)*. The smaller GHRH peptides in rat and mouse contain 43 and 42 residues respectively with approx 70% homology between rodent and human GHRH *(32,33)*. Similar to other species, the homology is greatest in the amino terminal residues. Because no amide donor is present at the carboxyl terminus of the GHRH peptide, both rat and mouse GHRH are nonamidated *(32,33)*.

In larger mammals, including humans, amidation of both the GHRH peptide and the carboxyl terminal peptide (GHRH-RP) occurs; a posttranslational modification commonly associated with biological function *(27,31)*. Although amidation does not occur in rat and mouse GHRH, synthetic rat GHRH$_{1-29}$ can become functional by

```
MetProLeuTrpValPhePhePheValIleLeuThrLeuSerAsnSerSerHisCysSer
```

```
ProProProProLeuThrLeuArgMetArgArg TyrAlaAspAlaIlePheThrAsn
                                    1   2   3   4   5   6   7   8
SerTyrArgLysValLeuGlyGlnLeuSerAla ArgLysLeuLeuGlnAspIleMetSer
 9  10  11  12  13  14  15  16  17  18  19  20  21  22  23  24  25  26  27  28
ArgGlnGlnGlyGluSerAsnGlnGluArgGlyAlaArgAlaArgLeuGly ArgGlnGlu
 29  30  31  32  33  34  35  36  37  38  39  40  41  42  43  44  45
AspSerMetTryAlaGluGlnLysGlnMetGluLeuGluSerIleLeuValAlaLeuLeu
```

```
GlnLysHisSerArgAsnSerGlnGly
```

Fig. 3. Amino acid sequence of preproGHRH. The GHRH and GHRH-RP polypeptides are highlighted and amino acids numbered. The terminal glycine of GHRH (amino acid 45) is used as an amide donor resulting in the mature 1–44 GHRH. Arrows depict other potential cleavage sites next to arginine residues. Proteolytic cleavage at these sites would result in the observed 37 and 40 amino acid GHRH variants.

C terminal amidation *(34)*. Similarly human GHRH biological activity can be retained in the C terminal shortened 1–29 synthetic form by amidation.

$GHRH_{1-44}$-NH_2 is rapidly metabolized by proteolytic cleavage at Ala^2-Asp^3 to the biologically inactive fragment $GHRH_{3-44}$-NH_2. The $t_{1/2}$ for this reaction is 17 min at 37°C in vitro and 6.8 min in vivo *(35)*. The enzyme catalyzing this reaction, dipeptidyl peptidase IV (DPP IV), is a membrane bound exoproteinase that is widely distributed in mammalian tissues *(36)*. In humans, DPP IV proteolysis is the major route of GHRH degradation, although trypsin-like cleavages occur at bonds 11–12 and 12–13 in plasma *(26)*. In vitro studies of rat serum and liver homogenates indicate that there are also several other cleavage sites *(37)*.

Prepro-GHRH contains a cryptic carboxyl terminal peptide (GHRH-RP) that has sequence homology to the biologically active peptides VIP and PACAP (Fig. 2). As it is believed that the GHRH, PRP/PACAP and PHI/VIP genes gene evolved from a single ancestral gene, it is possible that a second biologically active peptide product is encoded (Fig. 1). In support of this hypothesis, GHRH-RP also has a biologically identifiable action in rats testes where it has been shown to activate Sertoli cell expression of stem cell factor *(38)*.

ONTOGENY, LOCALIZATION, AND REGULATION OF GHRH GENE TRANSCRIPTION AND TRANSLATION

Hypothalamus

GHRH-containing neurons are primarily located in hypothalamic nuclei. In rat hypothalamus, the GHRH neurons involved in somatotroph regulation originate from the arcuate nucleus in the ventrolateral hypothalamus, and project to the external layer of the median eminence where they terminate in close proximity to the hypophysial portal circulation *(39–43)*. In primate hypothalamus, GHRH neurons have been localized to the corresponding anatomical area, the infundibular nucleus *(44,45)*. GHRH neurons are also found in the dorsomedial nucleus and the ventromedial nucleus of the hypothalamus *(46,47)*. In addition to this efferent pathway projecting to the median eminence, there are two other pathways. The first ascends to the anterior periventricular nucleus and the parvocellular paraventricular nucleus. The second has ascending branches to the medial preoptic area (MPOA) and the suprachiasmatic nuclei, and descending branches through the lateral hypothalamic area to the medial nucleus of the amygdala *(46,47)*. These pathways are not close to the hypophysial portal circulation and electrophysiological studies suggest they have neurotransmitter-like properties *(48)*.

The ontogeny of hypothalamic GHRH neurons has been studied in several species including humans. In rodents, GHRH immunoreactive neurons can be detected as early as gestational d 16 *(49)* whereas in the human fetus GHRH neurons have been identified by wk 18 of gestation *(50)*. Although GHRH neurons appear relatively late in the human gestation, anterior pituitary explant cultures from postconception wk 9 will secrete GH in response to GHRH, indicating a functionally intact axis *(51)*. As GH levels are detectable by 10 wk of gestation and are increasing before 18 wk *(52)*, this suggests several possibilities; GH regulation is independent of GHRH in early to mid gestation; unidentified hypothalamic GHRH neurons are present and functional in early gestation; or that GHRH produced from another site (such as the placenta) is acting on fetal somatotrophs. Placental GHRH has been demonstrated in amniotic fluid *(53)* and placental GHRH mRNA has been identified as early as postconception d 7 in rats *(54)*. Placental GHRH may therefore play a role in the early regulation of the fetal GH axis.

Several factors regulate hypothalamic GHRH gene transcription (Fig. 4). As in many endocrine systems, an inhibitory feedback effect of growth hormone and IGF-I on GHRH mRNA expression exists. In hypophysectomized rats, GHRH mRNA levels are increased five- to sixfold over those seen in intact animals *(55)*. Giving hypophysectomized animals growth hormone results in a decrease in GHRH mRNA levels, although they remain higher than in intact animals. Increased GHRH mRNA expression has also been observed in mice following immunoneutralization of GHRH with anti-GHRH sera *(56)*. Administration of anti-GHRH sera results in secondary growth hormone deficiency and decreased feedback inhibition on GHRH transcription. Following administration of either growth hormone or IGF-I to these mice, a reduction in GHRH mRNA levels is seen. However, similar to hypophysectomized animals, mRNA levels remained elevated compared to intact animals. This feedback inhibition by growth hormone and IGF-I explains the elevation in GHRH mRNA levels seen in other growth hormone deficient states. One specific example is the *lit/lit* mouse which has GH deficiency attributable to a defect in the GHRH receptor. GHRH mRNA levels are three times higher than those in heterozygous littermates *(32)*.

Thyroid hormone deficiency results in reduced growth hormone secretion and a variety of abnormalities in the GH axis *(57,58)*, including an increase in GHRH mRNA expression *(59,60)*. In hypothyroid rats, this increase in GHRH expression is reversed to a similar degree with either growth hormone or thyroxine replacement *(61)*, suggesting that the increase is secondary to the reduced growth hormone levels observed in hypothyroid states.

Rats demonstrate sexual dimorphism of GHRH mRNA expression with higher levels seen in male rats *(62)*. In rodents, androgens increase and estrogens decrease GHRH mRNA levels suggesting that sex steroid receptors influence GHRH transcription *(63,64)*. Although there are gender differences in growth hormone secretion in humans, it is

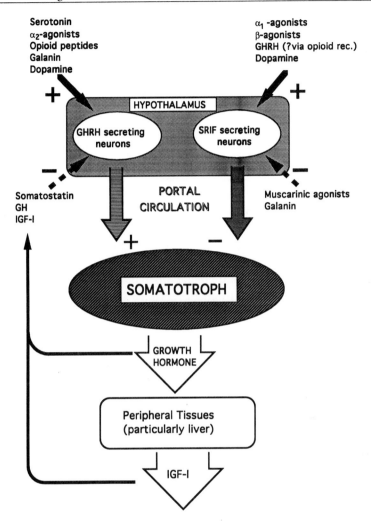

Fig. 4. Schematic model illustrating the various regulatory levels controlling GHRH release. Many hypothalamic neurons types have been shown to associate with GHRH neurons and to modulate GHRH release. Of particular importance in GHRH release is the hypothalamic communication between somatostatin (SRIF) secreting neurons and GHRH secreting neurons. Stimulation of somatostatin containing neurons causes suppression of GHRH. GHRH neurons also stimulate somatostatin containing neurons and this acts as a local negative feedback loop on GHRH release. Outside the hypothalamus, the main regulators of GHRH release are growth hormone (GH) and IGF-I, that function in a traditional, negative feedback manner. Dashed arrows indicate inhibitory effects and solid arrows indicate stimulatory effects.

unclear whether these are caused by changes in GHRH gene transcription, synthesis, or secretion, or by other factors, such as somatostatin *(65)*.

Growth hormone and IGF1 have important effects on carbohydrate, protein and fat metabolism and are altered in states of acute and chronic malnutrition *(66)*. It is therefore not surprising that nutritional status has been shown to affect the hypothalamic control of these hormones *(67)*. Acute food deprivation in rats results in low growth hormone levels. Hypothalamic GHRH mRNA levels decline beginning within 24 h of food deprivation and reach a nadir at 48 h *(68)*. Refeeding after 72 h of food deprivation restores GHRH mRNA levels within 48 h. Normalization of mRNA levels is dependent on the protein content of the food and protein-deficient, isocaloric diets fail to restore mRNA levels *(69)*. As GH inhibits GHRH expression, the reduced GH levels following acute food deprivation would be expected to increase GHRH expression. The reduced GHRH mRNA levels observed suggest this abnormality precedes and results in the decrease in GH levels.

In both humans and rats, morbid obesity is also associated with altered GH secretory dynamics with a reduction in GH pulsatility and reduced serum GH levels *(70)*. These changes may reflect abnormalities of the GH axis at varying levels, including resistance to GHRH action at the level of somatotrophs and increased somatostatinergic tone *(70,71)*. However, abnormalities also exist in GHRH production. In obese Zucker fatty rats, both hypothalamic GHRH peptide concentrations and GHRH mRNA levels were reduced *(71,72)*. This suggests that abnormal GHRH mRNA expression contributes to this animal model of obesity.

Abnormalities in glucose or insulin metabolism may also alter hypothalamic GHRH expression. Streptozotocin induced diabetic rats have a decrease in episodic GH secretion and markedly reduced hypothalamic GHRH mRNA levels that are restored with insulin therapy *(73)*.

Placenta

Transcription of placental GHRH mRNA occurs at a different transcription initiation site from the hypothalamic GHRH transcript and involves alternate splicing *(11,22)*. Since exons two to five are conserved, the preproGHRH peptide translated in placenta is identical to that from the hypothalamus *(14)*. GHRH peptides and mRNAs have been identified in rat, mouse, and human placentas *(11,14,74)*. Furthermore, GHRH gene transcription appears to be regulated during pregnancy. In rats, placental GHRH mRNA is detectable by gestational d 7 and increases until it peaks just prior to parturition *(54)*. A similar pattern has been observed in the mouse *(14)*.

Although the unique placental transcription site and promoter region suggest tissue specific regulation, few studies have addressed the factors involved. Both placental GHRH peptide and mRNA are reduced by the cytokines interleukin-6 (IL-6), IL-11, leukemia inhibitory factor, and oncostatin-M *(75)*. These cytokines all use the signal transducer gp130 in their receptor complex *(75)*. Activin-A, an activator of follicle stimulating hormone (FSH) secretion reduces placental GHRH mRNA expression and inhibits GHRH secretion within the placenta. Conversely, inhibin, an inhibitor of FSH secretion stimulates placental GHRH secretion *(76)*. Transforming growth factor β1 (TGFβ1) also inhibits placental GHRH release, although it affects neither gene transcription nor protein synthesis *(77)*. The physiological relevance of these findings is not yet established. However, IL-1, IL-6, and TNFα are present in human placental tissue and have also been implicated in regulating human chorionic gonadotropin (hCG) secretion *(78)*.

Gonads

GHRH mRNA expression and GHRH-like peptide have been demonstrated in testes and ovaries of both rats and humans *(11,17,21,79–82)*. In contrast to placental and hypothalamic GHRH mRNA, the predominant form found in rodent gonads is larger at approx 1750 nucleotides *(21,22)*. Characterization of the testicular transcript indicates a unique transcription start site approx 700 base pairs 5' to the placental transcription start site and a unique untranslated first exon *(22)*. The rodent ovarian GHRH mRNA transcript has not yet been fully sequenced, but is similar in size to that in testis *(21)*.

Gonadal localization of GHRH mRNA and a GHRH-like peptide has been performed using Northern blot analysis, *in situ* hybridization and immunohistochemistry. In rat testis, high expression of GHRH mRNA in spermatocytes, round spermatids, and to a lesser extent, Sertoli cells was demonstrated. No GHRH mRNA was observed in elongating spermatids, peritubular myoid cells, or Leydig cells *(83)*. A GHRH-like peptide has been localized to early and intermediate spermatid cells *(80,84)* and a GHRH-like peptide has also been detected in isolated Leydig cell cultures *(85)*.

GHRH receptor mRNA has also been recently localized to the testis using RT-PCR *(86)*. Expression of the GHRH receptor was most abundant in Sertoli and germ cells, with less, but detectable expression in Leydig cells. Interestingly, treatment of Sertoli cells with GHRH increased the expression of GHRH receptor mRNA in a dose-dependent manner *(86)*.

Ovarian localization of GHRH-like peptide in rat and bovine studies suggests it is found primarily within the follicle, and specifically within granulosa cells *(21,87)*. In humans, a GHRH-like peptide has also been isolated from ovarian tissue *(81)* and from follicular fluid *(88)*.

The ontogeny of GHRH mRNA has been examined in rat testis by dot blot hybridization *(89)*. GHRH mRNA was not detectable in late gestation (d 19), was present in small amounts by d 2 of life and remained at a similar level until d 19 when a rapid increase was observed. Adult levels were reached by d 42. Interestingly, GHRH mRNA expression was developmentally dependent on an intact hypothalamic-pituitary axis. Hypophysectomy on both d 21 and d 42 caused a marked diminution in testicular GHRH mRNA expression while hypophysectomy on d 65 resulted in a much smaller reduction. The reduced GHRH mRNA expression was not reversed by the subsequent administration of GH. This effect is similar to that observed with gonadotropin-dependent spermatogenesis. Once postpubertal spermatogenesis is established, an intact hypothalamic-pituitary-gonadal axis is not required to maintain GHRH mRNA expression *(89)*.

Many details involved in the regulation of GHRH transcription, translation and release in gonadal tissue remain to be explored. Given the different transcriptional initiation site in testis, transcriptional regulation is likely to be different from hypothalamic or placentally derived GHRH mRNA. Indeed, the finding of tissue-specific expression of GHRH in hypothalamic, placental and gonadal tissue raises the possibility that GHRH may have tissue-specific effects that are mediated via autocrine and paracrine actions.

GHRH RECEPTOR—STRUCTURE AND FUNCTION

Similar to other members of the glucagon-secretin family of polypeptides, GHRH binds to and activates a stimulatory G protein-coupled receptor. The receptors cloned from rat, mice, and human *(90,91)* are all 423 amino acids in length, whereas the porcine GHRH receptor is larger at 451 amino acids *(92)*. In rat pituitary, a larger isoform has also been characterized with a predicted length of 464 amino acids *(90,91)*. This larger variant represents the insertion of 41 amino acids into the third cytoplasmic loop of the receptor and arises by alternative RNA splicing to include an additional exon of 123 base pairs. The GHRH receptor has been localized to mouse chromosome 6 *(10)* and human chromosome 7p15 *(93)*.

Like other members of the G protein-coupled receptor family, the GHRH receptors all have seven transmembrane helix regions with three extracellular and three cytoplasmic loops. Among GHRH receptors, there is a high degree of species homology with 94% identity between mouse and rat and 82% between rodent and human receptors (23).

The GHRH receptor family includes the secretin, PTH, calcitonin, glucagon, VIP, GLP-1, PACAP, and the GIP receptors. Among members of this family, the GHRH receptor is most homologous with the VIP receptor at 47% identity, compared to 42, 35, and 28% for the secretin, calcitonin and PTH receptors, respectively (94).

Despite the sequence homology with other receptors, the GHRH receptor is specific for GHRH. Rat has a GHRH-binding affinity (K_d) between 0.011–0.4 nM (94–97). Of the other secretin-glucagon like peptides tested, only PACAP binds to the GHRH receptor, although its binding affinity is 100 times less than GHRH. Activation of the GHRH receptor by various ligands from the GHRH receptor family was assessed by cAMP generation (94). Similar to the binding studies, GHRH was highly specific for the GHRH receptor, with the closely related ligands secretin, VIP and PACAP generating 0, 12, and 18% of the cAMP response compared to that generated by GHRH.

GHRH RECEPTOR ONTOGENY, LOCALIZATION, AND REGULATION

GHRH receptor mRNA localization by Northern analyses (94,98), and RNA protection assays (99) indicates that it is expressed predominantly in the pituitary gland and hypothalamus. Using RT-PCR, GHRH receptor mRNA has been further localized to the periventricular, arcuate and ventromedial hypothalamic nuclei (99).

The ontogeny of hypothalamic GHRH receptor expression has recently been examined in rats (100). Pituitary GHRH receptor mRNA expression is highest in late fetal life, declining to a nadir by d 12 postnatally and reaching a second peak at d 30 (approximately the time of puberty). The levels then gradually decrease out to 1 yr. This pattern of GHRH receptor mRNA expression levels does not parallel growth hormone or pit-1 mRNA expression at similar ages indicating GHRH receptor expression is not likely to be developmentally regulated by these factors. The increase in GHRH receptor expression at puberty is similar to the pubertal increase in GHRH expression and suggests that sex steroids may modulate both GHRH and its receptors.

The pituitary GHRH receptor mRNA transcripts described have been of two sizes. In rats, the predominant form is ~2.5 kb with a 4 kb isoform also present (90). In mice, 2.0 and 2.1 kb transcripts are seen, whereas in the sheep 2.0 and 3.5 kb have been identified (23,94).

As GHRH is found in many tissues outside the hypothalamus and is expected to act in a paracrine or autocrine manner, GHRH receptors would also be predicted to be present in these tissues. As mentioned previously, a GHRH receptor mRNA was detected, predominantly in Sertoli and germ cells, with some expression seen in Leydig cells (83). GHRH binding has also been demonstrated in other tissues including human leukocytes (101).

GHRH receptors are regulated by GHRH and like other G protein ligands, chronic exposure to GHRH causes desensitization of pituitary GHRH receptors (102,103). This desensitization results from a reduced number of binding sites rather than reduced binding affinity (102). Using GHRH antisera to block endogenous GHRH action, it has been recently demonstrated that GHRH also negatively regulates pituitary GHRH receptor mRNA expression *(104)*. Rats treated with specific GHRH antisera had a 3.8-fold increase in GHRH receptor mRNA transcripts compared to controls.

It is also likely that the pituitary-specific POU domain protein, *pit-1* is involved in GHRH receptor gene expression *(98)*. *Pit-1*, a transcriptional regulatory protein, is important in the control of growth hormone, prolactin and TSH transcription. Deficiency results in somatotroph, lactotroph and thyrotroph hypoplasia. In the Snell dwarf mouse, which has defective *pit-1*, there is also a failure to express GHRH receptor mRNA. Using a reporter gene fused to the GHRH promotor, it has been shown that this failure of expression can be reversed by the addition of *pit-1* expression vectors *(91)*. As GHRH stimulates *pit-1* expression, the possibility for a positive feedback loop exists. However, the effect of *pit-1* on GHRH receptor transcription appears to be permissive and other factors such as GHRH binding are more important in downregulating GHRH receptor expression.

GHRH RECEPTOR SIGNAL TRANSDUCTION

GHRH receptor effects are mediated by activation of heterotrimeric Gs-proteins, resulting in both an increase in intracellular cAMP and intracellular Ca^{2+} ion influx *(105,106)*. Binding of GHRH to its receptor results in the displacement of GDP by GTP from the α_s subunit of the Gs-protein and subsequent Gs dissociation into an α_s subunit and β/γ heterodimer (Fig. 5). The α_s subunit activates adenylyl cyclase and increase cAMP production resulting in the activation of protein kinase A (PKA). PKA can phosphorylate and activate a variety of cellular substrates including the cAMP response element binding protein (CREB) which binds to DNA cAMP response elements (CREs) in promotor or enhancer regions to increase transcription *(107)*. The promotor of the regulatory transcription factor *pit-1* contains two CREB binding sites *(108)* and inhibition of these sites attenuates *pit-1* promotor activity *(109)*. In somatotrophs, *pit-1* increases the transcription of both growth hormone and GHRH receptor genes. Thus it is likely that stimulatory effects of GHRH on growth hormone and GHRH receptor expression are mediated indirectly by a cAMP dependent increase in *Pit-1* expression.

In somatotrophs as in other endocrine tissues, hormone release is triggered by a change in free intracellular Ca^{2+} *(110–112)*. PKA activation and subsequent ion channel phosphorylation has been implicated in the increase in intracellular Ca^{2+} concentration observed following administration of GHRH to somatotrophs in vitro *(110,111,113)*. Electrophysiological studies have shown GHRH increases intracellular free Ca^{2+} concentration within seconds, reaching a peak at approx 30 s *(110)*. This effect can be blocked by L-type calcium channel antagonists or by the addition of EDTA to the media suggesting Ca^{2+} influx is the source of the increased intracellular free Ca^{2+} *(110)*. There is no evidence that GHRH causes release of intracellular Ca^{2+} stores *(114)*.

The delay of 30 s until the peak intracellular Ca^{2+} current occurs suggests that secondary messengers are involved. Cuttler et al. have demonstrated that forskolin, an adenylyl cyclase activator, increases Ca^{2+} influx into somatotrophs while somatostatin inhibits Ca^{2+} influx *(111)*. This second messenger system, therefore, likely involves a PKA-dependent pathway *(111,115)*.

Although the delayed increase in Ca^{2+} influx seen following GHRH stimulation is probably secondary to the biochemical events resulting in PKA activation and the presumed phosphorylation of ion channels, an immediate effect (within seconds) is also

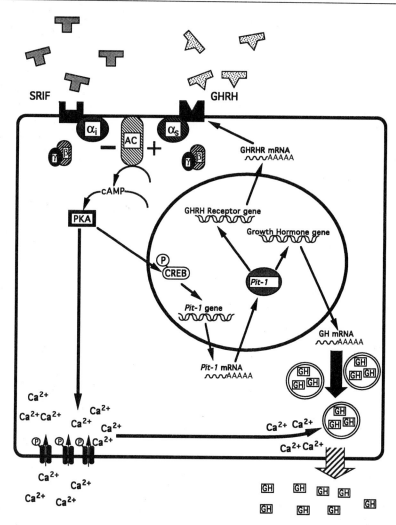

Fig. 5. Simplified schematic representation of GHRH signaling pathways in pituitary somato-trophs. GHRH, after binding to the GHRH receptor (GHRHR) activates a membrane-associated Gs protein, with GTP displacing bound GDP on the α_s subunit. The Gs protein dissociates into an activated α_s subunit and a β/γ heterodimer, with the activated α_s subunit stimulating adenylyl cyclase (AC) to increase cAMP accumulation. Somatostatin (SRIF), via a Gs protein, antagonizes GHRH stimulation of adenylyl cyclase activity and is the main modulator of GHRH in somatotrophs. Increasing cAMP activates protein kinase A (PKA) with phosphorylation of the DNA binding protein CREB and probable phosphorylation of calcium channels. PKA phosphorylation of calcium channels leads to an increase in free intracellular Ca^{2+}. The increase in intracellular Ca^{2+} stimulates exocytosis and the release of growth hormone into the systemic circulation. Phosphorylation also activates CREB, which increases the expression of another DNA binding protein, *pit-1*. This protein functions to increase transcription of both growth hormone (GH) and the GHRH receptor genes. The resultant increase in transcription, translation and synthesis of *pit-1* leads to an increase in transcription and ultimately increased intracellular growth hormone and GHRH receptor protein.

consistently observed and is associated with somatotroph depolarization *(116)*. This effect has been observed at concentrations of GHRH which have only minimally affected cAMP levels *(117)*. It, therefore, appears that an early initial influx of calcium occurs as a direct result of GHRH receptor activation, followed by a later and more prolonged increase in Ca^{2+} flux secondary to PKA mediated actions *(110)*. This increase in intracellular free Ca^{2+} stimulates exocytosis and GH release.

Activation of protein kinase C (PKC) has also been shown to increase GH release from somatotrophs *(118)*. PKC activation augments GHRH-mediated GH release and has been shown to increase cAMP accumulation *(119)*.

Recently, a receptor for the GH releasing peptides has been identified on somatotrophs. This is also a G protein-coupled receptor which is not a Gs subtype and may mediate the PKC actions on GH release observed in pituitary cell cultures *(120)*.

BIOLOGICAL EFFECTS OF GHRH

Pituitary and Growth Hormone Release

Less than two years after GHRH was isolated, its use in human subjects was first reported *(121–123)*. Intravenous $GHRH_{1-40}$ and $GHRH_{1-44}$ produced a rise in plasma growth hormone levels that peaked after 2–3 h. The potency of the two compounds was almost identical, with a maximal stimulatory dose of 1 μg/kg. A monophasic dose-response was observed at doses up to 1 μg/kg and a biphasic response was seen at higher doses (3.3 and 10.1 μg/kg). Subsequent studies using $GHRH_{1-29}$-NH_2 also confirmed that this shortened analog was equipotent to the native GHRH variants *(124)*. The hormonal response to GHRH is quite specific. Other than a variable, small increase in prolactin levels, no detectable increase in anterior pituitary or other enteropancreatic peptides was noted *(121)*.

Continuous infusions of GHRH for periods of 6–24 h also result in elevated growth hormone levels. However, at high GHRH doses (33 ng/kg/min), some attenuation of growth hormone release was seen *(125)*. The clinical significance of this observation is uncertain and may be secondary to receptor downregulation or a result of feedback inhibition by increased growth hormone secretion. However, infusions of GHRH in normal adult men for up to 14 d did not result in any attenuation of growth hormone release, with growth hormone secretion doubling compared to pretreatment levels *(126)*. Pathological conditions of chronic GHRH excess, such as ectopic production by pancreatic tumors, results in persistent elevation of growth hormone levels and subsequent acromegaly *(127)*. Thus, although some attenuation of the stimulatory GHRH effect on growth hormone release may occur following prolonged continuous exposure, somatotrophs remain responsive to GHRH.

The effects of excess GHRH have been examined using transgenic mice overexpressing GHRH. These mice have elevated growth hormone levels, grow more rapidly, and have eventual weights up to twice those of age and sex matched controls *(23)*. Young animals have evidence of pituitary hyperplasia which progresses to pituitary adenomas in older animals. Similar findings are observed in human patients with ectopic GHRH production. Patients typically have elevated growth hormone levels, acromegalic features, and evidence of pituitary hyperplasia *(128,129)*. Probable excess hypothalamic GHRH secretion has been reported in at least two children with gigantism; in one from birth or possibly prenatally and in a 7-yr-old child *(130,131)*. The pituitaries of these patients were enlarged and the histology showed massive somatotroph, lactotroph and mammosomatotroph hyperplasia. Areas of GH and prolactin secreting cell adenomatous transformation were also evident.

Because GHRH signal transduction is modulated via receptor-Gs-protein activation of cAMP/PKA, it would be expected that abnormalities occurring along this signal transduction cascade could also affect somatotrophs. Interestingly, these have been observed in patients with growth hormone secreting pituitary adenomas. Approximately 30–40% of these patients have missense mutations within codons 201 and 227 of the α_s subunit resulting in constitutive activation *(132,133)*. In the McCune-Albright syndrome, the underlying defects are somatic mutations in the Gs-protein similar to those in pituitary adenomas. These result in constitutive activation of Gs-proteins and secondary abnormalities of bone (polyostotic fibrous dysplasia), skin (cafe-au-lait-spots) and endocrine organs. In some patients, growth hormone excess secondary to α_s subunit constitutive activation has been reported *(134,135)*. Thus, GHRH excess or other abnormalities in the signal transduction pathway that lead to cAMP elevation will result in increased growth hormone release as well as trophic actions on somatotrophs and chronic excess can cause both pituitary hyperplasia and adenoma formation.

GHRH deficiency can be induced in neonatal rodents by exposure to monosodium glutamate (MSG), which causes a selective loss of arcuate nucleus neurons *(136,137)*. MSG-induced arcuate lesions produce impaired growth, hypogonadism, hypothyroidism and obesity. Arcuate nucleus neurons also produce many other neuropeptides, including gonadotropin releasing hormone (GnRH), neuropeptide Y, galanin, dynorphin, enkephalin, neurotensin, and somatostatin, which are sensitive to MSG exposure *(138)*. Although the growth failure in MSG treated mice is caused by GHRH deficiency, the other effects of MSG exposure may be secondary to deficiencies of these other neuropeptide containing neurons.

The only genetic model of GHRH deficiency described in the literature is the *Gsh-1* gene knockout mouse *(24)*. As described above, this *hox* gene encodes a transcriptional regulatory protein, whose absence in mice results in GHRH deficiency with a distinct phenotype (*see* GHRH Gene Structure). Anterior pituitary glands from these mice are one-third normal size and have a decreased number of somatotrophs and lactotrophs. These findings are consistent with the known trophic effect of GHRH on somatotrophs and suggest GHRH may also have a trophic effect on lactotrophs. Human studies to date have failed to demonstrate molecular abnormalities in GHRH peptide or gene expression *(139)*.

Although isolated GHRH deficiency has not been demonstrated, defective hypothalamic GHRH receptors have been identified in mice and humans *(10,91,140,141)*. The dwarf *little (lit)* mouse phenotype consists of postnatal growth failure and delayed pubertal maturation with biochemical evidence of growth hormone deficiency and high GHRH levels *(10,91)*. Pituitary histology reveals somatotroph hypoplasia. The condition is transmitted by an autosomal recessive mode of inheritance and has been shown to be caused by a missense mutation in the amino-terminal extracellular portion of the receptor, which converts an aspartic acid codon to a glycine codon at amino acid position 60 *(91)*. Recently, GHRH receptor defects have been identified as a cause for isolated growth hormone deficiency in humans *(140)*. However, it is likely that GHRH receptor defects will be an uncommon cause of growth hormone deficiency *(142)*.

Sleep Regulation

Other than its preeminent role in growth hormone regulation, GHRH is also a well documented humoral sleep factor (for recent reviews *see* refs. *143,144*). The effects of intracereboventricular (icv) GHRH administration have been studied in rats and rabbits. In rats, following a single icv injection of GHRH, locomotor activity decreases and time spent in nonrapid eye movement (NREM) sleep increases *(145,146)*. Rabbits, similarly, have a dose-dependent increase in NREM sleep with single icv injections of GHRH (0.01, 0.1, and 1.0 nmol/kg) *(146)*.

These findings are supported by studies involving GHRH inhibition, either using the competitive GHRH antagonist (N-Ac-Tyr^1, D-Arg^2)-GHRH$_{1-29}$-NH$_2$, or by passive immunization with anti-GHRH sera. In rats, icv injection of this competitive GHRH antagonist causes a dose-dependent suppression of NREMS over the following hour *(147)*. At the highest dose administered (14 nmol), NREMS was suppressed for 3 h, rapid eye movement sleep (REMS) was also decreased and plasma growth hormone levels were suppressed. Similarly, icv injection of anti-GHRH sera decreased both NREMS and REMS *(148)*. This effect was most noticeable 6–11 h after the injections.

In humans, the effect of exogenous GHRH depends on the timing of administration during sleep. When given soon after sleep begins, intravenous GHRH does not modify NREMS or REMS significantly *(149)*. However, GHRH administration during late sleep (specifically the third period of REMS) is followed by a marked decrease in wake time and an almost 10-fold increase in slow wave sleep *(150)*. Following sleep deprivation until 4:00 AM, administration of GHRH soon after sleep begins (during the first slow wave period) does not modify either slow wave or REMS, but decreases wake time. Interestingly, irrespective of the timing of GHRH administration, the total sleep period was increased significantly compared to control subjects receiving saline. These results suggest GHRH has effects on sleep patterns in humans which are more pronounced later in the sleep period. The primary effect of GHRH on human sleep may be to increase NREMS. An effect of GHRH on REMS has only been observed in rats and rabbits.

Although exogenously administered GHRH consistently modifies sleep patterns across species in a dose-dependent manner, further evidence is required to establish that endogenous GHRH has a role in sleep physiology. However, the observations that sleep patterns can be altered by antagonizing endogenous GHRH action using either anti-GHRH sera or a competitive GHRH antagonist, argues strongly that GHRH does indeed have a physiological role in the modulation of sleep. Using GHRH antibodies to block endogenous GHRH action, it has been shown that GHRH may also influence sleep recovery following sleep deprivation *(148)*. In sleep-deprived rats, GHRH antibodies inhibit sleep recovery and the expected increase in NREMS seen in sleep-deprived control animals does not occur. Indeed, the amount of NREMS decreases to levels similar to those observed in nonsleep deprived control animals.

GHRH belongs to a group of sleep promoting humoral agents including the cytokine interleukin-1 (IL-1). IL-1, similar to GHRH, increases NREMS duration in rats and rabbits following icv administration *(151–153)*. This effect of IL-1 is GHRH dependent and can be blocked by pretreating animals with anti-GHRH sera, suggesting GHRH at least in part mediates and is necessary for IL-1 action *(154)*.

GHRH effects might be indirectly mediated via GH release. Certainly, there is a close association between growth hormone release and sleep, with the major GH secretory bursts occurring in deep NREMS soon after sleep begins. However, there are no consistent data implicating GH as the mediator of the observed sleep promoting effects of GHRH in animals or humans and GHRH modulating effects on sleep are probably mediated by a direct CNS action.

Appetite Regulation and Food Intake

In rats and sheep, central administration of GHRH results in altered, circadian dependent feeding behavior (155–158). When GHRH is administered during a nonfeeding period of the circadian clock (daytime in rats who are nocturnal eaters), food intake is stimulated. In contrast when GHRH is administered during night time in rats, no effect on food intake is noted. It is likely this circadian-specific stimulation of food intake is dependent on an endogenous GHRH circadian rhythm as nocturnal food intake is associated with a concurrent increase in hypothalamic GHRH levels (159). Thus, the lack of effect on feeding of nocturnal GHRH administration may result from prior stimulation by endogenous GHRH.

Specific injection of GHRH into the suprachiasmatic nucleus-medial preoptic area (SC-MPOA) increases GHRH-induced feeding in a dose-dependent manner (160,161). Because the suprachiasmatic nuclei are the site of the circadian pacemaker, it is not surprising that GHRH action on food intake involves diurnal rhythmicity. To further examine photoperiod effects, GHRH antisera were injected into the SCN/ MPOA area of rats at various time points (159). GHRH antisera significantly reduced feeding when administered at dark-onset (when endogenous GHRH is increased), but did not affect feeding behavior when administered at other times during the day or night. These results suggest that endogenous GHRH is involved in the circadian regulation of feeding rats.

To establish whether GHRH affects the central circadian pacemaker directly, GHRH injections were placed directly into the suprachiasmatic nuclei of hamsters (162). GHRH caused a phase advancement in the circadian pacemaker of up to 150 min. This GHRH effect on circadian phase was present only during a sensitive 8-h period of the circadian cycle beginning at the time of activity onset.

Several observations suggest GHRH acts as a neurotransmitter rather than a hormone in mediating effects on feeding behavior. The doses of GHRH required to cause an effect on feeding behavior are small, ranging from 0.1 to 1.0 pmol (160). These doses are much lower than those required to stimulate growth hormone release (94,95). The SCN/MPOA also is not directly associated with the portal circulation suggesting a nonhormonal mode of action and electrophysiology studies on rat forebrain neurons indicate GHRH has neurotransmitter properties (46,163).

GHRH stimulation of feeding behavior is not only periodic, but is also macronutrient selective. Central GHRH administration causes a specific increase in protein intake with no change in carbohydrate or fat intake (164). As GHRH also modulates growth hormone release, it is conceivable that this protein selective appetite stimulation could optimize the anabolic effects of growth hormone.

Although there is a clear effect of GHRH on promoting circadian modulated feeding behavior in several animal species, this has not yet been shown conclusively in humans. However, Vaccarino et al. have investigated the effects of GHRH in anorexia nervosa (165). Patients receiving GHRH had a significant increase in food consumption following GHRH administration that was not macronutrient selective.

Immunomodulation

Several neuropeptides and hormones have important modulating effects on leukocyte function. These include VIP, somatostatin, growth hormone and IGF-I (166). There is increasing evidence demonstrating GHRH may also be an important immunomodulator.

GHRH in vitro stimulates [³H]thymidine uptake (a marker for DNA synthesis), [³H]uridine uptake (a marker for RNA synthesis) and GH mRNA production in leukocytes extracted from rat spleen and thymus *(101)*. Using peripheral blood lymphocytes, several studies have shown enhanced proliferation after treatment with $GHRH_{1-44}-NH_2$ or $GHRH_{1-29}-NH_2$ *(101,167,168)*. However, in high doses (>120 nM), GHRH inhibits lymphocyte proliferation suggesting a biphasic GHRH effect *(168)*. Other in vitro studies have shown enhanced lymphocyte chemotaxis, inhibition of natural killer (NK) cell activity, and increased histamine release from mast cells following application of GHRH *(169–172)*.

These effects are unlike those produced by GH, IGF-I, and somatostatin suggesting GHRH effects on leukocytes are direct and mediated via GHRH receptors *(173)*. Although GHRH appears to act on leukocytes independently of GH, it remains unclear whether GHRH is involved in GH release from these cells. Relatively low doses of GHRH (0.1–10 nM) fail to stimulate GH secretion while large doses of GHRH (100 nM) cause a modest increase in GH production in a small percentage of cells, suggesting no stimulatory effect of GHRH *(174,175)*. In contrast, antisense GHRH mRNA was shown to partially block (~60%) the expression of GH, suggesting GHRH may have at least a permissive effect on GH transcription *(176)*.

Although GHRH has pharmacologic effects on leukocytes, it remains uncertain whether GHRH has physiologic actions. Assuming GHRH action is mediated by an autocrine and/or paracrine mechanism, dose-response studies indicate GHRH levels would need to be in the nanomolar range to have a biological effect. This contrasts with the pituitary where picomolar amounts of GHRH are found in the portal circulation. As noted above, GHRH has been localized to numerous tissues and it is feasible that within these tissues, nanomolar concentrations of GHRH occur.

Placenta and Fetus

Placental GHRH may regulate the GH-IGF-I-IGF-II axis in the mother, fetus or placenta. It has been established that placental GH is the predominant growth hormone form in the human maternal circulation, with pituitary derived GH being suppressed in late gestation *(177,178)*. Maternal intravenous GHRH infusions and in vitro GHRH application to trophoblast cultures does not stimulate placental growth hormone release suggesting it is unlikely that placental GHRH modulates the synthesis and release of placental GH *(178,179)*.

The ontogeny of placental GHRH, IGF-I and IGF-II mRNA has been examined in rats *(54)*. Expression of GHRH and IGF-II mRNA is concurrent, gradually increasing throughout gestation. In contrast, IGF-I mRNA expression peaks at gestational d 10. This suggests that GHRH may modulate placental IGF-II expression.

The effects of placental GHRH on fetal GH, IGF-I and IGF-II are difficult to differentiate from fetal hypothalamic GHRH effects. Paradoxically, when anti-GHRH serum, known to cross the placenta, was administered prenatally (from d 7–19 of gestation) to pregnant rats, a slight, but significant increase in fetal growth was observed *(180)*. In contrast with this study, passive immunization of rats with anti-GHRH serum on one occasion at gestational d 16 had no effect on fetal growth but significantly impaired postnatal growth *(181)*. Somatotroph function at 10 and 30 d of age in these rats was also abnormal. A similar permanent impairment in postnatal growth was caused by passive immunization of rats with anti-GHRH serum soon after birth. These studies suggest that hypothalamic GHRH is required in late fetal/neonatal life for normal postnatal somatotroph function *(182)*.

Although placental and/or fetal hypothalamic GHRH may play a role in fetal growth, this effect is likely small. Rat models of GH deficiency including *gsh-1* deficiency are not associated with fetal growth impairment *(24,181,183)*. Similarly, transgenic mice overexpressing GHRH have birthweights no different than normal littermates and only postnatally have growth acceleration *(23)*. Taken together, these data suggest that placental GHRH does not play a major role in regulating fetal growth.

Gonads

Ovary

Although GHRH has been used successfully as an adjuvant in patients with infertility *(184)*, GHRH function in human ovaries remains to be clarified. Studies predominantly on rat and bovine ovarian tissue are expanding our understanding of GHRH's ovarian actions. Studies of rat granulosa cells in vitro indicate that GHRH enhances their maturation by amplifying the stimulatory effects of FSH. These GHRH actions are mediated at least in part by increased cAMP levels *(82,185)*. FSH effects, which are potentiated by GHRH, include increased granulosa cell steroidogenesis and increased luteinizing hormone (LH) receptor expression *(185)*. FSH also increases granulosa cell GHRH receptor expression and, as GHRH potentiates FSH actions, this suggests a positive intraovarian autoregulatory loop exists to accelerate follicular maturation *(82)*.

GHRH also increases the proliferation of in vitro bovine granulosa cells. This effect is augmented by the concurrent application of insulin and is independent of gonadotropin stimulation *(87)*. An increase in granulosa cell DNA synthesis by GHRH, independent of gonadotropins, has also been demonstrated in rats *(186)*. Hypothalamic GHRH stimulates the expression and release of both GH and, indirectly, IGF-I. As these hormones are also found within the ovary, it is possible that GHRH induced granulosa cell proliferation is mediated via stimulation of a local ovarian GH/IGF-I axis, although this remains to be confirmed.

Investigating the effect of GHRH on rat oocyte maturation, Apa et al. demonstrated that GHRH specifically accelerated meiotic maturation in Graafian follicles *(187)*. This effect is dependent on the presence of follicular cells; no effect was observed in denuded oocytes. Furthermore, this effect did not appear to be cAMP dependent and could be indirectly blocked by anti-GH sera supporting the hypothesis that GHRH can stimulate local growth hormone.

Ovulation involves follicular rupture; a process in which plasmin, a trypsin-like protease decreases the tensile strength of the follicular wall. Plasminogen is converted to plasmin by the protease, plasminogen activator (PA). FSH induces PA activity and it has recently been shown that GHRH also potentiates this FSH effect *(186)*.

Testis

GHRH is one of many peptides described in both human and animal testes. Little is known of testicular GHRH function in primates and most of the information regarding GHRH testicular effects is derived from rat studies. As described in Gonads of Ontogeny, Localization, and Regulation of GHRH Gene Transcription and Translation, testicular GHRH is abundant and predominantly localized to developing spermatogenic cells, whereas the GHRH receptor mRNA is expressed predominantly in Sertoli and germ cells, with lower levels of expression in Leydig cells. Although GHRH exposure to Leydig cell cultures enhances cAMP accumulation and increases LH-induced testosterone secretion, GHRH receptor expression suggests that Sertoli and germ cells are the main sites of GHRH action *(86)*. Indeed, GHRH exposure to Sertoli cell cultures potentiates the cAMP response to FSH *(84)*, and can alone under similar conditions increase Sertoli cell cAMP levels threefold compared to controls *(83)*.

Stem cell factor (also known as Steel factor, mast cell growth factor, or hemopoietic growth factor) and its receptor *c-kit* are also necessary for normal spermatogenesis *(188)*. Stem cell factor (SCF) is found primarily within Sertoli cells *(189)*, whereas the *c-kit* receptor mRNA is localized to primordial germ cells, spermatogonia, and Leydig cells *(190)*. Mutations of either SCF or its receptor result in abnormal germ cell migration and spermatogenesis *(191)*.

GHRH induces *c-fos* mRNA expression in Sertoli cell cultures and significantly increases SCF mRNA expression *(192)*. The nuclear proto-oncogene *c-fos* regulates the transcriptional activity of a wide variety of genes by forming heterodimers with members of the *jun* family and subsequently binding to AP-1 sites on DNA *(193)*. Absence of *c-fos* expression, as in mice with germline mutations of *c-fos* results in abnormal spermatogenesis *(194)*.

Sertoli cells are important regulators of spermatogenesis and communicate with germ cells, spermatids and mature sperm via several paracrine factors, one of which is SCF. In return, GHRH secreted from germ cells and spermatids can stimulate Sertoli cells to increase SCF and *c-fos* transcription as well as potentiate FSH effects on Sertoli cells. Thus, GHRH appears to form an autoregulatory loop with SCF, enabling two way communication between Sertoli cells, germ cells and spermatids. Disruption of Sertoli cell communication as with loss of function mutations in the SCF gene markedly impairs spermatogenesis *(191)*. Although the effects of gonadal GHRH deficiency have not been studied, the *gsh-1* knockout mouse has marked sexual infantilism and testes which are small, poorly vascularized, and located within the abdomen *(24,195)*. Microscopically these testes show hypocellular seminiferous tubules and maturation arrest of spermatogenic cells at the spermatid stage. It has recently been reported that GHRH mRNA expression is also markedly reduced in the testes from these mice, suggesting GHRH may also play an important role in testes *(195)*.

CONCLUSIONS

The insights gained from characterization of GHRH and its receptor have confirmed the fundamental role GHRH plays in growth regulation. Additionally, GHRH has a widespread distribution and the varying tissue-specific promotor and initiation sites that strongly suggest tissue-specific expression and function. The biological actions of GHRH in gonads and placenta confirm this tissue specificity. GHRH also functions within the hypothalamus as a neuromodulator and has effects on circadian rhythm, feeding behavior and sleep. These effects are reproducible in rodent studies, but need to be verified further in humans.

Perturbations in GHRH and GHRH receptor function demonstrate the importance of this hormone in growth regulation. Transgenic mice overexpressing GHRH have an overgrowth syndrome and also develop somatotroph hyperplasia and eventual pituitary adenoma formation. Similar pituitary changes have been seen in humans with ectopic GHRH excess. Hypothalamic lesions in mice, with destruction of GHRH neurons, result in extreme dwarfism, although no isolated GHRH deficiency has been described in either animals or humans. Mutations in the GHRH receptor have, however, been reported in both mice and humans and also result in marked dwarfism.

Outside the hypothalamus, GHRH has demonstrable actions in gonads and leukocytes. The immunomodulatory actions of GHRH occur at pharmacologic and possibly physiologic levels on leukocytes. These actions appear to be specific for GHRH and not mediated via GH or IGF-I. In the ovary, GHRH effects are directed at follicular development and ovulation, and are mediated by potentiating FSH. GHRH also mediates proliferative actions on granulosa cells, which do not involve FSH, and may involve stimulation of local GH or IGF-I expression. In testes, GHRH potentiates the effects of both LH on Leydig cells and FSH on Sertoli cells while the stimulation of SCF appears to be gonadotropin independent. It may also function as part of an autoregulatory loop involving SCF.

Thus, although GHRH is foremost a major regulator of pituitary somatotrophs, molecular and physiology studies have shown it has other functions, both centrally and in peripheral tissues. Future progress will certainly provide additional understanding about these diverse functions and further insights into the pathophysiology and treatment of GHRH dysfunction.

ACKNOWLEDGMENTS

The authors would like to thank Linda DiMeglio and Jane Peart for their helpful comments in preparing this manuscript. This work was supported by grants from the Riley Memorial Association, the Genentech Foundation and the National Institute of Health.

REFERENCES

1. Brazeau P, Vale W, Burgus R, et al. Hypothalamic polypeptide that inhibits the secretion of immunoreactive pituitary growth hormone. Science 1973;179:77–79.
2. Reichlin S. Growth and the hypothalamus. Endocrinology 1960;67:760–773.
3. Guillemin R, Brazeau P, Bohlen P, Esch F, Ling N, Wehrenberg WB. Growth hormone-releasing factor from a human pancreatic tumor that caused acromegaly. Science 1982;218(4572):585–587.
4. Rivier J, Spiess J, Thorner M, Vale W. Characterization of a growth hormone-releasing factor from a human pancreatic islet tumour. Nature 1982;300(5889):276–278.
5. Spiess J, Rivier J, Vale W. Characterization of rat hypothalamic growth hormone-releasing factor. Nature 1983;303(5917):532–535.
6. Ling N, Esch F, Bohlen P, Brazeau P, Wehrenberg WB, Guillemin R. Isolation, primary structure, and synthesis of human hypothalamic somatocrinin: growth hormone-releasing factor. Proc Natl Acad Sci USA 1984;81(14):4302–4306.
7. Campbell RM, Scanes CG. Evolution of the growth hormone-releasing factor (GRF) family of peptides. Growth Regulation 1992;2(4):175–191.
8. Mayo KE, Cerelli GM, Lebo RV, Bruce BD, Rosenfeld MG, Evans RM. Gene encoding human growth hormone-releasing factor precursor: structure, sequence, and chromosomal assignment. Proc Natl Acad Sci USA 1985;82(1):63–67.
9. Rao PN, Hayworth R, Akots G, Pettenati MJ, Bowden DW. Physical localization of chromosome 20 markers using somatic cell hybrid cell lines and fluorescence in situ hybridization. Genomics 1992;14(2):532–535.
10. Godfrey P, Rahal JO, Beamer WG, Copeland NG, Jenkins NA, Mayo KE. GHRH receptor of little mice contains a missense mutation in the extracellular domain that disrupts receptor function. Nature Genetics 1993;4(3):227–232.
11. Berry SA, Srivastava CH, Rubin LR, Phipps WR, Pescovitz OH. Growth hormone-releasing hormone-like messenger ribonucleic acid and immunoreactive peptide are present in human testis and placenta. J Clin Endocrinol Metab 1992;75(1):281–284.

12. Weigent DA, Blalock JE. Immunoreactive growth hormone-releasing hormone in rat leukocytes. J Neuro-immunol 1990;29(1–3):1–13.
13. Baird A, Wehrenberg WB, Bohlen P, Ling N. Immunoreactive and biologically active growth hormone-releasing factor in the rat placenta. Endocrinology 1985;117(4):1598–1601.
14. Suhr ST, Rahal JO, Mayo KE. Mouse growth-hormone-releasing hormone: precursor structure and expression in brain and placenta. Mol Endocrinol 1989;3(11):1693–1700.
15. Mizobuchi M, Frohman MA, Downs TR, Frohman LA. Tissue-specific transcription initiation and effects of growth hormone (GH) deficiency on the regulation of mouse and rat GH-releasing hormone gene in hypothalamus and placenta. Mol Endocrinol 1991;5(4):476–484.
16. Gonzalez-Crespo S, Boronat A. Expression of the rat growth hormone-releasing hormone gene in placenta is directed by an alternative promoter. Proc Natl Acad Sci USA 1991;88(19):8749–8753.
17. Berry SA, Pescovitz OH, Pescovitz OH, et al. Identification of a rat GHRH-like substance and its messenger RNA in rat testis. Production of monoclonal antibodies against human growth hormone releasing hormone and their use in an enzyme-linked immunosorbent assay (ELISA) [published erratum appears in J Immunol Methods 1987 Aug 3;101(2):287]. Endocrinology 1988;123(1):661–663.
18. Bosman FT, Van Assche C, Nieuwenhuyzen Kruseman AC, Jackson S, Lowry PJ. Growth hormone releasing factor (GRF) immunoreactivity in human and rat gastrointestinal tract and pancreas. J Histochem Cytochem 1984;32(11):1139–1144.
19. Bruhn TO, Mason RT, Vale WW. Presence of growth hormone-releasing factor-like immunoreactivity in rat duodenum. Endocrinology 1985;117(4):1710–1712.
20. Matsubara S, Sato M, Mizobuchi M, Niimi M, Takahara J. Differential gene expression of growth hormone (GH)-releasing hormone (GRH) and GRH receptor in various rat tissues. Endocrinology 1995;136(9):4147–4150.
21. Bagnato A, Moretti C, Ohnishi J, Frajese G, Catt KJ. Expression of the growth hormone-releasing hormone gene and its peptide product in the rat ovary. Endocrinology 1992;130(3):1097–1102.
22. Srivastava CH, Monts BS, Rothrock JK, Peredo MJ, Pescovitz OH. Presence of a spermatogenic-specific promoter in the rat growth hormone-releasing hormone gene. Endocrinology 1995;136(4):1502–1508.
23. Mayo KE, Godfrey PA, Suhr ST, Kulik DJ, Rahal JO. Growth hormone-releasing hormone: synthesis and signaling. Recent Prog Hormone Res 1995;50:35–73.
24. Li H, Zeitler PS, Valerius MT, Small K, Potter SS. Gsh-1, an orphan Hox gene, is required for normal pituitary development. EMBO J 1996;15(4):714–724.
25. Mayo KE, Vale W, Rivier J, Rosenfeld MG, Evans RM. Expression-cloning and sequence of a cDNA encoding human growth hormone-releasing factor. Nature 1983;306(5938):86–88.
26. Frohman LA, Downs TR, Chomczynski P, Brar A, Kashio Y. Regulation of growth hormone-releasing hormone gene expression and biosynthesis. Yale J Biol Med 1989;62(5):427–433.
27. Bloch B, Baird A, Ling N, Guillemin R. Immunohistochemical evidence that growth hormone-releasing factor (GRF) neurons contain an amidated peptide derived from cleavage of the carboxyl-terminal end of the GRF precursor. Endocrinology 1986;118(1):156–162.
28. Steiner DF, Quinn PS, Chan SJ, Marsh J, Tager HS. Processing mechanisms in the biosynthesis of proteins. Ann NY Acad Sci 1980;343:1–16.
29. Land H, Schutz G, Schmale H, Richter D. Nucleotide sequence of cloned cDNA encoding bovine arginine vasopressin-neurophysin II precursor. Nature 1982;295(5847):299–303.
30. Furutani Y, Morimoto Y, Shibahara S, et al. Cloning and sequence analysis of cDNA for ovine corticotropin-releasing factor precursor. Nature 1983;301(5900):537–540.
31. Frohman LA, Jansson JO. Growth hormone-releasing hormone. Endocrine Rev 1986;7(3):223–253.
32. Frohman MA, Downs TR, Chomczynski P, Frohman LA. Cloning and characterization of mouse growth hormone-releasing hormone (GRH) complementary DNA: increased GRH messenger RNA levels in the growth hormone-deficient lit/lit mouse. Mol Endocrinol 1989;3(10):1529–1536.
33. Mayo KE, Cerelli GM, Rosenfeld MG, Evans RM. Characterization of cDNA and genomic clones encoding the precursor to rat hypothalamic growth hormone-releasing factor. Nature 1985; 314(6010):464–467.
34. Kraicer J, French MB, Lussier BT, Moor BC, Brazlan P. A comparison of the biological activities of authentic rat GRF(1–43)OH with the analogue rat GRF(1–29)NH2. Can J Physiol Pharmacol 1991;69(2):181–184.
35. Frohman LA, Downs TR, Williams TC, Heimer EP, Pan YC, Felix AM. Rapid enzymatic degradation of growth hormone-releasing hormone by plasma in vitro and in vivo to a biologically inactive product cleaved at the NH2 terminus. J Clin Invest 1986;78(4):906–913.

36. Bongers J, Lambros T, Ahmad M, Heimer EP. Kinetics of dipeptidyl peptidase IV proteolysis of growth hormone-releasing factor and analogs. Biochim Biophys Acta 1992;1122(2):147–153.
37. Boulanger L, Roughly P, Gaudreau P. Catabolism of rat growth hormone-releasing factor(1-29) amide in rat serum and liver. Peptides 1992;13(4):681–689.
38. Breyer PR, Rothrock JK, Beaudry N, Pescovitz OH. A novel peptide from the growth hormone releasing hormone gene stimulates Sertoli cell activity. Endocrinology 1996;137(5):2159–2162.
39. Bloch B, Brazeau P, Ling N, et al. Immunohistochemical detection of growth hormone-releasing factor in brain. Nature 1983;301(5901):607,608.
40. Jacobowitz DM, Schulte H, Chrousos GP, Loriaux DL. Localization of GRF-like immunoreactive neurons in the rat brain. Peptides 1983;4(4):521–524.
41. VandePol CJ, Leidy JW, Jr., Finger TE, Robbins RJ. Immunohistochemical localization of GRF-containing neurons in rat brain. Neuroendocrinology 1986;42(2):143–147.
42. Merchenthaler I, Vigh S, Schally AV, Petrusz P. Immunocytochemical localization of growth hormone-releasing factor in the rat hypothalamus. Endocrinology 1984;114(4):1082–1085.
43. Merchenthaler I, Thomas CR, Arimura A. Immunocytochemical localization of growth hormone releasing factor (GHRF)-containing structures in the rat brain using anti-rat GHRF serum. Peptides 1984;5(6):1071–1075.
44. Bloch B, Brazeau P, Bloom F, Ling N. Topographical study of the neurons containing hpGRF immunoreactivity in monkey hypothalamus. Neurosci Lett 1983;37(1):23–28.
45. Leidy JW, Jr., Robbins RJ. Regional distribution of human growth hormone-releasing hormone in the human hypothalamus by radioimmunoassay. J Clin Endocrinol Metab 1986;62(2):372–378.
46. Sawchenko PE, Swanson LW, Rivier J, Vale WW. The distribution of growth-hormone-releasing factor (GRF) immunoreactivity in the central nervous system of the rat: an immunohistochemical study using antisera directed against rat hypothalamic GRF. J Compar Neurol 1985;237(1):100–115.
47. Meister B, Hokfelt T. The somatostatin and growth hormone-releasing factor systems. In: Nemeroff CB, ed. Neuroendocrinology. CRC, Boca Raton, FL, 1992.
48. Twery MJ, Moss RL. Effects of human pancreatic growth hormone-releasing hormone and fragments of rat hypothalamic growth hormone-releasing hormone on the activity of rat brain neurons. Neurosci Lett 1986;69(2):176–181.
49. Burgunder JM. Prenatal ontogeny of growth hormone releasing hormone expression in rat hypothalamus. Devel Neurosci 1991;13(6):397–402.
50. Bresson JL, Clavequin MC, Fellmann D, Bugnon C. Ontogeny of the neuroglandular system revealed with HPGRF 44 antibodies in human hypothalamus. Neuroendocrinology 1984;39(1):68–73.
51. Goodyer CG, Branchaud CL, Lefebvre Y. Effects of growth hormone (GH)-releasing factor and somatostatin on GH secretion from early to midgestation human fetal pituitaries. J Clin Endocrinol Metab 1993;76(5):1259–1264.
52. Kaplan SL, Grumbach MM, Aubert MLF. The ontogenesis of pituitary hormones and hypothalamic factors in the human fetus: maturation of central nervous system. Regulation of anterior pituitary function. Recent Prog Hormone Res 1976;32:161–243.
53. Mizobuchi M, Downs TR, Frohman LA. Growth hormone-releasing hormone immunoreactivity in mouse placenta, maternal blood, and amniotic fluid: molecular characterization and secretion from primary cell cultures in vitro. Endocrinology 1995;136(4):1731–1736.
54. Pescovitz OH, Johnson NB, Berry SA. Ontogeny of growth hormone releasing hormone and insulin-like growth factors-I and -II messenger RNA in rat placenta. Pediatric Res 1991;29(5):510–516.
55. Chomczynski P, Downs TR, Frohman LA. Feedback regulation of growth hormone (GH)-releasing hormone gene expression by GH in rat hypothalamus. Mol Endocrinol 1988;2(3):236–241.
56. Uchiyama T, Kaji H, Abe H, Chihara K. Negative regulation of hypothalamic growth hormone-releasing factor messenger ribonucleic acid by growth hormone and insulin-like growth factor I. Neuroendocrinology 1994;59(5):441–450.
57. Giustina A, Wehrenberg WB. Influence of thyroid hormones on the regulation of growth hormone secretion. Eur J Endocrinol 1995;133(6):646–653.
58. Bertherat J, Bluet-Pajot MT, Epelbaum J. Neuroendocrine regulation of growth hormone. Eur J Endocrinol 1995;132(1):12–24.
59. Williams T, Maxon H, Thorner MO, Frohman LA. Blunted growth hormone (GH) response to GH-releasing hormone in hypothyroidism resolves in the euthyroid state. J Clin Endocrinol Metab 1985;61(3):454–456.

60. Katakami H, Downs TR, Frohman LA. Decreased hypothalamic growth hormone-releasing hormone content and pituitary responsiveness in hypothyroidism. J Clin Invest 1986;77(5):1704–1711.

61. Downs TR, Chomczynski P, Frohman LA. Effects of thyroid hormone deficiency and replacement on rat hypothalamic growth hormone (GH)-releasing hormone gene expression in vivo are mediated by GH. Mol Endocrinol 1990;4(3):402–408.

62. Argente J, Chowen JA. Control of the transcription of the growth hormone-releasing hormone and somatostatin genes by sex steroids. Hormone Res 1993;40(1–3):48–53.

63. Zeitler P, Vician L, Chowen-Breed JA, et al. Regulation of somatostatin and growth hormone-releasing hormone gene expression in the rat brain. Metab Clin Exper 1990;39(9 Suppl 2): 46–49.

64. Zeitler P, Argente J, Chowen-Breed JA, Clifton DK, Steiner RA. Growth hormone-releasing hormone messenger ribonucleic acid in the hypothalamus of the adult male rat is increased by testosterone. Endocrinology 1990;127(3):1362–1368.

65. Veldhuis JD. Gender differences in secretory activity of the human somatotropic (growth hormone) axis. Eur J Endocrinol 1996;134(3):287–295.

66. Thissen JP, Ketelslegers JM, Underwood LE. Nutritional regulation of the insulin-like growth factors. Endocr Rev 1994;15(1):80–101.

67. Berelowitz M, Bruno JF, White JD. Regulation of hypothalamic neuropeptide expression by peripheral metabolism. Trends Endocr Metab 1992;3(4):127–132.

68. Bruno JF, Olchovsky D, White JD, Leidy JW, Song J, Berelowitz M. Influence of food deprivation in the rat on hypothalamic expression of growth hormone-releasing factor and somatostatin. Endocrinology 1990;127(5):2111–2116.

69. Bruno JF, Song JF, Berelowitz M. Regulation of rat hypothalamic preprogrowth hormone-releasing factor messenger ribonucleic acid by dietary protein. Endocrinology 1991;129(3):1226–1232.

70. Williams T, Berelowitz M, Joffe SN, et al. Impaired growth hormone responses to growth hormone-releasing factor in obesity. A pituitary defect reversed with weight reduction. N Engl J Med 1984;311(22):1403–1407.

71. Ahmad I, Finkelstein JA, Downs TR, Frohman LA. Obesity-associated decrease in growth hormone-releasing hormone gene expression: a mechanism for reduced growth hormone mRNA levels in genetically obese Zucker rats. Neuroendocrinology 1993;58(3):332–337.

72. Tannenbaum GS, Lapointe M, Gurd W, Finkelstein JA. Mechanisms of impaired growth hormone secretion in genetically obese Zucker rats: roles of growth hormone-releasing factor and somatostatin. Endocrinology 1990;127(6):3087–3095.

73. Tannenbaum GS. Growth hormone secretory dynamics in streptozotocin diabetes: evidence of a role for endogenous circulating somatostatin. Endocrinology 1981;108(1):76–82.

74. Margioris AN, Brockmann G, Bohler HC, Jr., Grino M, Vamvakopoulos N, Chrousos GP. Expression and localization of growth hormone-releasing hormone messenger ribonucleic acid in rat placenta: in vitro secretion and regulation of its peptide product. Endocrinology 1990;126(1):151–158.

75. Yamaguchi M, Miki N, Ono M, et al. Inhibition of growth hormone-releasing factor production in mouse placenta by cytokines using gp130 as a signal transducer. Endocrinology 1995;136(3): 1072–1078.

76. Yamaguchi M, Endo H, Tasaka K, Miyake A. Mouse growth hormone-releasing factor secretion is activated by inhibin and inhibited by activin in placenta. Biol Reproduc 1995;53(2):368–372.

77. Yamaguchi M, Endo H, Maeda T, et al. Transforming growth factor-beta 1 post-transcriptionally inhibits mouse growth hormone releasing factor secretion in placenta. Biochem Biophys Res Commun 1994;204(3):1206–1211.

78. Silen ML, Firpo A, Francus T, Klein RF, Lowry SF. The effect of interleukin-1 alpha and tumor necrosis factor alpha on the secretion of human chorionic gonadotropin by JAR human choriocarcinoma cells. Biochem Biophys Res Commun 1989;164(1):284–289.

79. Tsagarakis S, Ge F, Besser GM, Grossman A. Similar high molecular weight forms of growth hormone-releasing hormone are found in rat brain and testis. Life Sci 1991;49(22):1627–1634.

80. Pescovitz OH, Berry SA, Laudon M, et al. Localization and growth hormone (GH)-releasing activity of rat testicular GH-releasing hormone-like peptide. Endocrinology 1990;127(5):2336–2342.

81. Moretti C, Fabbri A, Gnessi L, et al. Immunohistochemical localization of growth hormone-releasing hormone in human gonads. J Endocrinol Invest 1990;13(4):301–305.

82. Bagnato A, Moretti C, Frajese G, Catt KJ. Gonadotropin-induced expression of receptors for growth hormone releasing factor in cultured granulosa cells. Endocrinology 1991;128(6):2889–2894.

83. Srivastava CH, Collard MW, Rothrock JK, Peredo MJ, Berry SA, Pescovitz OH. Germ cell localization of a testicular growth hormone-releasing hormone-like factor. Endocrinology 1993;133(1):83–89.

84. Fabbri A, Ciocca DR, Ciampani T, Wang J, Dufau ML. Growth hormone-releasing hormone in testicular interstitial and germ cells: potential paracrine modulation of follicle-stimulating hormone action on Sertoli cell function. Endocrinology 1995;136(5):2303–2308.

85. Ciampani T, Fabbri A, Isidori A, Dufau ML. Growth hormone-releasing hormone is produced by rat Leydig cell in culture and acts as a positive regulator of Leydig cell function. Endocrinology 1992;131(6):2785–2792.

86. Srivastava CH, Kelly MR, Monts BS, Wilson TM, Breyer PR, Pescovitz OH. Growth hormone-releasing hormone receptor mRNA is present in rat testis. Endocrine 1994;2:607–610.

87. Spicer LJ, Langhout DJ, Alpizar E, et al. Effects of growth hormone-releasing factor and vasoactive intestinal peptide on proliferation and steroidogenesis of bovine granulosa cells. Mol Cell Endocrinol 1992;83(1):73–78.

88. Moretti C, Fabbri A, Gnessi L, Forni L, Fraioli F, Frajese G. GHRH stimulates follicular growth and amplified FSH-induced ovarian folliculogenesis in women with anovulatory infertility. Proc Second Int Symp Reproduct Med, 1989.

89. Berry SA, Pescovitz OH. Ontogeny and pituitary regulation of testicular growth hormone-releasing hormone-like messenger ribonucleic acid. Endocrinology 1990;127(3):1404–1411.

90. Mayo KE. Molecular cloning and expression of a pituitary-specific receptor for growth hormone-releasing hormone. Mol Endocrinol 1992;6(10):1734–1744.

91. Lin SC, Lin CR, Gukovsky I, Lusis AJ, Sawchenko PE, Rosenfeld MG. Molecular basis of the little mouse phenotype and implications for cell type-specific growth [see comments]. Nature 1993; 364(6434):208–213.

92. Hsiung HM, Smith DP, Zhang XY, Bennett T, Rosteck PR, Jr., Lai MH. Structure and functional expression of a complementary DNA for porcine growth hormone-releasing hormone receptor. Neuropeptides 1993;25(1):1–10.

93. Wajnrajch MP, Chua SC, Green ED, Leibel RL. Human growth hormone-releasing hormone receptor (GHRHR) maps to a YAC at chromosome 7p15. Mammal Genome 1994;5(9):595.

94. Gaylinn BD, Harrison JK, Zysk JR, Lyons CE, Lynch KR, Thorner MO. Molecular cloning and expression of a human anterior pituitary receptor for growth hormone-releasing hormone. Mol Endocrinol 1993;7(1):77–84.

95. Carrick TA, Bingham B, Eppler CM, Baumbach WR, Zysk JR. A rapid and sensitive binding assay for growth hormone releasing factor. Endocrinology 1995;136(10):4701–4704.

96. Seifert H, Perrin M, Rivier J, Vale W. Growth hormone-releasing factor binding sites in rat anterior pituitary membrane homogenates: modulation by glucocorticoids. Endocrinology 1985;117(1): 424–426.

97. Seifert H, Perrin M, Rivier J, Vale W. Binding sites for growth hormone releasing factor on rat anterior pituitary cells. Nature 1985;313(6002):487–489.

98. Lin C, Lin SC, Chang CP, Rosenfeld MG. Pit-1-dependent expression of the receptor for growth hormone releasing factor mediates pituitary cell growth [see comments]. Nature 1992;360(6406): 765–768.

99. Takahashi T, Okimura Y, Yoshimura K, et al. Regional distribution of growth hormone-releasing hormone (GHRH) receptor mRNA in the rat brain. Endocrinology 1995;136(10):4721–4724.

100. Korytko AI, Zeitler P, Cuttler L. Developmental regulation of pituitary growth hormone-releasing hormone receptor gene expression in the rat. Endocrinology 1996;137(4):1326–1331.

101. Guarcello V, Weigent DA, Blalock JE. Growth hormone releasing hormone receptors on thymocytes and splenocytes from rats. Cell Immunol 1991;136(2):291–302.

102. Bilezikjian LM, Seifert H, Vale W. Desensitization to growth hormone-releasing factor (GRF) is associated with down-regulation of GRF-binding sites. Endocrinology 1986;118(5):2045–2052.

103. Wehrenberg WB, Seifert H, Bilezikjian LM, Vale W. Down-regulation of growth hormone releasing factor receptors following continuous infusion of growth hormone releasing factor in vivo. Neuroendocrinology 1986;43(2):266–268.

104. Miki N, Ono M, Murata Y, et al. Regulation of pituitary growth hormone-releasing factor (GRF) receptor gene expression by GRF. Biochem Biophys Res Commun 1996;224(2):586–590.

105. Brazeau P, Ling N, Esch F, Bohlen P, Mougin C, Guillemin R. Somatocrinin (growth hormone releasing factor) in vitro bioactivity; Ca++ involvement, cAMP mediated action and additivity of effect with PGE2. Biochem Biophys Res Commun 1982;109(2):588–594.

106. Bilezikjian LM, Vale WW. Stimulation of adenosine 3',5'-monophosphate production by growth hormone-releasing factor and its inhibition by somatostatin in anterior pituitary cells in vitro. Endocrinology 1983;113(5):1726–1731.

107. Gonzalez GA, Montminy MR. Cyclic AMP stimulates somatostatin gene transcription by phosphorylation of CREB at serine 133. Cell 1989;59(4):675–680.

108. McCormick A, Brady H, Theill LE, Karin M. Regulation of the pituitary-specific homeobox gene GHF1 by cell-autonomous and environmental cues. Nature 1990;345(6278):829–832.

109. Gaiddon C, Tian J, Loeffler JP, Bancroft C. Constitutively active G(S) alpha-subunits stimulate Pit-1 promoter activity via a protein kinase A-mediated pathway acting through deoxyribonucleic acid binding sites both for Pit-1 and for adenosine 3',5'-monophosphate response element-binding protein. Endocrinology 1996;137(4):1286–1291.

110. Chen C, Clarke IJ. Modulation of Ca2+ influx in the ovine somatotroph by growth hormone-releasing factor. Am J Physiol 1995;268(2 Pt 1):E204–212.

111. Cuttler L, Glaum SR, Collins BA, Miller RJ. Calcium signalling in single growth hormone-releasing factor-responsive pituitary cells. Endocrinology 1992;130(2):945–953.

112. Holl RW, Thorner MO, Leong DA. Intracellular calcium concentration and growth hormone secretion in individual somatotropes: effects of growth hormone-releasing factor and somatostatin. Endocrinology 1988;122(6):2927–2932.

113. Narayanan N, Lussier B, French M, Moor B, Kraicer J. Growth hormone-releasing factor-sensitive adenylate cyclase system of purified somatotrophs: effects of guanine nucleotides, somatostatin, calcium, and magnesium. Endocrinology 1989;124(1):484–495.

114. Chen C, Wu D, Clarke IJ. Signal transduction systems employed by synthetic GH-releasing peptides in somatotrophs. J Endocrinol 1996;148(3):381–386.

115. Naumov AP, Herrington J, Hille B. Actions of growth-hormone-releasing hormone on rat pituitary cells: intracellular calcium and ionic currents. Pflugers Archiv—Eur J Physiol 1994;427(5–6):414–421.

116. Chen C, Israel JM, Vincent JD. Electrophysiological responses of rat pituitary cells in somatotroph-enriched primary culture to human growth-hormone releasing factor. Neuroendocrinology 1989;50(6):679–687.

117. Login IS, Judd AM, MacLeod RM. Association of 45Ca2+ mobilization with stimulation of growth hormone (GH) release by GH-releasing factor in dispersed normal male rat pituitary cells. Endocrinology 1986;118(1):239–243.

118. Ohmura E, Friesen HG. 12-O-tetradecanoyl phorbol-13-acetate stimulates rat growth hormone (GH) release through different pathways from that of human pancreatic GH-releasing factor. Endocrinology 1985;116(2):728–733.

119. Ishizuka T, Morita H, Mune T, et al. Growth hormone secretion in human acromegalic pituitary adenomas: cyclic adenosine monophosphate and protein kinase C responses. Metab Clin Experiment 1996;45(2):206–210.

120. Howard AD, Feighner SD, Cully DF, et al. A receptor in pituitary and hypothalamus that functions in growth hormone release [see comments]. Science 1996;273(5277):974–977.

121. Thorner MO, Rivier J, Spiess J, et al. Human pancreatic growth-hormone-releasing factor selectively stimulates growth-hormone secretion in man. Lancet 1983;1(8314–8315):24–28.

122. Rosenthal SM, Schriock EA, Kaplan SL, Guillemin R, Grumbach MM. Synthetic human pancreas growth hormone-releasing factor (hpGRF1-44-NH2) stimulates growth hormone secretion in normal men. J Clin Endocrinol Metab 1983;57(3):677–679.

123. Gelato MC, Pescovitz O, Cassorla F, Loriaux DL, Merriam GR. Effects of a growth hormone releasing factor in man. J Clin Endocrinol Metab 1983;57(3):674–676.

124. Laron Z, Breddam K, Widmer F, Meldal M. Usefulness of the growth hormone-releasing hormone test regardless of which fragment is used (GHRH 1–44, 1–40 or 1–29). Amidation of growth hormone releasing factor (1–29) by serine carboxypeptidase catalysed transpeptidation. Israel J Med Sci 1991;27(6):343–345.

125. Vance ML, Kaiser DL, Evans WS, et al. Evidence for a limited growth hormone (GH)-releasing hormone (GHRH)-releasable quantity of GH: Effects of 6-hour infusions of GHRH on GH secretion in normal man. J Clin Endocrinol Metab 1985;60(2):370–375.

126. Vance ML, Kaiser DL, Martha PM, Jr., et al. Lack of in vivo somatotroph desensitization or depletion after 14 days of continuous growth hormone (GH)-releasing hormone administration in normal men and a GH-deficient boy. J Clin Endocrinol Metab 1989;68(1):22–28.

127. Melmed S, Ezrin C, Kovacs K, Goodman RS, Frohman LA. Acromegaly due to secretion of growth hormone by an ectopic pancreatic islet-cell tumor. N Engl J Med 1985;312(1):9–17.
128. Frohman LA, Szabo M. Ectopic production of growth hormone-releasing factor by carcinoid and pancreatic islet tumors associated with acromegaly. Prog Clin Biol Res 1981;74:259–271.
129. Ezzat S, Asa SL, Stefaneanu L, et al. Somatotroph hyperplasia without pituitary adenoma associated with a long standing growth hormone-releasing hormone-producing bronchial carcinoid. J Clin Endocrinol Metab 1994;78(3):555–560.
130. Moran A, Asa SL, Kovacs K, et al. Gigantism due to pituitary mammosomatotroph hyperplasia. N Engl J Med 1990;323(5):322–327.
131. Zimmerman D, Young WF, Jr., Ebersold MJ, et al. Congenital gigantism due to growth hormone-releasing hormone excess and pituitary hyperplasia with adenomatous transformation. J Clin Endocrinol Metab 1993;76(1):216–222.
132. Landis CA, Masters SB, Spada A, Pace AM, Bourne HR, Vallar L. GTPase inhibiting mutations activate the alpha chain of Gs and stimulate adenylyl cyclase in human pituitary tumours. Nature 1989;340(6236):692–696.
133. Adams EF, Lei T, Buchfelder M, Petersen B, Fahlbusch R. Biochemical characteristics of human pituitary somatotropinomas with and without gsp mutations: in vitro cell culture studies. J Clin Endocrinol Metab 1995;80(7):2077–2081.
134. Moran A, Pescovitz OH. Long-term treatment of gigantism with combination octreotide and bromocriptine in a child with McCune-Albright syndrome. Endocr J 1994;2:111–113.
135. Premawardhana LD, Vora JP, Mills R, Scanlon MF, Spada A, Vallar L. Acromegaly and its treatment in the McCune-Albright syndrome. G-protein oncogenes in acromegaly. Clin Endocrinol 1992; 36(6):605–608.
136. Olney JW, Adamo NJ, Ratner A. Monosodium glutamate effects. Science 1971;172(980):294.
137. Bloch B, Ling N, Benoit R, Wehrenberg WB, Guillemin R. Specific depletion of immunoreactive growth hormone-releasing factor by monosodium glutamate in rat median eminence. Nature 1984;307(5948):272,273.
138. Meister B, Ceccatelli S, Hokfelt T, Anden NE, Anden M, Theodorsson E. Neurotransmitters, neuropeptides and binding sites in the rat mediobasal hypothalamus: effects of monosodium glutamate (MSG) lesions. Exper Brain Res 1989;76(2):343–368.
139. Perez Jurado LA, Phillips JA 3rd, Francke U. Exclusion of growth hormone (GH)-releasing hormone gene mutations in familial isolated GH deficiency by linkage and single strand conformation analysis. J Clin Endocrinol Metab 1994;78(3):622–628.
140. Wajnrajch MP, Gertner JM, Harbison MD, Chua SC, Jr., Leibel RL. Nonsense mutation in the human growth hormone-releasing hormone receptor causes growth failure analogous to the little (lit) mouse. Nature Genet 1996;12(1):88–90.
141. Maheshwari H, Silverman BL, Dupuis JGB. Dwarfism of Sindh: A novel form of familial isolated GH deficiency linked to the locus for the GH releasing hormone receptor. 10th Int Congr Endocrinol, San Francisco, CA, 1996.
142. Cao Y, Wagner JK, Hindmarsh PC, Eble A, Mullis PE. Isolated growth hormone deficiency: testing the little mouse hypothesis in man and exclusion of mutations within the extracellular domain of the growth hormone-releasing hormone receptor. Pediat Res 1995;38(6):962–966.
143. Krueger JM, Obal F, Jr. Growth hormone-releasing hormone and interleukin-1 in sleep regulation. FASEB J 1993;7(8):645–652.
144. Krueger JM, Takahashi S, Kapas L, et al. Cytokines in sleep regulation. Adv Neuroimmunol 1995;5(2):171–188.
145. Ehlers CL, Reed TK, Henriksen SJ. Effects of corticotropin-releasing factor and growth hormone-releasing factor on sleep and activity in rats. Neuroendocrinology 1986;42(6):467–474.
146. Obal F, Jr., Alfoldi P, Cady AB, Johannsen L, Sary G, Krueger JM. Growth hormone-releasing factor enhances sleep in rats and rabbits. Am J Physiol 1988;255(2 Pt 2):R310–316.
147. Obal F, Jr., Payne L, Kapas L, Opp M, Krueger JM. Inhibition of growth hormone-releasing factor suppresses both sleep and growth hormone secretion in the rat. Brain Res 1991;557(1–2):149–153.
148. Obal F, Jr., Payne L, Opp M, Alfoldi P, Kapas L, Krueger JM. Growth hormone-releasing hormone antibodies suppress sleep and prevent enhancement of sleep after sleep deprivation. Am J Physiol 1992;263(5 Pt 2):R1078–1085.
149. Kupfer DJ, Jarrett DB, Ehlers CL. The effect of GRF on the EEG sleep of normal males. Sleep 1991;14(1):87,88.

150. Kerkhofs M, Van Cauter E, Van Onderbergen A, Caufriez A, Thorner MO, Copinschi G. Sleep-promoting effects of growth hormone-releasing hormone in normal men. Am J Physiol 1993;264(4 Pt 1):E594–598.
151. Opp MR, Krueger JM. Anti-interleukin-1 beta reduces sleep and sleep rebound after sleep deprivation in rats. Am J Physiol 1994;266(3 Pt 2):R688–695.
152. Opp MR, Krueger JM. Interleukin-1 is involved in responses to sleep deprivation in the rabbit. Brain Res 1994;639(1):57–65.
153. Imeri L, Opp MR, Krueger JM. An IL-1 receptor and an IL-1 receptor antagonist attenuate muramyl dipeptide- and IL-1-induced sleep and fever. Am J Physiol 1993;265(4 Pt 2):R907–913.
154. Obal F, Jr., Fang J, Payne LC, Krueger JM. Growth-hormone-releasing hormone mediates the sleep-promoting activity of interleukin-1 in rats. Neuroendocrinology 1995;61(5):559–565.
155. Vaccarino FJ, Bloom FE, Rivier J, Vale W, Koob GF. Stimulation of food intake in rats by centrally administered hypothalamic growth hormone-releasing factor. Nature 1985;314(6007):167,168.
156. Riviere P, Bueno L. Influence of regimen and insulinemia on orexigenic effects of GRF1-44 in sheep. Physiol Behav 1987;39(3):347–350.
157. Vaccarino FJ, Buckenham KE. Naloxone blockade of growth hormone-releasing factor-induced feeding. Regul Peptides 1987;18(3–4):165–171.
158. Feifel D, Vaccarino FJ. Feeding effects of growth hormone-releasing factor in rats are photoperiod sensitive. Behav Neurosci 1989;103(4):824–830.
159. Vaccarino FJ, Feifel D, Rivier J, Vale W. Antagonism of central growth hormone-releasing factor activity selectively attenuates dark-onset feeding in rats. J Neurosci 1991;11(12):3924–3927.
160. Dickson PR, Vaccarino FJ. Characterization of feeding behavior induced by central injection of GRF. Am J Physiol 1990;259(3 Pt 2):R651–657.
161. Vaccarino FJ, Hayward M. Microinjections of growth hormone-releasing factor into the medial pre-optic area/suprachiasmatic nucleus region of the hypothalamus stimulate food intake in rats. Regul Peptides 1988;21(1–2):21–28.
162. Vaccarino FJ, Sovran P, Baird JP, Ralph MR. Growth hormone-releasing hormone mediates feeding-specific feedback to the suprachiasmatic circadian clock. Peptides 1995;16(4):595–598.
163. Twery MJ, Moss RL. Sensitivity of rat forebrain neurons to growth hormone-releasing hormone. Peptides 1985;6(4):609–613.
164. Dickson PR, Vaccarino FJ. GRF-induced feeding: evidence for protein selectivity and opiate involvement. Peptides 1994;15(8):1343–1352.
165. Vaccarino FJ, Kennedy SH, Ralevski E, Black R. The effects of growth hormone-releasing factor on food consumption in anorexia nervosa patients and normals. Biol Psych 1994;35(7):446–451.
166. Campbell RM, Scanes CG. Endocrine peptides 'moonlighting' as immune modulators: roles for somatostatin and GH-releasing factor. J Endocrinol 1995;147(3):383–396.
167. Weigent DA, Riley JE, Galin FS, LeBoeuf RD, Blalock JE. Detection of growth hormone and growth hormone-releasing hormone-related messenger RNA in rat leukocytes by the polymerase chain reaction. Proc Soc Exper Biol Med 1991;198(1):643–648.
168. Valtorta A, Moretta A, Maccario R, Bozzola M, Severi F. Influence of growth hormone-releasing hormone (GHRH) on phytohemagglutinin-induced lymphocyte activation: comparison of two synthetic forms. GHRH and PHA-induced lymphocyte activation. Thymus 1991;18(1):51–59.
169. Pawlikowski M, Zelazowski P, Dohler K, Stepien H. Effects of two neuropeptides, somatoliberin (GRF) and corticoliberin (CRF), on human lymphocyte natural killer activity. Brain Behav Immun 1988;2(1):50–56.
170. Hattori N, Ikekubo K, Ishihara T, Moridera K, Hino M, Kurahachi H. Spontaneous growth hormone (GH) secretion by unstimulated human lymphocytes and the effects of GH-releasing hormone and somatostatin. J Clin Endocrinol Metab 1994;79(6):1678–1680.
171. Zelazowski P, Dohler KD, Stepien H, Pawlikowski M. Effect of growth hormone-releasing hormone on human peripheral blood leukocyte chemotaxis and migration in normal subjects. Neuroendocrinology 1989;50(2):236–239.
172. Estevez MD, Alfonso A, Vieytes MR, Louzao MC, Botana LM. Study of the activation mechanism of human GRF(1–29)NH2 on rat mast cell histamine release. Inflamm Res 1995;44(2):87–91.
173. Auernhammer CJ, Strasburger CJ. Effects of growth hormone and insulin-like growth factor I on the immune system. Eur J Endocrinol 1995;133(6):635–645.
174. Kao TL, Meyer WJd, Tanaka Y, Egawa M, Inoue S, Takamura Y. Inhibition of immunoreactive growth hormone secretion from lymphoid cell lines by dexamethasone: Effect of hypothalamic

administration of growth hormone-releasing factor (GRF) on feeding behavior in rats. Life Sci 1992;51(13):1033–1039.

175. Hattori N, Shimatsu A, Sugita M, Kumagai S, Imura H. Immunoreactive growth hormone (GH) secretion by human lymphocytes: augmented release by exogenous GH. Biochem Biophys Res Commun 1990;168(2):396–401.

176. Payne LC, Rohn W, Weigent DA. Lymphocyte-derived growth hormone releasing hormone is an autocrine modulator of lymphocyte-derived growth hormone. 76th Ann Meet Endocrine Society, 1994.

177. Frankenne F, Closset J, Gomez F, Scippo ML, Smal J, Hennen G. The physiology of growth hormones (GHs) in pregnant women and partial characterization of the placental GH variant. J Clin Endocrinol Metab 1988;66(6):1171–1180.

178. de Zegher F, Vanderschueren-Lodeweyckx M, Spitz B, et al. Perinatal growth hormone (GH) physiology: effect of GH-releasing factor on maternal and fetal secretion of pituitary and placental GH. J Clin Endocrinol Metab 1990;71(2):520–522.

179. Evain-Brion D, Alsat E, Mirlesse V, et al. Regulation of growth hormone secretion in human trophoblastic cells in culture. Hormone Res 1990;33(6):256–259.

180. Spatola E, Pescovitz OH, Marsh K, Johnson NB, Berry SA, Gelato MC. Interaction of growth hormone-releasing hormone with the insulin-like growth-factors during prenatal development in the rat. Endocrinology 1991;129(3):1193–1200.

181. Cella SG, Locatelli V, Broccia ML, et al. Long-term changes of somatotrophic function induced by deprivation of growth hormone-releasing hormone during the fetal life of the rat. J Endocrinol 1994;140(1):111–117.

182. Cella SG, De Gennaro Colonna V, Locatelli V, et al. Somatotropic dysfunction in growth hormone-releasing hormone-deprived neonatal rats: effect of growth hormone replacement therapy. Pediatric Res 1994;36(3):315–322.

183. Jansson JO, Ishikawa K, Katakami H, Frohman LA. Pre- and postnatal developmental changes in hypothalamic content of rat growth hormone-releasing factor. Endocrinology 1987;120(2):525–530.

184. Volpe A, Coukos G, Barreca A, Giordano G, Artini PG, Genazzani AR. Clinical use of growth hormone-releasing factor for induction of superovulation. Human Reprod 1991;6(9):1228–1232.

185. Moretti C, Bagnato A, Solan N, Frajese G, Catt KJ. Receptor-mediated actions of growth hormone releasing factor on granulosa cell differentiation. Endocrinology 1990;127(5):2117–2126.

186. Karakji EG, Tsang BK. Growth hormone releasing factor and vasoactive intestinal peptide stimulate rat granulosa cell plasminogen activator activity in vitro during follicular development. Mol Cell Endocrinol 1995;107(1):105–112.

187. Apa R, Lanzone A, Miceli F, et al. Growth hormone-releasing factor stimulates meiotic maturation in follicle- and cumulus-enclosed rat oocyte. Mol Cell Endocrinol 1995;112(2):195–201.

188. Pescovitz OH, Srivastava CH, Breyer PR, Monts BA. Paracrine control of spermatogenesis. Trends Endocrinol Metab 1994;5(3):126–131.

189. Rossi P, Albanesi C, Grimaldi P, Geremia R. Expression of the mRNA for the ligand of c-kit in mouse Sertoli cells. Biochem Biophys Res Commun 1991;176(2):910–914.

190. Manova K, Nocka K, Besmer P, Bachvarova RF. Gonadal expression of c-kit encoded at the W locus of the mouse. Development 1990;110(4):1057–1069.

191. Huang E, Nocka K, Beier DCTY, et al. The hematopoietic growth factor KL is encoded by the Sl locus and is the ligand of the c-kit receptor, the gene product of the W locus. Cell 1990;63(1):225–233.

192. Srivastava CH, Breyer PR, Rothrock JK, Peredo MJ, Pescovitz OH. A new target for growth hormone releasing-hormone action in rat: the Sertoli cell. Endocrinology 1993;133(3):1478–1481.

193. Cohen DR, Vandermark SE, McGovern JD, Bradley MP. Transcriptional regulation in the testis: a role for transcription factor AP-1 complexes at various stages of spermatogenesis. Oncogene 1993; 8(2):443–455.

194. Johnson RS, Spiegelman BM, Papaioannou V, et al. Pleiotropic effects of a null mutation in the c-fos proto-oncogene: The ontogeny of growth hormone in the human fetal pituitary. Cell 1992;71(4): 577–586.

195. Monts B, Li H, McFarland K, et al. Testicular effects of homologous inactivation of *GSH-1* in transgenic mice. 10th Int Congr Endocrinol, San Francisco, CA, 1996.

7

The Glomerular Physiology of Diabetic Nephropathy

David J. Klein, PhD, MD

CONTENTS

THE GLOMERULAR PHYSIOLOGY OF DIABETIC NEPHROPATHY
REFERENCES

THE GLOMERULAR PHYSIOLOGY OF DIABETIC NEPHROPATHY

The diabetic nephropathy (DN) develops in 30–40% of people with type I diabetes mellitus (DM) and is associated with a sixfold increase in mortality from the disease *(1)*. Its incidence peaks after approx 15 yr of postpubertal disease. Few subjects develop DN after 30 yr of disease.

The metabolic consequences of the diabetic state play an important role in the development of DN. This notion was supported by twin studies that showed that identical twins discordant for insulin-dependent diabetes mellitus (IDDM) had different glomerular basement membrane (GBM) widths *(2)*. Long-term exposure to hyperglycemia, as indicated by serum hemoglobin A1c determination, as well as the duration of overt disease were independent risk factors in the progression of DN *(3,4)*. In one study, the incidence of microalbuminuria, a marker of risk for DN, did not bear a linear relationship to hemoglobin A1. Its incidence exhibited a threshold at a hemoglobin A1 value of 10% (equivalent HgbA1c 8.0%), above which the relative risk per per cent change in its value was twice that below the cutoff. Thus, mechanisms of glomerular injury acting below the glycemic threshold are exacerbated by moderate to severe hyperglycemia. This review will present a summary of experimental evidence supporting several potential mechanisms whereby high concentrations of glucose may play a role in the progression of DN.

Genetic determinants for progression of DN to end stage renal disease have been suggested by studies that showed that renal failure tended to develop in families which already had a member with the disease *(5,6)*. There is an association between DN and both a family history of hypertension and increased Na-H countertransport *(7,8)*. Polymorphisms at various genetic loci have been associated with increased risk for DN. These have been identified in the angiotensin convening enzyme inhibitor (ACE), angiotensinogen, Type-IV collagen, and aldose reductase genes *(7,9–13)*. How the underlying DNA sequences responsible for genetic polymorphisms translate into differences in

From: *Molecular and Cellular Pediatric Endocrinology*
Edited by: S. Handwerger © Humana Press Inc., Totowa, NJ

113

molecular structure and function has yet to be determined. It is likely that these and other yet to be identified loci determine susceptibility to the DN by controlling compensatory mechanisms which act to prevent renal damage from exposure to high concentrations of glucose and other metabolic consequences of IDDM.

The physiologic changes which accompany glomerular ECM expansion in DN include an alteration in the ability of the nephron to effectively retain negatively charged substances in the blood (14). This is accompanied by an increase in glomerular capillary molecular pore size. Hyperfiltration (increased glomerular filtration rate, GFR) occurs early in the disease and is associated with an increased glomerular capillary filtration pressure and efferent arteriolar resistance (15). This stage is followed by a gradual, inexorable decline in renal function once DN has been established.

Incipient diabetic nephropathy has been defined as the excretion of between 30 and 200 µg/min of albumin in three separate timed urine collections. Overt diabetic nephropathy is persistent dipstick positive proteinuria. This nomenclature implies progression from one stage to the next. However, it is important to note that microalbuminuria does not progress in every case to proteinuria and renal failure. Nor does the absence of albumin from the urine signify the presence of normal renal function or mesangial volume on kidney biopsy. Microalbuminuria definitively predicts progression to proteinuria and renal failure only when accompanied by hypertension and/or decreased GFR (16).

The specificity of microalbuminuria as an indicator of progression to overt DN has been brought into question by two recent studies. One 5-yr followup study of patients with 17.5 years average disease duration and persistent microalbuminuria showed that DN developed in only 19% of patients, whereas 33% reverted to normal over a period (17). Although the average GFR decreased more in patients who progressed to DN, diminished renal function was not detected in all proteinuric subjects. Progressors had a significantly higher hemoglobin A1c values, mean blood pressures, and incidence of proliferative retinopathy than did nonprogressors. Cholesterol concentrations also appeared to be a risk factor for DN progression in some studies. Another 4-yr followup study showed that 30% of normotensive, persistently microalbuminuric subjects with similar disease duration progressed to DN (18). These results may differ from earlier reports which showed higher rates progression to overt DN in microalbuminuric subjects (85%) because of disparities in metabolic control (hemoglobin A1 was not determined in earlier studies) or because of differences in the length of follow up (which would bring the progression rate to approx 50% in the more recent studies). It thus appears that microalbuminuria is a relatively insensitive and nonspecific indicator of the risk of progression to DN. New tests that better predict the underlying renal pathology are clearly needed. Mesangial volume remains the gold standard for studies designed to predict outcome of various interventions designed to affect progression of DN.

Pharmacological normalization of glomerular capillary and systemic hypertension with angiotensin converting enzyme (ACE) inhibitors slows the progression to end stage renal disease in overt DN associated with established renal failure (19). In animals, treatment with agents that lower glomerular capillary filtration pressure from the onset of diabetes was associated with diminished glomerulosclerosis, despite equivalent metabolic control (20,21). ACE inhibitors were more effective than other agents or combination of agents in sustaining lower glomerular capillary hypertension (15,21). Lowering blood pressure with agents that failed to affect this parameter, was less effective in preventing diabetic glomerulosclerosis.

Treatment of microalbuminuric diabetic humans without renal failure or hypertension with ACE inhibitors remains controversial. Antihypertensive therapy diminished microalbuminuria itself, but had no effect on GFR in 4- and 5-yr follow-up studies *(18,22)*. Because of its rapid amelioration with ACE inhibitors, it appears that microalbuminuria reflects functional (hemodynamic/physiologic) rather than structural changes. It remains unknown whether or not this is associated with reversal or slower progression of the pathologic changes and renal functional abnormalities in humans without overt renal failure. The preliminary report of a long-term comparison of ACE inhibitor and calcium channel blockers treatment in subjects with albuminuria and hypertension has shown that, whereas the former treatment may be associated with diminished albumin clearance, GFR decreased more rapidly *(23)*. These findings bring to light the necessity of using long-term progression of renal functional and/or structural abnormalities when comparing the efficacy of various treatment strategies. It must also be kept in mind that the overwhelming influence, and perhaps permissive effects, of hyperglycemia on disease progression may confound our ability to discern any differences. This is particularly true when relatively insensitive indicators of disease progression are employed as endpoints. A fundamental knowledge of glomerular molecular dynamics in response to the diabetic state and to variations in glucose concentrations in vitro will enable the development of more sensitive tools designed to specifically reflect the underlying pathophysiologic changes that occur in the DN.

Glomerular Extracellular Matrix Structure

The glomerular ECM is comprised of the GBM and the mesangium. Despite being a continuous structure, each of these ECMs has a unique molecular composition. This is because each region has distinct associated cell types that synthesize a unique mixture of ECM components. These cells have been isolated and maintain many of their properties in culture. The mesangial stalk contains intrinsic, contractile cells and is bounded on its capillary surface by fenestrated microvascular endothelial cells, whereas epithelial cell podocytes interdigitate along the urinary aspect of the GBM. Together, the glomerular ECM and these cellular elements form a filtrate from capillary blood that is selective on the basis of both molecular radius and intrinsic molecular charge *(24)*.

The GBM contains Type-IV or basement membrane collagens whose triple helices are comprised of either the ubiquitous chain types ($\alpha1$ and $\alpha2$) or unique GBM chains ($\alpha3$ and $\alpha5$). The mesangium contains only $\alpha1$ and $\alpha2$ Type-IV collagens. Abnormalities in the gene structure of the unique GBM Type-IV collagens underly Goodpasture's and Alport's Syndromes *(25)*. Laminin and entactin are also present in the GBM, whereas fibronectin appears to be mainly a mesangial ECM component in humans. ECM components often have a modular structure with domains which interact with other ECM molecules (i.e., through heparin or thrombospondin binding domains), which mediate chemotactic responses, or which interact with cell surfaces (i.e., RGD containing peptides bind to cell surface ECM receptors designated integrins). These interactions not only maintain ECM connectivity, but also foster interaction between the ECM and the cellular cytoskeleton. This continuous network acts to signal the intracellular compartment of occurrences in the ECM.

Proteoglycans (PG) are distributed in a netlike array along the GBM *(26,27)*. Their highly negatively charged glycosaminoglycan (GAG) chains, which are predominantly HS, are thought to contribute to the charge barrier to plasma ultrafiltration *(28)*. One

GBM HS containing PG, perlecan, has been fully characterized (27,29–32). Perlecan is synthesized as a high-mol-wt precursor that is processed to several glycoprotein products present in GBM and mesangium (33). A basement membrane associated chondroitin sulfate (CS) PG (bamacan) has recently been identified (34). Its mesangial localization in kidney is consistent with previous histochemical descriptions the distribution of glomerular CS PGs.

PGs play an important role in maintaining extracellular matrix (ECM) integrity, in cell-ECM interactions, in organogenesis, and in specific cellular functions such as secretion and growth factor action (35,36). The PG protein core contains a domain structure that varies with PG function and tissue localization. GAG chains ($n = 1$–120/PG) consist of repeat disaccharide units (a hexosamine and a uronic acid, $n = 50$–150/chain) covalently attached via an invariant tetrasaccharide linkage region to the protein core (37). Consensus GAG attachment sites are comprised of Ser-Gly residues flanked by acidic amino acids (i.e., DA_SGD_GLG_SGD_VG_SGD_T in perlecan). The immediate peptide sequence surrounding this site, however, is not the sole determinant of which GAG (CS or HS) attaches or its degree of modification. These are a function of cell type and incubation conditions (i.e., the presence of growth factors) (38–44). Specific regional modifications of GAG sequence by sulfation (of hydroxyl and amino groups) and epimerization (C6 carboxyl groups) mediate particular PG functions. For example, antithrombin binds to an HS hexasaccharide with a 6-O-sulfate on residue 2 and a 3-O-sulfate on residue 4 (45–47). Distinct oligosaccharides are recognized by the heparin binding domains of each basic fibroblast growth factor (bFGF) and contribute to cell-specific response to this family of growth factors (48–50).

ECM PGs appear in the interstitium or as a component of specialized matrices such as basement membranes. Aggrecan and versican belong to a family of modular CS PGs in cartilage and aorta that form link protein stabilized macroaggregates on a hyaluronic acid backbone (51–53). They retain water in the ECM, acting like a "coiled spring" to resist compressive forces. The small leucine-rich interstitial CS PGs (SLRPs), decorin and biglycan, are differentially regulated during development and by growth factors (54,55). Each has a unique tissue distribution. Decorin binds at regular intervals along collagen chains, mediates collagen fibrillogenesis and participates in cell proliferation as well as modulation of transforming growth factor-β (TGF-β and bFGF action (56–60). The HS PG perlecan is not only important in basement membrane formation and function but also binds bFGF (61–63). Members of the collagen gene family which bear GAG side chains are closely associated with collagen II fibrils and help maintain an expanded fibrillar structure in ECM (64,65).

Cell surface PGs of the glypican family are covalently attached to plasma membrane lipids via phosphatidylinositol linkages, which targets the PG to the apical surface (66–74). The protein cores of syndecans, which are primarily basolateral in polarized cells, are themselves intercalated in the plasma membrane. The cDNAs of five syndecans have been characterized. The amino acid sequences of their transmembrane and cytoplasmic domains have a high degree of homology, while their ectodomains are unique (42). Because of this and their conserved gene structure, syndecan genes were thought to have evolved from a common ancestor, after gene duplication (75,76). The expression of cell surface PGs are developmentally regulated (68,77–83). They promote an anticoagulant environment on endothelial cell surfaces, cell adhesion and motility, tumor cell invasion, antigen recognition, modulate serpin and growth factor activity, and provide a link between the ECM and the cellular cytoskeleton *(84–89)*.

Differential growth factor affinity for ECM and cell surface PGs may modulate growth factor distribution and activity *(90–92)*. Not only may PGs act as low-affinity receptors that help concentrate the growth factor at the cell surface, but they may also prevent growth factor degradation and participate in feedback regulation of their synthesis *(66,90–107)*. Interactions of PGs with other components of the ECM, such as thrombospondin, may modulate growth factor (TGF-β) activation and by these means impart control over cell proliferation *(108)*.

Abnormalities of Glomerular Extracellular Matrix Metabolism in Diabetes

Decreased renal function in DN is associated with accumulation of ECM in the renal glomerulus. This results in reduction in the capillary filtration surface area *(109)*. Whereas a thickened GBM is characteristic of DN, mesangial volume is the parameter that best correlates with abnormalities in renal function in diabetes by electron microscopic morphometric analysis.

A change in ECM composition accompanies its expansion in DN. Abnormalities in GBM charge density are associated with both animal model and human proteinuric states, including the congenital nephrotic syndrome and the DN *(27,29,30)*. Whereas most ECM components accumulate in the diabetic mesangium, GBM from diabetic humans and streptozotocin-induced diabetic (STZ) rats contain less HS PG *(30,110–117)*. A relative decrease in GBM HS PG in DN has been postulated to perturb the GBM charge barrier and engender a compensatory increase in synthesis of other ECM components *(118,119)*. Bamacan has been shown to have an abnormal localization in the GBM in early STZ induced diabetes *(120)*. The role played by this "mesangialization" of the GBM in DN will be an important avenue of future research.

Immunofluorescent microscopic studies of kidney biopsy material from diabetic humans showed that although the unique GBM Type-IV collagen chains (α3, α4, and α5) accumulate, staining for the more common α1 and α2 Type-IV chains was decreased in the expanded mesangium and GBM *(121)*. The increase in the α2: α3 Type-IV collagen ratio, which occurs in diabetic glomerulosclerosis, reflects the preferential expansion of the mesangium over the peripheral GBM. Thus, expression of each collagen chain pair appears to be uniquely regulated during renal morphogenesis and in disease states.

Whereas an association between loss of anionic sites (PG) and albuminuria exists in the DN, there is only a minor loss of these sites in subjects with incipient nephropathy *(117)*. This, along with the fact that physiologic studies show a rapidly reversible alteration in glomerular pore size, points to the possibility that decreased GBM HS PG content is not primarily responsible for the early, reversible alterations in glomerular physiology present in DN. In established DN, profound and possibly irreversible alterations in relative GBM PG content are paramount. Intermittent perturbations in ECM synthesis resulting from episodes of hyperglycemia may result in transiently altered ECM processing and accumulation of ECM with an abnormal composition. The rate of ECM accumulation will depend upon the degree of this chronic, intermittent exposure to hyperglycemia. The ability to compensate for these abnormalities by altering either glomerular physiology (GFR) and/or by altering glomerular structure (glomerular hypertrophy) may also help to determine the individual the rate of progression of DN.

Why Is GBM HS PG Decreased by Diabetes?

Decreased GBM HS PG may result from disturbances in PG protein core processing (turnover), in posttranslational modification of its GAG chains, and/or in PG interactions with other ECM components. Alterations in GBM function result not only from structural abnormalities in individual GBM components, but may also be caused by changes in the noncovalent interactions that bind its various constituents in a regular structure. It is important to note that GBM assembly is not a static process since the half-life of several of its components can be measured in hours or days.

In vivo studies have shown that, after correcting for the decreased specific activity of [^{35}S]sulfate in diabetic sera, *de novo* glomerular ^{35}S-PG synthesis was not diminished in STZ or in Zucker diabetic rats, and may be increased *(122,123)*. Total kidney perlecan mRNA was unchanged in a rat model of Type-II diabetes, but the ratio of perlecan to Type-IV collagen mRNA was decreased and correlated with the degree of albuminuria *(124)*. A transient decrease was followed by increased expression of perlecan mRNA in STZ diabetic rat kidneys, while expression of other ECM products increased steadily with increasing disease duration when compared with controls *(125)*. Mice over-expressing the growth hormone (GH) gene developed a glomerulosclerosis similar to that seen in DN and exhibited increased kidney perlecan expression *(126)*. In conclusion, it is most likely that total PG synthesis is not decreased by diabetes, but that alterations in proportionate accumulation or processing may occur. It will be important to study the effects of diabetes on the expression of individual PGs.

Altered PG sulfation may perturb the charge barrier to plasma ultrafiltration, modify PG-ECM interactions, or cause abnormalities in growth factor signaling *(40,89,98,127–130)*. Whereas STZ diabetes decreased the activity of liver enzymes that control PG sulfation, studies in tissues directly affected by disease complications have shown conflicting results *(123,127,130–132)*. This may stem from the inability to completely separate individual PGs from cell culture supernatants using conventional biochemical means *(133–135)*. Disturbed ECM interactions may also result from changes in the GAG side chain type (i.e., CS/DS vs HS) or number *(136)*. It appears that the same protein core can acquire different GAG types and/or differentially modified chains not only as a function of the protein core, but also depending upon cell type and substrate availability. These differential effects may account for the organ specific nature of various metabolic injuries that are engendered by diabetic milieu. Organ (cell type) and PG type specific alterations in PG production may regulate growth factor action and cellular function by altering ECM-cell surface-cytoskeletal interactions.

Since cell surface PGs act as coreceptors for bFGF, transforming growth factor-β (TGF-β), and insulin-like growth factor (IGF) binding protein (BP) 3, changes in GAG structure may affect relative binding to cell surface and ECM PGs, where they are "stored." Effects on growth factor action may be amplified since their (TGF-β) expression is inhibited in a negative feedback manner by PG *(40,89,98,127–130)*.

The Role of Growth Factors in DN

TGF-β Mediated Control of ECM Production Has Been Implicated in DN

TGF-β is a disulfide-linked 25 kDa homodimer which is synthesized as a latent precursor and secreted noncovalently bound to latency-associated peptide *(137)*. Its extracellular activation is mediated by exposure to an acid microenvironment (i.e., tissue injury), by plasmin, by mannose-6-phosphate receptor binding, or by association with thrombospondin (TSP). Thus, measurement of TGF-β protein or its mRNA does not necessarily reflect growth factor *bioactivity (138)*.

Members of the TGF-β superfamily are involved in organ development *(139,140)*. Competition for early growth response (EGR) binding to the TGF-β promoter by the Wilm's Tumor associated transcription factor in the kidney and nerve growth factor in neurons promote organ development *(141,142)*. Regulatory elements in the TGF-β gene promoter are also involved in growth factor autoregulation and in cell proliferation *(142–151)*. Endothelial cell proliferation in response to vascular injury is associated with a transient increase in EGR (which displaces Sp-1 from the TGF-β) followed by PDGF expression *(152)*. Thus, autoregulation of EGR and TGF-β activity is important in mitogen-induced growth and growth factor-induced differentiation.

TGF-β action is regulated in a negative feedback manner by several leucine-rich PGs (biglycan and decorin) and its binding to perlecan in the ECM has been implicated in growth factor storage *(96,99,107,153,154)*. A cell surface PG, betaglycan, is itself a low-affinity TGF-β receptor *(102,155–157)*. Each of the three TGF-β receptors participates in either growth factor-mediated control of ECM synthesis or its regulation of cell proliferation and decreased numbers of TGF-β receptor II are present on certain cancer cells *(158–162)*. Importantly, TGF-β controls PG sulfation, an effect that may engender secondary changes in response to other growth factors (such as IGF-I or bFGF) whose effects are also mediated in part by HS PG binding *(41,50,89,98,105,163–165)*.

Altered ECM metabolism in experimental glomerulonephritis and in the DN may involve tissue specific changes TGF-β expression or action *(137,166–174)*. In a recent study by Ziyadeh et al. infusion of neutralizing anti-TGF-β antibodies attenuated the kidney hypertrophy and ECM expression induced in mice with STZ induced diabetes *(175)*. These in vivo studies implicate TGF-β and its autoregulation by ECM in the pathogenesis of DN.

TGF-β expression was increased in TGF-receptor bearing renal cells exposed to high glucose concentrations, in vitro *(176,177)*. Mesangial cells also exhibited increased expression of collagen (Types-IV and -I) and plasminogen activator inhibitor (PAI-1) expression under these conditions *(173,178–182)*. High glucose concentrations may modulate TGF-β activity either at the level of growth factor expression (mediated by either PG [decorin] mediated feedback control or by c-myc), activation (through control of plasminogen activator inhibitor (PAI-1) or TSP), receptor binding, or signal transduction through the MAPK family *(183)*. The promoter regions of both ECM (PAI-1, perlecan, and stromelysin) and growth factor related genes (including TGF-β and c-myc themselves) contain TGF-β responsive sequences *(174,184–197)*. These regulatory elements have been proposed to bind nuclear factor-I (Type-I collagen) or are AP-1 sites (PAI-1, stromelysin). TGF-β responsive promoters in the stromelysin and decorin genes appeared to be transcriptional repressors, whereas those in the PAI-1 gene were found to enhance transcription *(186,191)*.

INVOLVEMENT OF THE GROWTH HORMONE (GH)/INSULIN-LIKE GROWTH FACTOR-I (IGF-I) AXIS IN DN

The IGFs are comprised of two primary proteins, IGF-I and IGF-II, that are structurally homologous to insulin and are expressed in almost all mammalian tissues *(198,199)*. Their actions are protean and include insulin-like metabolic effects, growth factor mitogenic properties and differentiation enhancement actions. IGF-I binds to specific tyrosine kinase receptors, which are highly homologous to those for insulin and use a similar signal transduction pathway, includes insulin receptor substrate-1 *(200)*. The biologic activity of the IGFs is modulated by a family of binding proteins (BPs). Translational and posttranslational processing of IGF BPs, including proteolytic cleavage and ECM sequestration, regulate IGF-I action. IGFBP-3 binds specifically and with high affinity to cell surfaces, appearing to utilize heparin binding domains on the carboxyterminal region of the protein *(89)*. IGF BPs 1 and 2 contain RGD peptide sequences which mediate binding to cell surface ECM receptors (integrins).

Epidemiologic studies suggest that the hormonal changes of puberty are permissive in the progression of DN *(201,202)*. There is a strong correlation between microalbuminuria and duration of diabetes since puberty rather than total disease duration *(203)*. No pre-pubertal patients displayed microalbuminuria despite the same duration of diabetes as the postpubertal patients. Because the association of diabetes complications and puberty appears incontrovertible, considerable effort has focused on examining the effects of the hormones that increase during puberty, e.g., sex steroids and the GH/IGF axis. Though sex steroids appear to influence insulin sensitivity, there is little evidence that complications of diabetes are influenced directly by sex steroid exposure. However, the link between GH/IGF and nephropathy is particularly convincing.

Secretion of GH and the GH dependent peptide, IGF-I, increase by approximately two- to fourfold during puberty and IDDM children have a substantially greater increase in GH secretion during that time *(204)*. Elevated GH and low IGF-I levels are induced by poor metabolic control in diabetes. Either when the GH deficient state is associated with diabetes or when it is induced by pituitary ablation, there is improved metabolic control associated with amelioration and/or a lower incidence of diabetic retinopathy *(205–207)*. GH deficient children with IDDM had a decreased incidence of microvascular complications compared to a control population without GH deficiency and similar metabolic control *(208)*.

Animal models have been employed to investigate GH/IGF actions on the kidney and changes related to diabetes *(209–211)*. The renal collecting ducts are the predominant sites of IGF-I and IGF-I mRNA production *(212–215)*. However, IGF-I receptors were not detected on collecting duct cells but on proximal tubule and mesangial cells, suggesting that IGF-I may act in a juxtacrine manner *(214)*. Several studies showed that increased IGF-I mRNA and protein expression is involved in the early renal hypertrophic stage of DN, an effect that occurs only in postpubertal animals *(209,210,215–217)*. Diabetes-induced renal hypertrophy is blocked by somatostatin analog treatment *(218)*. Hypophysectomy in rats decreased renal ECM PG synthesis, an effect that was reversible by IGF-I infusion. This is consistent with studies which revealed that IGF-I selectively increased PG production in an ex vivo renal perfusion system and in isolated mesangial cells *(see below) (129,219)*. Finally, several studies have revealed changes in IGF BPs in diabetes. Serum IGF BP 1 levels are reciprocally related to metabolic control and serum IGF BP 3 is diminished in diabetic humans *(220)*. Kidney IGF BP 2 is increased by STZ diabetes and diabetic rat kidney membranes accumulated IGF binding proteins 1 and 3 *(221)*. These changes may result in altered tissue specific regulation of IGF action.

Transgenic mice overexpressing GH develop mesangial expansion and glomerulo-sclerotic lesions, which are pathologically similar to those seen in DN *(126,210,222,223)*.

This is in contrast to transgenic animals moderately overexpressing IGF-I, which appear not to evolve any major renal pathology. These findings may be explained by the occurrence of compensatory changes in IGF BPs (GH excess produces increased IGFBP-3 expression where IGF-I overexpression leads to low levels of IGFBP-3 because IGF-I acts as a feedback inhibitor of pituitary GH secretion). GH antagonist overexpression inhibits the development of the STZ-induced DN, a lesion which is exacerbated in GH overexpressing animals *(217)*. The effects observed in GH transgenic animals might reflect perturbations that are related to the site of GH overproduction and/or that are independent of those mediated through the IGF system. This is supported by studies that show that human retinal microvascular endothelial cell proliferation is stimulated by GH *(224)*.

We have described the presence of several PGs on mesangial cell surfaces and have shown that total PG synthesis is stimulated by IGF-I *(135,219)*. Incubation in high concentrations of glucose abrogated the IGF-I mediated increase in PG synthesis but further stimulated protein synthesis. Rat mesangial cells have abundant receptors for IGF-I and IGF-I receptor mRNA abundance is increased in mesangial cells from diabetic mice *(203)*. IGF-I stimulated rat mesangial cell proliferation, ECM production, and amino acid and glucose uptake *(203,225,226)*. Recently, IGFBP-3 mRNA and protein has been shown to be induced in cultured human mesangial cells by exposure to TGF-β coincident with an IGFBP-4 protease *(293)*. This is of particular interest because TGF-β is speculated to be a mediator of ECM expansion in DN. Taken together, these data implicate a role for abnormalities in growth factor response, including GH1IGF, in the pathogenesis of ECM accumulation in DN.

Could Glucose Itself Cause the Complications of Diabetes?

Glucose may play a direct role in diabetic complications by causing structural alterations in ECM molecules (i.e., glycation), by changing the concentration of various intracellular metabolites which are important in substrate-mediated control of ECM synthesis (i.e., sorbitol or hexosamines), or by modulating signal transduction pathways (i.e., protein kinase C). High concentrations of glucose increased synthesis of many ECM components, of enzymes which control ECM metabolism (plasminogen activator and its inhibitor) and of ECM receptors (integrins) in human umbilical cord endothelial cells *(227–232)*. The effect of glucose on ECM synthesis in renal cells in response to growth factors has been described above.

Long-term exposure of bovine microvascular endothelial cells to high concentrations of glucose increased incorporation of [^{35}S]sulfate into PG without affected PG charge *(133)*. Interestingly, several studies have shown that while the effects of glucose on ECM synthesis occur rapidly after transfer to media containing increased glucose concentrations, these effects do not immediately disappear once the cells are returned to a normal metabolic environment *(228,233)*. Thus, cells "remember" past metabolic exposures (perhaps the result of ECM or nuclear protein glycation, *see below*). A direct effect of glucose on ECM production was supported by transfection of the glucose transporter GLUT 1 into a line of spontaneously immortalized rat mesangial cells *(234)*. Cells expressing human GLUI 1 had increased glucose utilization accompanied by increased collagen accumulation. These effects were apparent when the cells were incubated in normal concentrations and mimicked the effects of adding high concentrations of glucose to cells transfected with a control vector.

The Role of Advanced Glycation Endproducts in Diabetic Complications

The formation of advanced glycation endproducts (AGEs) has been proposed to play an important role in the pathogenesis of the long-term complications of diabetes *(235)*. The term "advanced glycation endproducts" refers to a complex mixture of molecules only a small percentage of which have been definitively identified and are quantifiable (i.e., pentosadine). Their formation can be measured using antibodies to these products or by excitation spectroscopy. They evolve by a series of slow, nonenzymatic, concentration (hemoglobin Alc) dependent posttranslational reactions of ECM, circulating, as well as intracellular proteins with glucose or its metabolic intermediates. AGE formations begins with the formation of a Shiff base between sugar alcohol adducts and amino groups on proteins which may then undergo an irreversible Amadori rearrangement with the formation of a covalent bond. Amadori products then undergo a series of modifications, including condensations, rearrangements, and fragmentations to form AGEs. Reactive AGE-forming intermediates may arise from oxidative reactions ("glycoxidation") of free sugars or from initial Schiff base by condensation with protein amino groups, rather than just from the "classical" Amadori rearrangement products. These resultant cross links increase during the normal aging process and in diabetes *(236)*.

The effects of AGE modification on protein function and processing are the subject of intense investigation. AGE formation in the ECM interferes with normal basement membrane assembly by disturbing the noncovalent interaction between various ECM components, such as fibronectin and PGs *(237)*. AGE modified peptides appear in the circulation from protein catabolism and accumulate in the ECM and in intracellular compartments. AGE-specific receptors have been identified on various cell types, including macrophage/monocytes and mesangial cells *(238)*. Binding of AGE-modified peptides to cell surfaces alters cytokine secretion, ECM production, and cellular proliferation *(239–243)*. AGE modified low-density lipoproteins do not bind normally to their receptors, which prolongs their half lives in renal failure and in diabetes *(244)*. These effects may be responsible in part for the increased incidence of macrovascular disease in subjects with diabetes and renal failure.

The role of AGEs in diabetic complications has been further supported by work that showed avoidance of AGE formation using aminoguanidine (AG) prevented the expansion of the glomerular mesangium and GBM width in DN *(235,236,243,245–247)*. AG may inhibit AGE formation through its nucleophilic hydrazine group by reacting with carbonyls of Amadori intermediates or by its guanidinium moiety reacting with dicarbonyls. However, it has been recently found to be a poor inhibitor of the reactions that occur subsequent to Amadori product formation, with novel inhibitors of the latter reaction series being described (vitamins B1 and B6 are inhibitory in vitro at levels well above physiologic concentrations) *(248,249)*. Inhibition of AGE reactivity with tissues using specific antibodies prevented the formation of glomerulosclerotic lesions *(250)*. Most recently, Rumble et al. have proposed that AGE formation may be responsible for the increased expression of TGF-β and Type-IV collagen deposition in diabetic mesenteric arteries *(251)*.

Despite these positive findings, one recent study employing STZ diabetes of 6 mo duration found that AG prevented albuminuria and the decreased collagen solubility in diabetes but failed to ameliorate the increased glomerular volume, GBM thickening, or increased vascular permeability of the DN, attributing some of the AG effects to its transient quenching of nitric oxide and to the multifactorial nature of the glomerular injury in DN *(252,253)*. The nature of injury inflicted by AGEs requires further using knowledge gained from the characterization of specific AGEs and inhibition of their formation or activity with novel agents.

EXTRACELLULAR GLUCOSE MODULATES CELLULAR PROLIFERATION

High concentrations of glucose inhibit mesangial cell proliferation *(219,224,243,254–256)*, an effect also described in other cell types *(224,257)*. One study showed slowing at several phases of the endothelial cell cycle *(257)*. Decreased endothelial cell proliferation in response to vascular injury may allow ingress into the vascular media of atherogenic substances, thus promoting macrovascular disease in diabetes. Although evidence suggests a role for increased cellular proliferation and response to growth factors early in the STZ diabetes, with later macrophage infiltration *(258)*, there is little data supporting an increase in cellular components in established human DN.

HS PG was found to be antiproliferative in mesangial and several other cell types *(93,259–263)*, whereas CS PG allows cellular multiplication *(84,264)*. We showed that a glypican-related melanoma cell surface HS PG binds to the heparin-binding domain of FN and that CS PG plays an important role in tumor cell adhesion and invasiveness *(84,85)*. PGs may control the proliferative environment by modulating interactions between ECM and cell surface receptors or by altering cellular sensitivity to, or availability of, growth factors *(35,97,100,106,108,172,219,241,264–269)*.

TGF-β may be involved in the antiproliferative effects of glucose *(172)*. It inhibits cellular proliferation by inducing p53 expression. This tumor suppressor retards progression through the G1 phase of the cell cycle by stimulating cdk inhibitor synthesis (p21$^{Cip/Kip}$ and p16^{Ink}), which in turn decreases cdk4 synthesis, cdk4/cyclin activity, and retinoblastoma gene product phosphorylation *(270,271)*. Growth factor autoinduction may be involved in regulation of both ECM synthesis and differentiation since p53 also induces endothelial cell TSP synthesis, which, in the presence of cell surface PGs, activates TGF-β and promotes angiogenesis *(272,273)*. TGF-β mediated inhibition of cell proliferation is also promoted by suppression of c-myc expression *(184,274,275)*.

Despite these findings, several recent studies caste some doubt upon the primary role of increased TGF-β activity in the DN. One study showed that high glucose concentrations induced TGF-β *like* effects on cell proliferation which were not associated with increased growth factor *activity (276)*. This was corroborated by the studies which showed that decorin overexpression in colon cancer cells caused TGF-β *independent* reduction in cell proliferation and increased the number of quiescent cells *(59,60)*.

THE ROLE OF INCREASED PROTEIN KINASE C (PKC) ACTIVITY IN DIABETIC COMPLICATIONS

PKC signal transduction is mediated via serine and threonine phosphorylation reactions. The subsequent reaction cascade influences cellular contractility, hormonal/growth factor signaling (vasopressin and angiotensin II), and vascular permeability. Growth factor activation of PKC or adhesion-mediated, increases in its activity may be mediated by dimerization of the cell surface PG syndecan 4 *(277,278)*. Increased cellular glucose metabolism resulting from increases in extracellular glucose concentrations may also provide the more proximal signal for PKC activation. High extracellular glucose concentrations increased translocation of PKC from the cytosol to the cell membrane and increased diacyl glycerol (DAG) mass *(279–282)*. Increased PKC activity was associated with alterations in ECM metabolism and vascular permeability *(281,283–290)*. Recently, inhibition of a specific PKC isoform (β2) was associated with normalization of PKC activity in diabetic rat retina and kidney as well as with functional normalization of albumin excretion, renal hyperfiltration, and retinal blood flow *(291)*. Whether or not prevention of functional changes in glomerular and retinal function is associated with forestalling permanent tissue alterations associated with diabetic complications will be an important topic of future research in this arena *(292)*.

The relative contribution and interactions between the various possible mechanisms for glomerular ECM accumulation in DN described above are an important area for future research. It is most likely that there is a complex intersection of each of these avenues of "glucose toxicity" that merges into the final common pathway of organ changes in DN. As more specific agents, which regulate metabolism in each of these pathways become available, their relative contributions may become more apparent. The benefits of such treatments may be masked by the overwhelming contribution of control of blood glucose concentrations (whether by direct or indirect effects) to the pathogenesis of diabetic complications. Whereas it is readily apparent that maintenance of near normoglycemia prevents the long-term complications of diabetes, it becomes feasible to control glucose levels in a relatively effortless manner. In the average subject with diabetes, interventions aimed at prevention of the secondary effects of high glucose concentrations will be warranted.

REFERENCES

1. Andersen AR, Christiansen JS, Andersen JK, Kreiner S, Deckert T. Diabetic nephropathy in Type 1 (insulin-dependent) diabetes: an epidemiological study. Diabetologia 1983;25:499–501.
2. Steffes MW, Sutherland DE, Goetz FC, Rich SS, Mauer SM. Studies of kidney and muscle biopsy specimens from identical twins discordant for type I diabetes mellitus. N Engl J Med 1985;312: 1282–1287.
3. Krolewski AS, Laffel LM, Krolewski M, Quinn M, Warram JH. Glycosylated hemoglobin and the risk of microalbuminuria in patients with insulin-dependent diabetes mellitus [see comments]. N Engl J Med 1995;332:1251–1255.
4. DCCT Res Group. The effect of intensive treatment of diabetes on the development and progression of long-term complications in insulin-dependent diabetes mellitus. N Engl J Med 1993;329: 977–986.
5. Seaquist ER, Goetz FC, Rich S, Barbosa JJ. Familial clustering of diabetic kidney disease. N Engl J Med 1989;320:1161–1165.
6. Quinn M, Angelico MC, Warram JH, Krolewski AS. Familial factors determine the development of diabetic nephropathy in patients with IDDM. Diabetologia 1996;39:940–945.
7. Krolewski AS, Canessa M, Warram JH, et al. Predisposition to hypertension and susceptibility to renal disease in insulin-dependent diabetes mellitus. N Engl J Med 1988;318:140–145.
8. Mangili R, Bending JJ, Scott G, Lai LK, Gupta A, Viberti G. Increased sodium-lithium countertransport activity in red cells of patients with insulin-dependent diabetes and nephropathy. N Engl J Med 1988;318:146–150.
9. Heesom AE, HIbberd ML, Millward A, Demaine AG. Polymorphisms in the 5' end of the aldose reductase gene is strongly associated with the development of diabetic nephropathy in type I diabetes. Diabetes 1997;46:287–291.
10. Doria A, Onuma T, Gearin G, Freire MB, Warram JH, Krolewski AS. Angiotensinogen polymorphism M235T, hypertension, and nephropathy in insulin-dependent diabetes. Hypertension 1996; 27:1134–1139.
11. Sweeney FP, Siczkowski M, Davies JE, Quinn PA, McDonald J, Krolewski B, Krolewski AS, Ng LL. Phosphorylation and activity of Na+/H+ exchanger isoform 1 of immortalized lymphoblasts in diabetic nephropathy. Diabetes 1995;44:1180–1185.

12. Doria A, Warram JH, Krolewski AS. Genetic predisposition to diabetic nephropathy. Evidence for a role of the antiotensin I-converting enzyme gene. Diabetes 1994;43:690–695.

13. Doria A, Laffel LMB, Warram JH, Pouyssegur J, Krolewski AS. Increased expression of the sodium/ hydrogen exchanger gene in lymphocytes from insulin dependent diabetic patients (IDD) with nephropathy. J Am Soc Nephrol 1991;2:288.

14. Nakamura Y, Myers BD. Charge selectivity of proteinuria in diabetic glomerulopathy. Diabetes 1988;37:1202–1211.

15. Zatz R, Dunn BR, Meyer TW, Anderson S, Rennke HG, Brenner BM. Prevention of diabetic glomerulopathy by pharmacological amelioration of glomerular capillary hypertension. J Clin Invest 1986;77:1925–1930.

16. Chavers BM, Bilous RW, Ellis EN, Steffes MW, Mauer SM. Glomerular lesions and urinary albumin excretion in type I diabetes without overt proteinuria [see comments]. N Engl J Med 1989;320: 966–970.

17. Almdal T, Norgaard K, Feldt-Rasmussen B, Deckert T. The predictive value of microalbuminuria in IDDM. A five-year follow-up study [see comments]. Diabetes Care 1994;17:120–125.

18. Mathiesen ER, Hommel E, Giese J, Parving HH. Efficacy of captopril in postponing nephropathy in normotensive insulin dependent diabetic patients with microalbuminuria. Br Med J 1991;303:81–87.

19. Lewis EJ, Hunsicker LG, Bain RP, Rohde RD. The effect of angiotensin-converting enzyme inhibition on diabetic nephropathy. N Engl J Med 1993;329:1456–1462.

20. Fujihara CK, Padilha RM, Zatz R. Glomerular abnormalities in long term experimental diabetes: role of hemodynamic and nonhemodynamic factors and effects of antihypertensive therapy. Diabetes 1992;41:286–293.

21. Anderson S, Rennke HG, Garcia DL, Brenner BM. Short and long term effects of antihypertensive therapy in the diabetic rat. Kidney Int 1989;36:526–536.

22. Viberti G, Mogensen CE, Groop LC, Pauls JF. Effect of captopril on progression to clinical proteinuria in patients with insulin-dependent diabetes mellitus and microalbuminuria. JAMA 1994;271:275–279.

23. Rossing P, Tarnow L, Boelskifte S, Jensen BR, Nielsen FS, Parving HH. Differences between nisoldipine and lisinopril on glomerular filtration rates and albuminuria in hypertensive IDDM patients with diabetic nephropathy during the first year of treatment. Diabetes 1997;46:481–487.

24. Renoke HG, Patel Y, Venkatachalam MA. Role of molecular charge in glomerular permeability: tracer studies with cationized ferritins. J Cell Biol 1975;67:638–646.

25. Hudson BG, Reeders ST, Tryggvason K. Type IV collagen: Structure, gene organization, and role in human diseases. Molecular basis of Goodpasture and Alport syndromes and diffuse leiomyomatosis. J Biol Chem 1993;268:26,033–26,036.

26. Kanwar YS, Linker A, Farquhar MG. Increased permeability of the glomerular basement membrane to ferritin after removal of glycosaminoglycans (heparan sulfate) by enzyme digestion. J Cell Biol 1980;86:688–693.

27. Vernier RL, Klein DJ, Sisson SP, Mahan JD, Oegema TR, Jr., Brown DM. Heparan sulfate—rich anionic sites in the human glomerular basement membrane. Decreased concentration in congenital nephrotic syndrome. N Engl J Med 1983;309:1001–1009.

28. Kanwar YS, Farquhar MG. Presence of heparan sulfate in the glomerular basement membrane. Proc Natl Acad Sci USA 1979;76:1303–1307.

29. Vernier RL, Steffes MW, Sisson-Ross S, Mauer SM. Heparan sulfate proteoglycan in the glomerular basement membrane in type 1 diabetes mellitus. Kidney Int 1992;41:1070–1080.

30. Shimomura H, Spiro RG. Studies on macromolecular components of human glomerular basement membrane and alterations in diabetes. Decreased levels of heparan sulfate proteoglycan and laminin. Diabetes 1987;36:374–381.

31. Iozzo RV, Cohen IR, Grässel S, Murdoch AD. The biology of perlecan: The multifaceted heparan sulphate proteoglycan of basement membranes and pericellular matrices. Biochem J 1994;302:625–639.

32. Cohen IR, Grässel S, Murdoch AD, Iozzo RV. Structural characterization of the complete human perlecan gene and its promoter. Proc Natl Acad Sci USA 1993;90:10,404–10,408.

33. Klein DJ, Brown DM, Oegema TR, Jr., Brenchley PE, Anderson JC, Dickinson MA, Horigan EA, Hassell JR. Glomerular basement membrane proteoglycans are derived from a large precursor. J Cell Biol 1988;106:963–970.

34. Wu RR, Couchman JR. cDNA cloning of the basement membrane chondroitin sulfate proteoglycan core protein, bamacan: a five domain structure including coiled coil motifs. J Cell Biol 1997;136:433–444.

35. Ruoslahti E. Proteoglycans in cell regulation. J Biol Chem 1989;264:13,369–13,372.

36. Iozzo RV, Murdoch AD. Proteoglycans of the extracellular environment: clues from the gene and protein side offer novel perspectives in molecular diversity and function. FASEB J 1996;10:598–614.
37. Hay EE. Cell Biology of the Extracellular Matrix. Plenum, New York, 1992.
38. Mann DM, Yamaguchi Y, Bourdon MA, Ruoslahti E. Analysis of glycosaminoglycan substitution in decorin by site-directed mutagenesis. J Biol Chem 1990;265:5317–5323.
39. Kato M, Wang H, Bernfield MR, Gallagher JT, Turnbull JE. Cell surface syndecan-1 on distinct cell types differs in fine structure and ligand binding of its heparan sulfate chains. J Biol Chem 1994;269:18,881–18,890.
40. Sanderson RD, Turnbull JE, Gallagher JT, Lander AD. Fine structure of heparan sulfate regulates syndecan-1 function and cell behavior. J Biol Chem 1994;269:13,100–13,106.
41. Rapraeger AC. Transforming growth factor (type beta) promotes the addition of chondroitin sulfate chains to the cell surface proteoglycan (syndecan) of mouse mammary epithelia. J Cell Biol 1989;109:2509–2518.
42. Bernfield MR, Kokenyesi R, Kato M, Hinkes MT, Spring J, Gallo RL, Lose EJ. Biology of the syndecans: A family of transmembrane heparan sulfate proteoglycans. Annu Rev Cell Biol 1992;8:365–393.
43. Kokenyesi R, Bernfield MR. Core protein structure and sequence determine the site and presence of heparan sulfate and chondroitin sulfate on syndecan-1. J Biol Chem 1994;269:12,304–12,309.
44. Shworak NW, Shirakawa M, Colliec-Jouault S, Liu J, Mulligan RC, Birinyi LK, Rosenberg RD. Pathway-specific regulation of the synthesis of anticoagulantly active heparan sulfate. J Biol Chem 1994;269:24,941–24,952.
45. Atha DH, Stephens AW, Rimon A, Rosenberg RD. Sequence variation in heparin octasaccharides with high affinity for antithrombin III. Biochem 1984;23:5801–5812.
46. Atha DH, Stephens AW, Rosenberg RD. Evaluation of critical groups required for the binding of heparin to antithrombin. Proc Natl Acad Sci USA 1984;81:1030–1034.
47. Atha DH, Lormeau JC, Petitou M, Rosenberg RD, Choay J. Contribution of monosaccharide residues in heparin binding to antithrombin III. Biochem 1985;24:6723–6729.
48. Choay J, Petitou M, Lormeau JC, Sinay P, Casu B, Gatti G. Structure-activity relationship in heparin: a synthetic pentasaccharide with high affinity for antithrombin m and eliciting high anti-factor Xa activity. Biochem Biophys Res Commun 1983;116:492–499.
49. Turnbull JE, Fernig DG, Ke Y, Wilkinson MC, Gallagher JT. Identification of the basic fibroblast growth factor binding sequence in fibroblast heparan sulfate. J Biol Chem 1992;267:10,337–10,341.
50. Guimond S, Maccarana M, Olwin BB, Lindahl U, Rapraeger AC. Activating and inhibitory heparin sequences for FGF-2 (basic FGF). Distinct requirements for FGF-1, FGF-2, and FGF-4. J Biol Chem 1993;268:23,906–23,914.
51. Krusius T, Ruoslahti E. Primary structure of an extracellular matrix proteoglycan core protein deduced from cloned cDNA. Proc Natl Acad Sci USA 1986;83:7683–7687.
52. Tanaka T, Har-El R, Tanzer ML. Partial structure of the gene for chicken cartilage proteoglycan core protein. J Biol Chem 1988;263:15,831–15,835.
53. Doege KJ, Sasaki M, Kimura T, Yamada Y. Complete coding sequence and deduced primary structure of the human cartilage large aggregating proteoglycan, aggrecan. Human-specific repeats, and additional alternatively spliced forms. J Biol Chem 1991;266:894–902.
54. Cizmeci-Smith G, Asundi V, Stahl RC, Teichman LJ, Chernousov M, Cowan K, Carey DJ. Regulated expression of syndecan in vascular smooth muscle cells and cloning of rat syndecan core protein cDNA. J Biol Chem 1992;267:15,729–15,736.
55. Cizmeci-Smith G, Stahl RC, Showalter LJ, Carey DJ. Differential expression of transmembrane proteoglycans in vascular smooth muscle cells. J Biol Chem 1993;268:18,740–18,747.
56. Sawhney RS, Hering TM, Sandell LJ. Biosynthesis of small proteoglycan II (decorin) by chondrocytes and evidence for a procore protein. J Biol Chem 1991;266:9231–9240.
57. Fisher LW, Termine JD, Young MF. Deduced protein sequence of bone small proteoglycan I (biglycan) shows homology with proteoglycan II (decorin) and several nonconnective tissue proteins in a variety of species. J Biol Chem 1989;264:4571–4576.
58. Vogel KG, Paulsson M, Heinegard D. Specific inhibition of type I and type II collagen fibrillogenesis by the small proteoglycan of tendon. Biochem J 1984;223:587–597.
59. Mauviel, A, Santra M, Chen YQ, Uitto J, Iozzo RV. Transcriptional regulation of decorin gene expression. Induction by quiescence and repression by tumor necrosis factor-alpha. J Biol Chem 1995;270:11,692–11,700.

60. Santra, M, Skorski T, Calabretta B, Lattime EC, Iozzo RV. De novo decorin gene expression suppresses the malignant phenotype in human colon cancer cells. Proc Natl Acad Sci USA 1995;92: 7016–7020.
61. Aviezer, D, Hecht D, Safran M, Eisinger M, David G, Yayon A. Perlecan, basal lamina proteoglycan, promotes basic fibroblast growth factor-receptor binding, mitogenesis, and angiogenesis. Cell 1994;79:1005–1013.
62. Noonan DM, Fulle A, Valente P, Cai S, Horigan E, Sasaki M, Yamada Y, Hassell JR. The complete sequence of perlecan, a basement membrane heparan sulfate proteoglycan, reveals extensive similarity with laminin A chain, low density lipoprotein-receptor, and the neural cell adhesion molecule. J Biol Chem 1991;266:22,939–22,947.
63. Noonan DM, Horigan EA, Ledbetter SR, Vogeli G, Sasaki M, Yamada Y, Hassell JR. Identification of cDNA clones encoding different domains of the basement membrane heparan sulfate proteoglycan. J Biol Chem 1988;263:16,379–16,387.
64. Muragaki, Y, Mariman EC, van Beersum SE, Perala M, van Mourik JB, Warman ML, Olsen BR, Hamel BC. A mutation in the gene encoding the alpha 2 chain of the fibril-associated collagen IX COL9A2, causes multiple epiphyseal dysplasia (EDM2). Nature Genet 1996;12:103–105.
65. Mallein-Gerin, F, Ruggiero F, Quinn TM, Bard F, Grodzinsky AJ, Olsen BR, Van der Rest M. Analysis of collagen synthesis and assembly in culture by immortalized mouse chondrocytes in the presence or absence of alpha 1 (IX) collagen chains. Exp Cell Res 1995;219:257–265.
66. Pilia G, Hughes-Benzie RM, MacKenzie A, Baybayan P, Chen EY, Huber R, Neri G, Cao A, Forabosco A, Schlessinger D. Mutations in GPC3, a glypican gene, cause the Simpson-Golabi-Behmel overgrowth syndrome [see comments]. Nature Genet 1996;12:241–247.
67. Weksberg R, Squire JA, Templeton DM. Glypicans: a growing trend [news;comment]. Nature Genet 1996;12:225–227.
68. Watanabe K, Yamada H, Yamaguchi Y. K-glypican: a novel GPI-anchored heparan sulfate proteoglycan that is highly expressed in developing brain and kidney. J Cell Biol 1995;130:1207–1218.
69. Stipp CS, Litwack ED, Lander AD. Cerebroglycan: An integral membrane heparan sulfate proteoglycan that is unique to the developing nervous system and expressed specifically during neuronal differentiation. J Cell Biol 1994;124:149–160.
70. Karthikeyan L, Maurel P, Rauch U, Margolis RK, Margolis RU. Cloning of a major heparan sulfate proteoglycan from brain and identification as the rat form of glypican. Biochem Biophys Res Commun 1992;188:395–401.
71. Mertens G, Cassiman JJ, Van den Berghe H, Vermylen J, David G. Cell surface heparan sulfate proteoglycans from human vascular endothelial cells. Core protein characterization and antithrombin III binding properties. J Biol Chem 1992;267:20,435–20,443.
72. Woods A, Höök M, Kjellén L, Smith CG, Rees DA. Relationship of heparan sulfate proteoglycans to the cytoskeleton and extracellular matrix of cultured fibroblasts. J Cell Biol 1984;99:1743–1753.
73. David G, Lories V, Decock P, Marynen B, Cassiman J-J, Van den Berghe H. Molecular cloning of a phosphatidylinositol-anchored membrane heparan sulfate proteoglycan from human lung fibroblasts. J Cell Biol 1990;111:3165–3176.
74. Lisanti MP, Sargiacomo M, Graeve L, Saltiel AR, Rodriguez-Boulan E. Polarized apical distribution of glycosyl-phosphatidylinositol-anchored proteins in a renal epithelial cell line. Proc Natl Acad Sci USA 1988;85:9557–9561.
75. Hinkes MT, Goldberger OA, Neumann PE, Kokenyesi R, Bernfield MR. Organization and promoter activity of the mouse syndecan-1 gene. J Biol Chem 1993;268:11,440–11,448.
76. Baciu PC, Acaster C, Goetinck PF. Molecular cloning and genomic organization of chicken syndecan-4. J Biol Chem 1994;269:696–703.
77. Brauker JH, Trautman MS, Bernfield MR. Syndecan, a cell surface proteoglycan, exhibits a molecular polymorphism during lung development. Dev Biol 1991;147:285–292.
78. Trautman MS, Kimelman J, Bernfield MR. Developmental expression of syndecan, an integral membrane proteoglycan, correlates with cell differentiation. Development 1991;111:213–220.
79. Vainio S, Jalkanen M, Vaahtokari A, Sahlberg C, Mali M, Bernfield MR, Thesleff I. Expression of syndecan gene is induced early, is transient, and correlates with changes in mesenchymal cell proliferation during tooth organogenesis. Dev Biol 1991;147:322–333.
80. Vainio S, Jalkanen M, Bernfield MR, Saxen L. Transient expression of syndecan in mesenchymal cell aggregates of the embryonic kidney. Dev Biol 1992;152:221–232.

81. Bernfield MR, Hinkes MT, Gallo RL. Developmental expression of the syndecans: Possible function and regulation. Development 1993;119 Suppl.:205–212.

82. Kim CW, Goldberger OA, Gallo RL, Bernfield MR. Members of the syndecan family of heparan sulfate proteoglycans are expressed in distinct cell-, tissue-, and development-specific patterns. Mol Biol Cell 1994;5:797–805.

83. Filmus J, Church JG, Buick RN. Isolation of a cDNA corresponding to a developmentally regulated transcript in rat intestine. Mol Cell Biol 1988;8:4243–4249.

84. Faassen AE, Schrager JA, Klein DJ, Oegema TR, Jr., Couchman JR, McCarthy JB. A cell surface chondroitin sulfate proteoglycan, immunologically related to CD44, is involved in type I collagen-mediated melanoma cell motility and invasion. J Cell Biol 1992;116:521–531.

85. Drake SL, Klein DJ, Mickelson DJ, Oegema TR, Jr., Furcht LT, McCarthy JB. Cell surface phosphatidylinositol-anchored heparan sulfate proteoglycan initiates mouse melanoma cell adhesion to a fibronectin-derived heparin-binding synthetic peptide. J Cell Biol 1992;117:1331–1341.

86. Saunders S, Jalkanen M, O'Farrel S, Bernfield MR. Molecular cloning of syndecan, an integral membrane proteoglycan. J Cell Biol 1989;108:1547–1556.

87. Carey DJ, Todd MS. A cytoskeleton-associated plasma membrane heparan sulfate proteoglycan in Schwann cells. J Biol Chem 1986;261:7518–7525.

88. Priglinger U, Geiger M, Bielek E, Vanyek E, Binder BR. Binding of urinary protein C inhibitor to cultured human epithelial kidney tumor cells (TCL-598). The role of glycosaminoglycans present on the luminal cell surface. J Biol Chem 1994;269:14,705–14,710.

89. Smith EP, Lu L, Chernausek SD, Klein DJ. Insulin-like growth factor-binding protein-3 (IGFBP-3) concentration in rat Sertoli cell-conditioned medium is regulated by a pathway involving association of IGFBP-3 with cell surface proteoglycans. Endocrinology 1994;135:359–364.

90. Moscatelli D. Basic fibroblast growth factor (bFGF) dissociates rapidly from heparan sulfates but slowly from receptors. J Biol Chem 1992;267:25,803–25,809.

91. Saksela L, Moscatelli D, Sommer A, Rifkin DB. Endothelial cell-derived heparan sulfate binds basic fibroblast growth factor and protects it from proteolytic degradation. J Cell Biol 1988;107:743–751.

92. Kiefer MC, Stephans JC, Crawford K, Okino K, Barr PJ. Ligand-affinity cloning and structure of a cell surface heparan sulfate proteoglycan that binds basic fibroblast growth factor. Proc Natl Acad Sci USA 1990;87:6985–6989.

93. Castellot JJ, Jr., Hoover RL, Harper PA, Karnovsky MJ. Heparin and glomerular epithelial cell-secreted heparin-like species inhibit mesangial-cell proliferation. Am J Pathol 1985;120:427–435.

94. Guillonneau X, Tassin J, Berrou E, Bryckaert M, Courtois Y, Mascarelli F. In vitro changes in plasma membrane heparan sulfate proteoglycans and in perlecan expression participate in the regulation of fibroblast growth factor 2 mitogenic activity. J Cell Physiol 1996;166:170–187.

95. Schlessinger J, Lax I, Lemmon M. Regulation of growth factor activation by proteoglycans: what is the role of the low affinity receptors? [Review]. Cell 1995;83:357–360.

96. Hildebrand A, Romaris M, Rasmussen LM, Heinegard D, Twardzik DR, Border WA, Ruoslahti E. Interaction of the small interstitial proteoglycans biglycan, decorin and fibromodulin with transforming growth factor beta. Biochem J 1994;302:527–534.

97. Li LY, Safran M, Aviezer D, Bohlen P, Seddon AP, Yayon A. Diminished heparin binding of a basic fibroblast growth factor mutant is associated with reduced receptor binding, mitogenesis, plasminogen activator induction, and in vitro angiogenesis. Biochem 1994;33:10,999–11,007.

98. Rapraeger AC, Guimond S, Krufka A, Olwin BB. Regulation by heparan sulfate in fibroblast growth factor signaling. Methods Enzymol 1994;245:219–240.

99. Fukushima D, Bützow R, Hildebrand A, Ruoslahti E. Localization of transforming growth factor β binding site in betaglycan. Comparison with small extracellular matrix proteoglycans. J Biol Chem 1993;268:22,710–22,715.

100. Mali M, Elenius K, Miettinen HM, Jalkanen M. Inhibition of basic fibroblast growth factor-induced growth promotion by overexpression of syndecan-1. J Biol Chem 1993;268:24,215–24,222.

101. Schonherr E, Jarvelainen HT, Kinsella MG, Sandell LJ, Wight TN. Platelet-derived growth factor and transforming growth factor-beta 1 differentially affect the synthesis of biglycan and decorin by monkey arterial smooth muscle cells. Arterioscler Thromb 1993;13:1026–1036.

102. Andres JL, DeFalcis D, Noda M, Massague J. Binding of two growth factor families to separate domains of the proteoglycan betaglycan. J Biol Chem 1992;267:5927–5930.

103. Elenius K, Määttä A, Salmivirta M, Jalkanen M. Growth factors induce 3 T3 cells to express bFGF-binding syndecan. J Biol Chem 1992;267:6435–6441.

104. Ornitz DM, Yayon A, Flanagan JG, Svahn CM, Levi E, Leder P. Heparin is required for cell-free binding of basic fibroblast growth factor to a soluble receptor and for mitogenesis in whole cells. Mol Cell Biol 1992;12:240–247.

105. Rapraeger AC, Krufka A, Olwin BB. Requirement of heparan sulfate for bFGF-mediated fibroblast growth and myoblast differentiation. Science 1991;252:1705–1708.

106. Ruoslahti E, Yamaguchi Y. Proteoglycans as modulators of growth factor activities. Cell 1991;64: 867–869.

107. Yamaguchi Y, Mann DM, Ruoslahti E. Negative regulation of transforming growth factor-β by the proteoglycan decorin. Nature (Lond) 1990;346:281–284.

108. Vogel T, Guo N, Krutzsch HC, Blake DA, Hartman J, Mendelovitz S, Panet A, Roberts DD. Modulation of endothelial cell proliferation, adhesion, and motility by recombinant heparin-binding domain and synthetic peptides from the type I repeats of thrombospondin. J Cell Biochem 1993;53:74–84.

109. Mauer SM, Steffes MW, Ellis EN, Sutherland DER, Brown DM, Goetz FC. Structural-functional relationships in diabetic nephropathy. J Clin Invest 1984;74:1143–1155.

110. Zhu D, Kim Y, Steffes MW, Groppoli TJ, Butkowski RJ, Mauer SM. Glomerular distribution of type IV collagen in diabetes by high resolution quantitative immunochemistry. Kidney Int 1994;45: 425–433.

111. Falk RJ, Scheinman JI, Mauer SM, Michael AF. Polyantigenic expansion of basement membrane constituents in diabetic nephropathy. Diabetes 1983;32(suppl 2):34–39.

112. Parthasarathy N, Spiro RG. Effect of diabetes on the glycosaminoglycan component of the human glomerular basement membrane. Diabetes 1982;31:738–741.

113. Kanwar YS, Rosenzweig LF, Linker A, Jakubowski ML. Decreased de novo synthesis of glomerular proteoglycans in diabetes: Biochemical and autoradiographic evidence. Proc Natl Acad Sci USA 1983;80:2272–2275.

114. Brown DM, Klein DJ, Michael AF, Oegema TR, Jr. 35S-glycosaminoglycan and 35S-glycopeptide metabolism by diabetic glomeruli and aorta. Diabetes 1982;31:418–425.

115. Cohen MP, Surma ML. [35S]sulfate incorporation into glomerular basement membrane glycosaminoglycans is decreased in experimental diabetes. Lab Clin Med 1981;98:715–722.

116. Klein DJ, Brown DM, Oegema TR, Jr. Glomerular proteoglycans in diabetes. Partial structural characterization and metabolism of de novo synthesized heparan-35SO4 and dermatan-35SO4 proteoglycans in streptozocin-induced diabetic rats. Diabetes 1986;35:1130–1142.

117. Vernier RL, Steffes MW, Sisson-Ross S, Mauer SM. Heparan sulfate proteoglycan in the glomerular basement membrane in type 1 diabetes mellitus. Kidney Int 1992;41:1070–1080.

118. Rohrbach DH, Wagner CW, Star VL, Martin GR, Brown KS, Yoon JW. Reduced synthesis of basement membrane heparan sulfate proteoglycan in streptozotocin-induced diabetic mice. J Biol Chem 1983;258:11,672–11,677.

119. Templeton DM. Retention of glomerular basement membrane-proteoglycans accompanying loss of anionic site staining in experimental diabetes. Lab Invest 1989;61:202–211.

120. McCarthy KJ, Abrahamson DR, Bynum KR, St. John PL, Couchman JR. Basement membrane-specific chondroitin sulfate proteoglycan is abnormally associated with the glomerular capillary basement membrane of diabetic rats. J Histochem Cytochem 1994;42:473–484.

121. Yagame M, Kim Y, Zhu D, Suzuki D, Eguchi K, Nomoto Y, Sakai H, Groppoli T, Steffes MW, Mauer SM. Differential distribution of type IV collagen chains in patients with diabetic nephropathy in non-insulin-dependent diabetes mellitus. Nephron 1995;70:42–48.

122. Fioretto PF, Keane WF, Kasiske BL, O'Donnell MP, Klein DJ. Alterations in glomerular proteoglycan metabolism in experimental non-insulin dependent diabetes mellitus. J Am Soc Nephrol 1993;3:1694–1704.

123. Klein DJ, Oegema TR, Jr., Brown DM. Release of glomerular heparan-35SO4 proteoglycan by heparin from glomeruli of streptozocin-induced diabetic rats. Diabetes 1989;38:130–139.

124. Ledbetter SR, Copeland EJ, Noonan DM, Vogeli G, Hassell JR. Altered steady-state mRNA levels of basement membrane proteins in diabetic mouse kidneys and thromboxane synthase inhibition. Diabetes 1990;39:196–203.

125. Fukui M, Nakamura T, Ebihara I, Shirato I, Tomino Y, Koide H. ECM gene expression and its modulation by insulin in diabetic rats. Diabetes 1992;41:1520–1527.

126. Doi T, Striker LJ, Kimata K, Peten EP, Yamada Y, Striker GE. Glomerulosclerosis in mice transgenic for growth hormone. Increased mesangial extracellular matrix is correlated with kidney mRNA levels. J Exp Med 1991;173:1287–1290.

127. Whiteside C, Templeton DM. Increased microalbuminuria in diabetic rats is independent of angiotensin II or glomerular proteoglycan synthesis. Canadian J Physiol Pharmacol 1992;70:1096–1103.

128. Matic M, Leveugle B, Fillit HM. Tumor necrosis factor-alpha alters the metabolism of endothelial cell proteoglycans. Autoimmunity 1994;18:275–284.

129. Lelongt B, Makino H, Kanwar YS. Status of glomerular proteoglycans in aminonucleoside nephrosis. Kidney Int 1987;31:1299–1310.

130. Kjellen L, Bielefeld D, Höök M. Reduced sulfation of liver heparan sulfate in experimentally diabetic rats. Diabetes 1983;32:337–342.

131. Unger E, Pettersson I, Eriksson UJ, Lindahl U, Kjellen L. Decreased activity of the heparan sulfate-modifying enzyme glucosaminyl N-deacetylase in hepatocytes from streptozotocin-diabetic rats. J Biol Chem 1991;266:8671–8674.

132. Cohen MP, Surma ML. Effect of diabetes on in vivo metabolism of [35S]-labeled glomerular basement membrane. Diabetes 1984;33:8–12.

133. Klein DJ, Cohen RM, Rymaszewski Z. Proteoglycan synthesis by bovine myocardial endothelial cells is increased by long term exposure to high concentrations of glucose. J Cell Physiol 1995;165:493–502.

134. Klein DJ, Oegema TR, Jr., Fredeen TS, van der Woude F, Kim Y, Brown DM. Partial characterization of proteoglycans synthesized by human glomerular epithelial cells in culture. Arch Biochem Biophys 1990;277:389–401.

135. Klein DJ, Brown DM, Kim Y, Oegema TR, Jr. Proteoglycans synthesized by human glomerular mesangial cells in culture. J Biol Chem 1990;265:9533–9543.

136. Rosenberg RD, Shworak NW, Liu J, Schwartz JJ, Zhang L. Heparan sulfate proteoglycans of the cardiovascular system: specific structures emerge but how is synthesis regulated? J Clin Invest 1997;99:2062–2070.

137. Roberts AB, McCune BK, Sporn MB. IGF-beta: regulation of extracellular matrix. [Review]. Kidney Int 1992;41:557–559.

138. Abe M, Harpel JG, Metz CN, Nunes I, Loskutoff DJ, Rifkin DB. An assay for transforming growth factor-beta using cells transfected with a plasminogen activator inhibitor-1 promoter-luciferase construct. Anal Biochem 1994;216:276–284.

139. Kingsley DM. The TGF-β superfamily: New members, new receptors, and new genetic tests of function in different organisms. Genes Dev 1994;8:133–146.

140. Wall NA, Hogan BLM. TGF-β related genes in development. Curr Opin Genet Dev 1994;4:517–522.

141. Dey BR, Sukhatme VP, Roberts AB, Sporn MB, Rauscher FJ, Kim SJ. Repression of the transforming growth factor-beta 1 gene by the Wilms' tumor suppressor WT1 gene product. Mol Endocrinol 1994;8:595–602.

142. Kim SJ, Park K, Rudkin BB, Dey BR, Sporn MB, Roberts AB. Nerve growth factor induces transcription of transforming growth factor-beta 1 through a specific promoter element in PC12 cells. J Biol Chem 1994;269:3739–3744.

143. Geiser AG, Busam KJ, Kim SJ, Lafyatis R, O'Reilly MA, Webbink R, Roberts AB, Sporn MB. Regulation of the transforming growth factor-beta 1 and -beta 3 promoters by transcription factor Spl. Gene 1993;129:223–228.

144. Romeo DS, Park K, Roberts AB, Sporn MB, Kim SJ. An element of the transforming growth factor-beta 1 5'-untranslated region represses translation and specifically binds a cytosolic factor. Mol Endocrinol 1993;7:759–766.

145. O'Reilly MA, Geiser AG, Kim SJ, Bruggeman LA, Luu AX, Roberts AB, Sporn MB. Identification of an activating transcription factor (ATF) binding site in the hymen transforming growth factor-beta 2 promoter. J Biol Chem 1992;267:19,938–19,943.

146. Geiser AG, Kim SJ, Roberts AB, Sporn MB. Characterization of the mouse transforming growth factor-beta 1 promoter and activation by the Ha-ras oncogene. Mol Cell Biol 1991;11:84–92.

147. Kim SJ, Lee HD, Robbins PD, Busam K, Sporn MB, Roberts AB. Regulation of transforming growth factor beta 1 gene expression by the product of the retinoblastoma-susceptibility gene. Proc Natl Acad Sci USA 1991;88:3052–3056.

148. Birchenall-Roberts MC, Ruscetti FW, Kasper J, Lee HD, Friedman R, Geiser A, Sporn MB, Roberts AB, Kim SJ. Transcriptional regulation of the transforming growth factor beta 1 promoter by v-src gene products is mediated through the AP-1 complex. Mol Cell Biol 1990;10:4978–4983.

149. Kim SJ, Glick A, Sporn MB, Roberts AB. Characterization of the promoter region of the human transforming growth factor-beta 1 gene. J Biol Chem 1989;264:402–408.

150. Kim SJ, Jeang KT, Glick AB, Sporn MB, Roberts AB. Promoter sequences of the human transforming growth factor-beta 1 gene responsive to transforming growth factor-beta 1 autoinduction. J Biol Chem 1989;264:7041–7045.

151. Kim SJ, Denhez F, Kim KY, Holt JT, Sporn MB, Roberts AB. Activation of the second promoter of the transforming growth factor-beta 1 gene by transforming growth factor-beta 1 and phorbol ester occurs through the same target sequences. J Biol Chem 1989;264:19,373–19,378.

152. Khachigian LM, Lindner V, Williams AJ, Collins T. Egr-l-induced endothelial gene expression: a common theme in vascular injury. Science 1996;271:1427–1431.

153. Border WA, Noble NA, Yamamoto T, Harper JR, Yamaguchi Y, Pierschbacher MD, Ruoslahti E. Natural inhibitor of transforming growth factor-beta protects against scarring in experimental kidney disease. Nature (Lond) 1992;360:361–364.

154. Nakamura T, Miller D, Ruoslahti E, Border WA. Production of extracellular matrix by glomerular epithelial cells is regulated by transforming growth factor-beta 1. Kidney Int 1992;41:1213–1221.

155. López-Casillas F, Cheifetz S, Doody J, Andres JL, Lane WS, Massague J. Structure and expression of the membrane proteoglycan betaglycan, a component of the TGF-beta receptor system. Cell 1991;67:785–795.

156. Lopez-Casillas F, Payne HM, Andres JL, Massagué J. Betaglycan can act as a dual modulator of TGF-beta access to signaling receptors: mapping of ligand binding and GAG attachment sites. J Cell Biol 1994;124:557–568.

157. Lopez-Casillas F, Wrana JL, Massague J. Betaglycan presents ligand to the TGF beta signaling receptor. Cell 1993;73:1435–1444.

158. Markowitz S, Wang J, Myeroff L, Parsons R, Sun L, Lutterbaugh J, Fan RS, Zborowska E, Kinzler KW, Vogelstein B, Brattain M, Wilson JKV. Inactivation of the type II TGF-beta receptor in colon cancer cells with microsatellite instability. Science 1995;268:1336–1338.

159. Carcamo J, Weis FM, Ventura F, Wieser R, Wrana JL, Attisano L, Massague J. Type I receptors specify growth-inhibitory and transcriptional responses to transforming growth factor beta and activin. Mol Cell Biol 1994;14:3810–3821

160. Park KC, Kim SJ, Bang YJ, Park JG, Kim NK, Roberts AB, Sporn MB. Genetic changes in the transforming growth factor β (TGF-β) type II receptor gene in human gastric cancer cells: Correlation with sensitivity to growth inhibition by TGF-β. Proc Natl Acad Sci USA 1994;91:8772–8776.

161. Sun L, Wu G, Willson JK, Zborowska E, Yang J, Rajkarunanayake I, Wang J, Gentry LE, Wang XF, Brattain MG. Expression of transforming growth factor beta type II receptor leads to reduced malignancy in human breast cancer MCF-7 cells. J Biol Chem 1994;269:26,449–26,455.

162. Wrana JL, Attisano L, Wieser R, Ventura F, Massague J. Mechanism of activation of the TGF-beta receptor. Nature (Lond) 1994;370:341–347.

163. Border WA, Okuda S, Languino LR, Ruoslahti E. Transforming growth factor-beta regulates production of proteoglycans by mesangial cells. Kidney Int 1990;37:689–695.

164. Bassols A, Massague J. Transforming growth factor beta regulates the expression and structure of extracellular matrix chondroitin/dermatan sulfate proteoglycans. J Biol Chem 1988;263:3039–3045.

165. Rapraeger AC. The coordinated regulation of heparan sulfate, syndecans and cell behavior. Curr Opin Cell Biol 1993;5:844–853.

166. Border WA, Okuda S, Languino LR, Sporn MB, Ruoslahti E. Suppression of experimental glomerulonephritis by antiserum against transforming growth factor beta 1. Nature (Lond) 1990;346:371–374.

167. Okuda S, Languino LR, Ruoslahti E, Border WA. Elevated expression of transforming growth factor-beta and proteoglycan production in experimental glomerulonephritis. Possible role in expansion of the mesangial extracellular matrix [published erratum appears in J Clin Invest 1990 Dec;86(6):2175]. J Clin Invest 1990;86:453–462.

168. Yamamoto T, Nakamura T, Noble NA, Ruoslahti E, Border WA. Expression of transforming growth factor beta is elevated in human and experimental diabetic nephropathy. Proc Natl Acad Sci USA 1993;90:1814–1818.

169. Isaka Y, Fujiwara Y, Ueda N, Kaneda Y, Kamada T, Imai E. Glomerulosclerosis induced by in vivo transfection of transforming growth factor-β or platelet-derived growth factor gene into the rat kidney. J Clin Invest 1993;92:2597–2601.

170. Sharrna K, Ziyadeh FN. Renal hypertrophy is associated with upregulation of TGF-beta 1 gene expression in diabetic BB rat and NOD mouse. Am J Physiol 1994;267:Pt 2:F1094-1.

171. Sharma K, Ziyadeh FN. Hyperglycemia and diabetic kidney disease. The case for transforming growth factor-beta as a key mediator. [Review]. Diabetes 1995;44:1139–1146.

172. Wolf G, Sharma K, Chen Y, Ericksen M, Ziyadeh FN. High glucose-induced proliferation in mesangial cells is reversed by autocrine TGF-beta. Kidney Int 1992;42:647–656.

173. Yamamoto T, Noble NA, Miller DE, Border WA. Sustained expression of TGF-beta 1 underlies development of progressive kidney fibrosis. Kidney Int 1994;45:916–927.

174. Sawdey MS, Loskutoff DJ. Regulation of murine type 1 plasminogen activator inhibitor gene expression in vivo. Tissue specificity and induction by lipopolysaccharide, tumor necrosis factor-alpha, and transforming growth factor-beta. J Clin Invest 1991;88:1346–1353.

175. Sharma K, Jin Y, Guo J, Ziyadeh FN. Neutralization of TGF-beta by anti-TGF-beta antibody attenuates kidney hypertrophy and the enhanced extracellular matrix gene expression in STZ-induced diabetic mice. Diabetes 1996;45:522–530.

176. Rocco MV, Chen Y, Goldfarb S, Ziyadeh FN. Elevated glucose stimulates TGF-beta gene expression and bioactivity in proximal tubule. Kidney Int 1992;41:107–114.

177. MacKay K, Striker LJ, Stauffer JW, Doi T, Agodoa LY, Striker GE. Transforming growth factor-beta. Murine glomerular receptors and responses of isolated glomerular cells. J Clin Invest 1989;83: 1160–1167.

178. Ziyadeh FN, Sharma K, Ericksen M, Wolf G. Stimulation of collagen gene expression and protein synthesis in murine mesangial cells by high glucose is mediated by autocrine activation of transforming growth factor-beta. J Clin Invest 1994;93:536–542.

179. Tada H, Tsukamoto M, Ishii H, Isogai S. A high concentration of glucose alters the production of tPA, uPA and PAI-1 antigens from human mesangial cells. Diabetes Res Clin Pract 1994;24:33–39.

180. Wilson HM, Reid FJ, Brown PA, Power DA, Haites NE, Booth NA. Effect of transforming growth factor-beta 1 on plasminogen activators and plasminogen activator inhibitor-1 in renal glomerular cells. Exp Nephrol 1993;1:343–350.

181. Hagege J, Peraldi MN, Rondeau E, Adida C, Delarue F, Medcalf R, Schleuning WD, Sraer JD. Plasminogen activator inhibitor-1 deposition in the extracellular matrix of cultured human mesangial cells. Am J Pathol 1992;141:117–128.

182. Peraldi MN, Rondeau E, Medcalf RL, Hagege J, Lacave R, Delarue F, Schleuning WD, Sraer JD. Cell-specific regulation of plasminogen activator inhibitor 1 and tissue type plasminogen activator release by human kidney mesangial cells. Biochim Biophys Acta 1992;1134:189–196.

183. Shibuya H, Yamaguchi K, Shirakabe K, Tonegawa A, Gotoh Y, Ueno N, Irie K, Matsumoto K. TAB1: An activator of the TAK1 MAPKKK in TGF-β signal transduction. Science 1996;272:1179–1182.

184. Pietenpol JA, Munger K, Howley PM, Stein RW, Moses HL. Factor-binding element in the human c-myc promoter involved in transcriptional regulation by transforming growth factor beta 1 and by the retinoblastoma gene product. Proc Natl Acad Sci USA 1991;88:10,227–10,231.

185. Kreisberg JI, Garoni JA, Radnik R, Ayo SH. High glucose and TGFβ₁ stimulate fibronectin gene expression through a cAMP response element. Kidney Int 1994;46:1019–1024.

186. Keeton MR, Curriden SA, van Zonneveld AJ, Loskutoff DJ. Identification of regulatory sequences in the type 1 plasminogen activator inhibitor gene responsive to transforming growth factor beta. J Biol Chem 1991;266:23,048–23,052.

187. Sawdey M, Podor TJ, Loskutoff DJ. Regulation of type 1 plasminogen activator inhibitor gene expression in cultured bovine aortic endothelial cells. Induction by transforming growth factor-beta, lipopolysaccharide, and tumor necrosis factor-alpha. J Biol Chem 1989;264:10,396–10,401.

188. Keski-Oja J, Raghow R, Sawdey M, Loskutoff DJ, Postlethwaite AE, Kang AH, Moses HL. Regulation of mRNAs for type-1 plasminogen activator inhibitor, fibronectin, and type I procollagen by transforming growth factor-beta. Divergent responses in lung fibroblasts and carcinoma cells. J Biol Chem 1988;263:3111–3115.

189. Prendergast GC, Diamond LE, Dahl D, Cole MD. The c-myc-regulated gene mrl encodes plasminogen activator inhibitor 1. Mol Cell Biol 1990;10:1265–1269.

190. Fisher LW, Heegaard AM, Vetter U, Vogel W, Just W, Termine JD, Young MF. Human biglycan gene. Putative promoter, intron-exon junctions, and chromosomal localization. J Biol Chem 1991; 266:14,371–14,377.

191. Santra M, Danielson KG, Iozzo RV. Structural and functional characterization of the human decorin gene promoter. J Biol Chem 1994;269:579–587.

192. Liu Y, Michalopoulos GK, Zarnegar R. Structural and functional characterization of the mouse hepatocyte growth factor gene promoter. J Biol Chem 1994;269:4152–4160.

193. Marigo V, Volpin D, Vitale G, Bressan GM. Identification of a TGF-β responsive element in the human elastin promoter. Biochem Biophys Res Commun 1994;199:1049–1056.

194. MacLellan WR, Lee T-C, Schwartz RJ, Schneider MO. Transforming growth factor-β response elements of the skeletal β-actin gene. Combinatorial action of serum response factor, YY1, and the SV40 enhancer-binding protein, TEF-1. J Biol Chem 1994;269:16,754–16,760.

195. Campbell CE, Flenniden AN, Skup D, Williams BRG. Identification of a serum-and phorbol ester-responsive element in the murine tissue inhibitor of metalloproteinase gene. J Biol Chem 1991;266:7199–7206.

196. Horton WE, Jr, Higginbotham JD, Chandrasekhar S. Transforming growth factor-beta and fibroblast growth factor act synergistically to inhibit collagen II synthesis through a mechanism involving regulatory DNA sequences. J Cell Physiol 1989;141:8–15.

197. Kerr LD, Miller DB, Matrisian LM. TGF-β inhibition of transin/stromelysin gene expression is mediated through a Fos binding sequence. Cell 1990;61:267–278.

198. Jones JI, Clemmons DR. Insulin-like growth factors and their binding proteins: biological actions. [Review]. Endocr Rev 1995;16:3–34.

199. LeRoith D. Insulinlike growth factors. N Engl J Med 1997;336:336–340.

200. Myers MG, Jr., Sun XJ, Cheatham B, Jachna BR, Glasheen EM, Backer JM, White MF. IRS-1 is a common element in insulin and insulin-like growth factor-I signaling to the phosphatidylinositol 3'-kinase. Endocrinol J 1993;32:1421–1430.

201. Rogers DG, White NH, Shalwitz RA, Palmberg P, Smith ME, Santiago JV. The effect of puberty on the development of early diabetic microvascular disease in insulin-dependent diabetes. Diabetes Res Clin Pract 1987;3:39–44.

202. Kostraba JN, Dorman JS, Orchard TJ, Becker DJ, Ohki Y, Ellis D, Doft BH, Lobes LA, LaPorte RE, Drash AL. Contribution of diabetes duration before puberty to development of microvascular complications in IDDM subjects. Diabetes Care 1989;12:686–693.

203. Lawson ML, Sochett EB, Chait PG, Balfe JW, Daneman D. Effect of puberty on markers of glomerular hypertrophy and hypertension in IDDM. Diabetes 1996;45:51–55.

204. Amiel SA, Sherwin RS, Hintz RL, Gertner JM, Press CM, Tamborlane WV. Effect of diabetes and its control on insulin-like growth factors in the young subject with type I diabetes. Diabetes 1984;33:1175–1179.

205. Alzaid A, Dinneen SF, Melton LJ, Rizza RA. The role of growth hormone in the development of diabetic retinopathy. Diabetes Care 1994;17:531–534.

206. Pousen JE. Houssay phenomenon in man: recovery from retinopathy in case of diabetes with Simmonce's disease. Diabetes 1953;2:7–12.

207. Plumb M, Nath K, Seaquist ER. Hypopituitarism stabilizes the renal and retinal complications of diabetes mellitus. Am J Nephrol 1992;12:265–267.

208. Merimee TJ. A follow up study of vascular disease in growth hormone deficient dwarfs with diabetes. N Engl J Med 1978;298:1217–1222.

209. Bach LA, Rechler MM. Insulin-like growth factors and diabetes. [Review]. Diabetes Metab Rev 1992;8:229–257.

210. Flyvbjerg A, Landau D, Domene H, Hernandez L, Gronbaek H, LeRoith D. The role of growth hormone, insulin-like growth factors (IGFs), and IGF-binding proteins in experimental diabetic kidney disease. [Review]. Metab Clin Exper 1995;44:67–71.

211. Chin E, Zhou J, Bondy C. Anatomical relationships in the patterns of insulin-like growth factor (IGF)-I, IGF binding protein-1, and IGF-I receptor gene expression in the rat kidney. Endocrinology 1992;130:3237–3245.

212. Rabkin R, Brody M, Lu LH, Chan C, Shaheen AM, Gillett N. Expression of the genes encoding the rat renal insulin-like growth factor-I system. J Am Soc Nephrol 1995;6:1511–1518.

213. Rogers SA, Ryan G, Hammerman MR. Insulin-like growth factors I and II are produced in the metanephros and are required for growth and development in vitro. J Cell Biol 1991;113:1447–1453.

214. Rogers SA, Miller SB, Hammerman MR. Insulin-like growth factor I gene expression in isolated rat renal collecting duct is stimulated by epidermal growth factor. J Clin Invest 1991;87:347–351.

215. Hise MK, Li L, Mantzouris N, Rohan RM. Differential mRNA expression of insulin-like growth factor system during renal injury and hypertrophy. Am J Physiol 1995;269:F817–F824.

216. Sayed-Ahmed N, Muchaneta-Kubara EC, Besbas N, Shortland J, Cope GH, El Nahas AM. Insulin-like growth factor-I and experimental diabetic kidney disease. Exp Nephrol 1993;1:364–371.

217. Chen NY, Chen WY, Bellush L, Yang CW, Striker IJ, Striker GE, Kopchick JJ. Effects of streptozotocin treatment in growth hormone (GH) and GH antagonist transgenic mice. Endocrinology 1995;136:660–667.

218. Flyvbjerg A, Marshall SM, Frystyk J, Hansen KW, Harris AG, Orskov H. Octreotide administration in diabetic rats: effects on renal hypertrophy and urinary albumin excretion. Kidney Int 1992;41:805–812.

219. Moran A, Brown DM, Kim Y, Klein DJ. Effects of IGF-I and glucose on protein and proteoglycan synthesis by human fetal mesangial cells in culture. Diabetes 1991;40:1346–1354.

220. Batch JA, Baxter RC, Werther G. Abnormal regulation of insulin-like growth factor binding proteins in adolescents with insulin-dependent diabetes. J Clin Endocrinol Metab 1991;73:964–968.

221. Gelato MC, Alexander D, Marsh K. Differential tissue regulation of insulinlike growth factor binding proteins in experimental diabetes mellitus in the rat. Diabetes 1992;41:1511–1519.

222. Doi T, Striker LJ, Gibson CC, Agodoa LY, Brinster RL, Striker GE. Glomerular lesions in mice transgenic for growth hormone and insulinlike growth factor-I. I. Relationship between increased glomerular size and mesangial sclerosis. Am J Pathol 1990;137:541–552.

223. Doi T, Striker LJ, Gibson CC, Agodoa LYC, Brinster RL, Striker GE. Glomerular lesions in mice transgenic for growth hormone and insulinlike growth factor-I. Am J Pathol 1990;137:541–552.

224. Rymaszewski Z, Cohen RM, Chomczynskii P. Human growth hormone stimulates proliferation of human retinal microvascular endothelial cells in vitro. Proc Natl Acad Sci USA 1991;88:617–621.

225. Kikkawa R, Haneda M, Togawa M, Koya D, Kajiwara N, Shigeta Y. Differential modulation of mitogenic and metabolic actions of insulin-like growth factor I in rat glomerular mesangial cells in high glucose culture. Diabetologia 1993;36:276–281.

226. Feld SM, Hirschberg R, Artishevsky A, Nast C, Adler SG. Insulin-like growth factor I induces mesangial proliferation and increases mRNA and secretion of collagen. Kidney Int 1995;48:45–51.

227. Cagliero E, Maiello M, Boeri D, Roy S, Lorenzi MJ. Increased expression of basement membrane components in human endothelial cells cultured in high glucose. J Clin Invest 1988;82:735–738.

228. Roy S, Sala R, Cagliero E, Lorenzi MJ. Overexpression of fibronectin induced by diabetes or high glucose: phenomenon with a memory. Proc Natl Acad Sci USA 1990;87:404–408.

229. Maiello M, Boeri D, Podesta F, Cagliero E, Vichi M, Odetti P, Adezati L, Lorenzi MJ. Increased expression of tissue plasminogen activator and its inhibitor and reduced fibrinolytic potential of human endothelial cells cultured in elevated glucose. Diabetes 1992;41:1009–1015.

230. Roy S, Maiello M, Lorenzi MJ. Increased expression of basement membrane collagen in human diabetic retinopathy. J Clin Invest 1994;93:438–442.

231. Roth T, Podesta F, Stepp MA, Boeri D, Lorenzi MJ. Integrin overexpression induced by high glucose and by human diabetes: Potential pathway to cell dysfunction in diabetic microangiopathy. Proc Natl Acad Sci USA 1993;90:9640–9644.

232. Ayo SH, Radnik RA, Goroni J, Glass WF, Kreisberg JI. High glucose causes an increase in extracellular matrix proteins in culture mesangial cells. Am J Pathol 1990;136:1339–1348.

233. Danne T, Spiro MJ, Spiro RG. Effect of high glucose on type IV collagen production by cultured glomerular epithelial, endothelial, and mesangial cells. Diabetes 1993;42:170–177.

234. Heilig CW, Concepcion LA, Riser BL, Freytag SO, Zhu M, Cortes P. Overexpression of glucose transporters in rat mesangial cells cultured in a normal glucose milieu mimics the diabetic phenotype. J Clin Invest 1995;96:1802–1814.

235. Brownlee M, Cerami A, Vlassara H. Advanced glycosylation end products in tissue and the biochemical basis of diabetic complications. N Engl J Med 1988;318:1315–1321.

236. Brownlee M, Vlassara H, Kooney T, Ulrich P, Cerami A. Aminoguanidine prevents diabetes-induced arterial wall protein cross-linking. Science 1986;232:1629–1632.

237. Tarsio JF, Wigness B, Rhode TD, Rupp WM, Buchwald H, Furcht L. Non-enzymatic glycation of fibronectin and alterations in the molecular association of cell matrix and basement membrane components in diabetes mellitus. Diabetes 1985;34:477–484.

238. Vlassara H, Brownlee M, Cerami A. High affinity receptor mediated uptake and degradation of glucose modified proteins: a potential mechanism for the removal of senescent macromolecules. Proc Natl Acad Sci USA 1985;82:5588–5592.

239. Yang C-W, Vlassara H, Peten EP, He C-J, Striker GE, Striker LJ. Advanced glycation end products up-regulate gene expression found in diabetic glomerular disease. Proc Natl Acad Sci USA 1994;91:9436–9440.

240. Doi T, Vlassara H, Kirstein M, Yamada Y, Striker G, Striker LJ. Receptor-specific increase in extracellular matrix production in mouse mesangial cells by advanced glycosylation end products is mediated via platelet-derived growth factor. Proc Natl Acad Sci USA 1992;89:2873–2877.

241. Kirstein M, Aston C, Hintz R, Vlassara H. Receptor-specific induction of insulin-like growth factor I in human monocytes by advanced glycosylation end product-modified proteins. J Clin Invest 1992;90:439–446.
242. Kirstein M, Brett J, Radoff S, Ogawa S, Stern D, Vlassara H. Advanced protein glycosylation induces transendothelial human monocyte chemotaxis and secretion of platelet-derived growth factor: role in vascular disease of diabetes and aging. Proc Natl Acad Sci USA 1990;87:9010–9014.
243. Crowley ST, Brownlee M, Edelstein D, Satriano JA, Mori T, Singhal PC, Schlondorff DO. Effects of nonenzymatic glycosylation of mesangial matrix on proliferation of mesangial cells. Diabetes 1991;40:540–547.
244. Bucala R, Makita Z, Vega G, Grundy S, Koschinsky T, Cerami A, Vlassara H. Modification of low density lipoprotein by advanced glycation end products contributes to the dyslipidemia of diabetes and renal insufficiency. Proc Natl Acad Sci USA 1994;91:9441–9445.
245. Soulis-Liparota T, Cooper M, Papazoglou D, Clarke B, Jerums G. Retardation by aminoguanidine of development of albuminuria, mesangial expansion, and tissue fluorescence in streptozocin-induced diabetic rat. Diabetes 1991;40:1328–1334.
246. Kihara M, Schmelzer JD, Poduslo JF, Curran GL, Nickander KK, Low PA. Aminoguanidine effects on nerve blood flow, vascular permeability, electrophysiology, and oxygen free radicals. Proc Natl Acad Sci USA 1991;88:6107–6111.
247. Soulis T, Cooper ME, Vranes D, Bucala R, Jerums G. Effects of aminoguanidine in preventing experimental diabetic nephropathy are related to the duration of treatment. Kidney Int 1997;50:627–654.
248. Booth AA, Khalifah RG, Todd P, Hudson BG. In vitro kinetic studies of formation of antigenic advanced glycation end products (AGEs). Novel inhibition of postAmadori glycation pathways. J Biol Chem 1997;272:5430–5437.
249. Khalifah RG, Todd P, Booth AA, Yang SX, Mott JD, Hudson BG. Kinetics of nonenzymatic glycation of ribonuclease A leading to advanced glycation end products. Paradoxical inhibition by ribose leads to facile isolation of protein intermediate for rapid post Amadori studies. Biochem 1996;35:4645–4554.
250. Cohen MP, Sharma K, Jin Y, Hud E, Wu VY, Tomaszewski J, Ziyadeh FN. Prevention of diabetic nephropathy in db/db mice with glycated albumin antagonists. A novel treatment strategy. J Clin Invest 1995;95:2338–2345.
251. Rumble JR, Cooper ME, Soulis T, Cox A, Wu L, Youssef S, Jasik M, Jerums G, Gilbert RE. Vascular hypertrophy in experimental diabetes. Role of advanced glycation end products. J Clin Invest 1997;99:1016–1027.
252. Bucala R, Tracey KJ, Cerami A. Advanced glycosylation products quench nitric oxide and mediate defective endothelium-dependent vasodilatation in experimental diabetes. J Clin Invest 1991;87:432–438.
253. Nyengaard JR, Chang K, Berhorst S, Reiser KM, Williamson JR, Tilton RG. Discordant effects of guanidines on renal structure and function and on regional vascular dysfunction and collagen changes in diabetic rats. Diabetes 1997;46:94–106.
254. Skolnik EY, Yang Z, Makita Z, Radoff S, Kirstein M, Vlassara H. Human and rat mesangial cell receptors for glucose-modified proteins: potential role in kidney tissue remodelling end diabetic nephropathy. J Exp Med 1991;174:931–939.
255. Cohen MP, Ziyadeh FN. Amadori glucose adducts modulate mesangial cell growth and collagen gene expression. Kidney Int 1994;45:475–484.
256. Nahman NS, Jr., Leonhart KL, Cosio FG, Hebert CL. Effects of high glucose on cellular proliferation and fibronectin production by cultured human mesangial cells. Kidney Int 1992;41:396–402.
257. Lorenzi MJ, Nordberg JA, Toledo S. High glucose prolongs cell-cycle traversal of cultured human endothelial cells. Diabetes 1987;36:1261–1267.
258. Young BA, Johnson RJ, Alpers CE, Eng E, Gordon K, Floege J, Couser WG, Seidel K. Cellular events in the evolution of experimental diabetic nephropathy. Kidney Int 1995;47:935–944.
259. Wang A, Fan M-Y, Templeton DM. Growth modulation and proteoglycan turnover in cultured mesangial cells. J Cell Physiol 1994;159:295–310.
260. Li W, Shen S, Khatami M, Rockey JH. Stimulation of retinal capillary pericyte protein and collagen synthesis in culture by high glucose concentration. Diabetes 1984;33:784–789.
261. Castellot JJ, Jr., Favreau LV, Karnovsky MJ, Rosenberg RD. Inhibition of vascular smooth muscle cell growth by endothelial cell-derived heparin. Possible role of a platelet endoglycosidase. J Biol Chem 1982;257:11,256–11,260.

262. Castellot JJ, Jr., Hoover RL, Karnovsky MJ. Glomerular endothelial cells secrete a heparinlike inhibitor and a peptide stimulator of mesangial cell proliferation. Am J Pathol 1986;125:493–500.
263. Kitamura M, Mitarai T, Maruyama N, Nagasawa R, Yoshida H, Sakai O. Mesangial cell behavior in a three-dimensional extracellular matrix. Kidney Int 1991;40:653–661.
264. Kinsella MG, Wight TN. Modulation of sulfated proteoglycan synthesis by bovine aortic endothelial cells during migration. J Cell Biol 1986;102:679–687.
265. Williams SP, Mason RM. Modulation of proteoglycan synthesis by bovine vascular smooth muscle cells during cellular proliferation and treatment with heparin. Arch Biochem Biophys 1991;287:386–396.
266. Yamaguchi Y, Ruoslahti E. Expression of human proteoglycan in Chinese hamster ovary cells inhibits cell proliferation. Nature (Lond) 1990;336:244–246.
267. Vainio S, Thesleff I. Sequential induction of syndecan, tenascin and cell proliferation associated with mesenchymal cell condensation during early tooth development. Differentiation 1992;50:97–105.
268. McClain DA, Paterson AJ, Roos MD, Wei X, Kudlow J. Glucose and glucosamine regulate growth factor gene expression in vascular smooth muscle cells. Proc Natl Acad Sci USA 1992;89:8150–8154.
269. Ruoslahti E, Reed JC. Anchorage dependence, integrins, and apoptosis. [Review]. Cell 1994;77:477,478.
270. Ewen ME, Sluss HK, Whitehouse LL, Livingston DM. TGF-β inhibition of Cdk4 synthesis is linked to cell cycle arrest. Cell 1993;74:1009–1020.
271. Reynisdóttir I, Polyak K, Iavarone A, Massagué J. Kip/Cip and Ink4 Cdk inhibitors cooperate to induce cell cycle arrest in response to TGF-β. Genes Dev 1995;9:1831–1845.
272. Schultz-Cherry S, Ribeiro S, Gentry L, Murphy-Ullrich JE. Thrombospondin binds and activates the small and large forms of latent transforming growth factor-beta in a chemically defined system. J Biol Chem 1994;269:26,775–26,782.
273. Dameron KM, Volpert OV, Tainsky MA, Bouck N. Control of angiogenesis in fibroblasts by p53 regulation of thrombospondin-1. Science 1994;265:1582–1584.
274. Pietenpol JA, Stein RW, Moran E, Yaciuk P, Schlegel R, Lyons RM, Pittelkow MR, Munger K, Howley PM, Moses HL. TGF-beta 1 inhibition of c-myc transcription and growth in keratinocytes is abrogated by viral transforming proteins with pRB binding domains. Cell 1990;61:777–785.
275. Pietenpol JA, Holt JT, Stein RW, Moses HL. Transforming growth factor beta 1 suppression of c-myc gene transcription: role in inhibition of keratinocyte proliferation. Proc Natl Acad Sci USA 1990;87:3758–3762.
276. Cagliero E, Roth T, Taylor AW, Lorenzi MJ. The effects of high glucose on human endothelial cell growth and gene expression are not mediated by transforming growth factor-beta Lab Invest 1995;73:667–673.
277. Oh E, Woods A, Couchman JR. Syndecan-4 proteoglycan regulates the distribution and activity of protein kinase C. J Biol Chem 1997;272:8133–8136.
278. Oh E, Woods A, Couchman JR. Multimerization of the cytoplasmic domain of Syndecan-4 is required for its ability to activate protein kinase C. J Biol Chem 1997;272:11,805–11,811.
279. Inoguchi T, Battan R, Handler E, Sportsman JR, Heath W, King GL. Preferential elevation of protein kinase C isoform beta II and diacylglycerol levels in the aorta and heart of diabetic rats: differential reversibility to glycemic control by islet cell transplantation. Proc Natl Acad Sci USA 1992;89:11,059–11,063.
280. Williams B, Schrier RW. Characterization of glucose-induced in situ protein kinase C activity in cultured vascular smooth muscle cells. Diabetes 1992;41:1464–1472.
281. Ayo SH, Radnik R, Garoni JA, Troyer DA, Kreisberg JI. High glucose increases diacylglycerol mass and activates protein kinase C in mesangial cell cultures. Am J Physiol 1991;261:F571–F577.
282. Craven PA, DeRubertis FR. Protein kinase C is activated in glomeruli from streptozotocin diabetic rats. Possible mediation by glucose. J Clin Invest 1989;83:1667–1675.
283. Templeton DM, Fan MY. Posttranscriptional effects of glucose on proteoglycan expression in mesangial cells. Metabolism: Clinical & Experimental 1996;45:1136–1146.
284. Sharma K, Danoff TM, DePiero A, Ziyadeh FN. Enhanced expression of inducible nitric oxide synthase in murine macrophages and glomerular mesangial cells by elevated glucose levels: possible mediation via protein kinase C. Biochem Biophys Res Commun 1995;207:80–88.
285. Studer RK, Negrete H, Craven PA, DeRubertis FR. Protein kinase C signals thromboxane induced increases in fibronectin synthesis and TGF-beta bioactivity in mesangial cells. Kidney Int 1995;48:422–430.

286. Fisher EJ, McLennan SV, Yue DK, Turtle JR. Cell-associated proteoglycans of retinal pericytes and endothelial cells: Modulation by glucose and ascorbic acid. Microvasc Res 1994;48:179–189.
287. Fumo P, Kuncio GS, Ziyadeh FN. PKC and high glucose stimulate collagen alpha 1 (IV) transcriptional activity in a reporter mesangial cell line. Am J Physiol 1994;267:(Pt 2):F632–F638.
288. Studer RK, Craven PA, DeRubertis FR. Thromboxane stimulation of mesangial cell fibronectin synthesis is signalled by protein kinase C and modulated by cGMP. Kidney Int 1994;46:1074–1082.
289. Somers CE, Mosher DF. Protein kinase C modulation of fibronectin matrix assembly. J Biol Chem 1993;268:22,277–22,280.
290. Wolf BA, Williamson JR, Easom RA, Chang K, Sherman WR, Turk J. Diacylglycerol accumulation and microvascular abnormalities induced by elevated glucose levels. J Clin Invest 1991;87:31–38.
291. Ishii H, Jirousek MR, Koya D, Takagi C, Xia P, Clermont A, Bursell SE, Kern TS, Ballas LM, Heath WF, Stramm LE, Feener EP, King GL. Amelioration of vascular dysfunctions in diabetic rats by an oral PKC beta inhibitor. Science 1996;272:728–731.
292. Porte D, Jr., Schwartz MW. Diabetes complications: why is glucose potentially toxic? Science 1996;272:699,700.
293. Ma JX, Catanese VM. TGF-beta and IGF-I regulate distinct subsets of IGF binding proteins in human mesangial cells by distinct mechanisms: evidence for separate pathways controlling mesangial cellularity and matrix expansion. Endocrinology 1996;2:464.

8 P450c17—The Qualitative Regulator of Steroidogenesis

Walter L. Miller, MD

Contents

QUANTITATIVE AND QUALITATIVE REGULATION OF STEROIDOGENESIS

The pathways of steroid hormone synthesis are well established, and the molecular identities of the responsible steroidogenic enzymes have been elucidated (Fig. 1) (for review, *see* refs. *1, 2*). The first step in the synthesis of all steroid hormone is the conversion of cholesterol to pregnenolone by the cholesterol side-chain cleavage system, which is found in the mitochondria in the adrenal cortex, gonads, placenta, and brain. Three pairs of electrons from NADPH are passed through a flavoprotein termed ferredoxin reductase (more commonly "adrenodoxin reductase") to an iron/sulfur protein termed ferredoxin (adrenodoxin) and thence to cytochrome P450scc (where scc denotes side-chain cleavage). P450scc is the enzymatic moiety that binds cholesterol and uses the three pairs of electrons sequentially to catalyze 20α-hydroxylation, 22-hydroxylation, and C20,22 bond scission to yield pregnenolone, which is then rapidly converted to other steroids. The conversion of cholesterol to pregnenolone is the quantitative regulator of steroidogenesis. The chronic, long-term steroidogenic capacity of a cell is determined

From: *Molecular and Cellular Pediatric Endocrinology*
Edited by: S. Handwerger © Humana Press Inc., Totowa, NJ

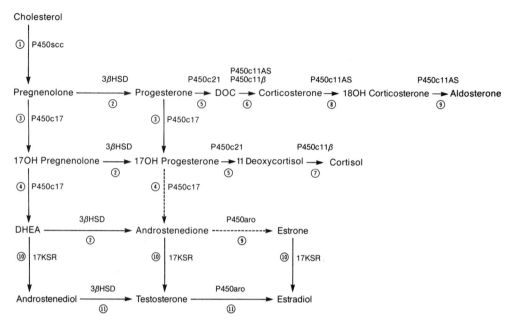

Fig. 1. Pathways of human adrenal steroidogenesis. Reaction 1: Mitochondrial cytochrome P450scc catalyzes 20α-hydroxylation, 22-hydroxylation, and scission of the C20–22 carbon bond of cholesterol, producing pregnenolone. Reaction 2: Type II 3β-HSD, a non-P450 short-chain dehydrogenase enzyme, catalyzes 3β-hydroxysteroid dehydrogenase and isomerase activities. Reaction 3: P450c17 catalyzes the 17α-hydroxylation of pregnenolone to 17OH-pregnenolone and of progesterone to 17OH-progesterone. Reaction 4: The 17,20-lyase activity of P450c17 converts 17OH-pregnenolone to DHEA, but negligible amounts of 17OH-progesterone are converted to Δ^4 androstenedione. Reaction 5: P450c21 catalyzes the 21-hydroxylation of both progesterone and 17OH-progesterone. Reactions 6, 8, and 9: In the adrenal zona glomerulosa, DOC is sequentially converted to corticosterone, 18OH-corticosterone and aldosterone by a single enzyme, P450c11AS (AS denotes Aldosterone Synthase). DOC is also converted to corticosterone by P450c11β in the zona fasciculata. Reaction 7: P450c11β catalyzes the conversion of 11-deoxycortisol to cortisol. Reactions 10 and 11 are found in the gonads. Reaction 10: Several isozymes of 17β-HSD mediate both 17-ketosteroid reductase and 17β-hydroxysteroid dehydrogenase activities; Type I converts estrone to estradiol and Type III converts DHEA to androstenediol, and androstenedione to testosterone. The reverse 17-ketosteroid reductase activities are catalyzed by the Type II and IV enzymes. Reaction 11: Testosterone is converted to estradiol by P450arom (aromatase).

primarily by transcription of the gene for P450scc, which determines how much P450scc enzyme is present *(3)*. The acute, short-term response of a cell to tropic hormones, which determines how much steroid is released, is determined by the action of the steroidogenic acute regulatory protein (StAR) *(4–7)*.

By contrast, the qualitative regulator of steroidogenesis is P450c17. P450c17 is a microsomal (Type II) cytochrome P450 enzyme that receives electrons from NADPH through the intermediacy of a flavoprotein, termed P450 oxidoreductase that is structurally unrelated to the adrenodoxin reductase of mitochondria, and which does not need an iron/sulfur protein intermediate. The same P450 oxidoreductase carries electrons to P450c17 and P450c21 (steroid 21-hydroxylase) and to the hepatic drug-metabolizing P450 enzymes. In the absence of P450c17, such as in the zona glomerulosa of the adrenal

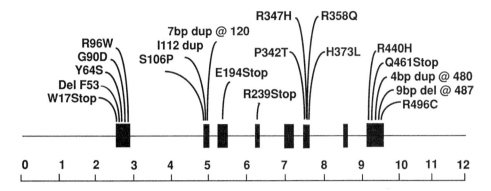

Fig. 2. Mutations of the gene for P450c17 that cause 17α-hydroxylase deficiency. The exons are shown as boxes and the scale is in kilobases. The references to the original descriptions of each of these mutations are found in refs. *14–16*. The mutations R347H and R358Q cause isolated 17,20 lyase deficiency.

cortex, pregnenolone will be converted to other C-21, 17-deoxy steroids, proceeding down the mineralocorticoid pathway to aldosterone. If the 17α-hydroxylase activity of P450c17 is present, such as in the zona fasciculata of the human adrenal, pregnenolone will undergo 17α-hydroxylation and proceed down the C-21 glucocorticoid pathway to cortisol. If the 17,20 lyase activity of P450c17 is also present then the steroid C17-20 bond will be cleaved, converting the 21-carbon steroid 17-hydroxypregnenolone to the 19-carbon 17-ketosteroid dehydroepiandrosterone, leading to androgens and subsequently to estrogens. Thus the nature of the P450c17 enzyme that distributes pregnenolone down these three alternative pathways is of considerable interest.

P450c17—ONE ENZYME, TWO ACTIVITIES

It was originally thought that each steroidogenic activity, such as 17α-hydroxylase and 17,20 lyase, had to be catalyzed by separate enzymes. It was known that plasma concentrations of DHEA and DHEA-sulfate (DHEA-S) would rise in older children and fall in the elderly independently of the concentrations of cortisol, suggesting that the 17,20 lyase activity needed for DHEA synthesis was regulated independently of the 17α-hydroxylase activity needed for cortisol synthesis. Also, cases of apparent isolated deficiency of 17,20 lyase activity were reported, further suggesting that 17α-hydroxylase and 17,20 lyase activities were catalyzed by different enzymes. However, several groups found that these two activities copurify with the P450c17 from adrenal or testicular microsomes from several species *(8–12)*. The presence of both activities in this single enzyme was confirmed by transfecting cells with either bovine *(13)* or human *(14)* P450c17 cDNA expression vectors and showing that the transfected cells made a single P450c17 protein and that the cells acquired both 17α-hydroxylase and 17,20 lyase activities. Cloning of the cDNA from human adrenals and testes and nuclease protection experiments *(15)* established that there was only one species of human P450c17 mRNA, and subsequent gene cloning confirmed that the human genome has only one P450c17 gene *(16)* lying on chromosome 10q24.3 *(17–19)*. Furthermore, about 20 mutations of the single human P450c17 gene have been described that ablate both 17α-hydroxylase and 17,20 lyase activity (Fig. 2) *(20–22)*, providing functional genetic evidence that there is only a single gene for human P450c17. Thus a single human P450c17 gene encodes a single species of mRNA that is identical in both the adrenals and gonads, and that mRNA encodes only a single P450c17 amino acid sequence that catalyzes both 17α-hydroxylase and 17,20 lyase activities.

TISSUE-SPECIFIC DIFFERENCES
AND THE ROLE OF ELECTRON DONORS

The 17,20 lyase activity is very high in testicular Leydig cells and ovarian theca cells so that virtually all steroidal precursors are converted to C19 sex steroids. By contrast, the adrenal zona fasciculata produces large amounts of 17 hydroxy C21 steroids (especially cortisol), and very little sex steroid. When it became clear that there was no separate 17,20 lyase enzyme and that the same P450c17 protein catalyzed 17α-hydroxylase and 17,20 lyase activities in both the adrenal and gonad, other explanations had to be sought for the high 17,20 lyase activity of testicular P450c17. One possibility was that the ratio of 17α-hydroxylase to 17,20 lyase activity was regulated by the amount of available P450 oxidoreductase (the flavoprotein that carries electrons to P450c17), as addition of purified hepatic P450 oxidoreductase to either adrenal or testicular microsomes or to purified P450c17 increased the ratio of lyase to hydroxylase activity *(23)*. Consistent with this, the molar ratio of P450 oxidoreductase to P450c17 is three- to fourfold higher in testes than in adrenals. Cytochrome b_5 increases 17,20 lyase, but not 17α-hydroxylase activity *(24–26)* through an allosteric mechanism, and not by functioning as an alternative election donor *(27)*.

We have examined the role of P450 oxidoreductase in the 17,20 lyase activity of human P450c17 by transfection experiments in nonsteroidogenic monkey kidney COS-1 cells *(28)*. P450c17 catalyzed 17α-hydroxylase activity with both pregnenolone and progesterone as substrates, and also catalyzed 17,20 lyase activity with 17OH pregnenolone as substrate, but did not catalyze the conversion of 17OH progesterone to Δ^4 androstenedione. Cotransfection of vectors expressing P450c17 and P450 oxidoreductase increased the 17,20 lyase activity with 17OH-pregnenolone as substrate, but still did not yield detectable 17,20 lyase activity with 17α-hydroxyprogesterone as substrate, showing that the 17,20 lyase activity of human P450c17 is strongly preferential for Δ^5 substrates. Our data in genetically manipulated yeast shows that human P450c17 catalyzes 17,20 lyase activity 100 times more efficiently with $\Delta 5$ than with $\Delta 4$ substrates *(27)*. Thus, 17OH progesterone is not converted to androstenedione in significant amounts in the human adrenal or gonad. Thus, the molar abundance of the electron donors for P450c17 can influence the relative ratio of 17α-hydroxylase and 17,20 lyase activities, and cytochrome b_5 allosterically facilitates election donation for the 17,20 lyase step.

ADRENARCHE

"Adrenarche" refers to the prepubertal rise in the secretion of adrenal androgens, principally DHEA and DHEA-S, that occurs only in human beings and other higher primates *(29)*. Concentrations of these steroids are very low in early childhood, then begin to rise at about age 8 without an associated change in the circulating concentrations of cortisol and ACTH *(29–31)*. This increased adrenal androgen secretion is independent of GnRH and gonadotropins, and is seen in patients who lack functional gonads *(32)*. Serum concentrations of DHEA and DHEA-S continue to rise after puberty, peaking in

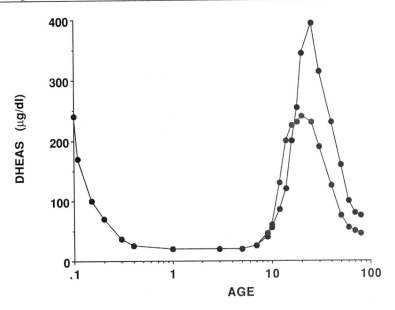

Fig. 3. Age-dependent changes in the concentration of DHEA-S (note log scale). Values are the same for both sexes until age 10–12, when female values begin to rise before male values, however, male values reach substantially higher levels in your adulthood. Data drawn from various sources.

early adulthood, and then fall with advancing age; by 60–70 yr the levels return to those seen in early adrenarchal, prepubertal children of 6–10 yr *(33)* (Fig. 3).

The mechanism of adrenarche is unknown. It has been suggested that a pituitary peptide stimulates DHEA secretion in the adrenal zona reticularis, analogous to the action of angiotensin II on the zona glomerulosa or of ACTH on the zona fasciculata, but no such adrenal androgen stimulating hormone has been found. Others have suggested that adrenarche might be mediated by intra-adrenal events, such as an ACTH-induced increase in P450c17 protein *(34)*. Measurements of the ratios of 17OH pregnenolone to pregnenolone and of DHEA to 17OH pregnenolone suggest that the 17α-hydroxylase activity in the adrenals of normal cycling women and postmenopausal women are equivalent, but that 17,20 lyase activity is reduced in postmenopausal women, suggesting that the diminution in serum DHEA levels in advancing age is caused by an intra-adrenal event *(35)*. Thus, the unsolved phenomenon of adrenarche shows that adrenal 17,20 lyase activity can be regulated independently of 17α-hydroxylase activity.

SERINE PHOSPHORYLATION OF P450c17 INCREASES 17,20 LYASE ACTIVITY—A MECHANISM FOR ADRENARCHE?

Although the 17,20 lyase activity of P450c17 can be substantially influenced by the molar abundance of redox partners such as P450 oxidoreductase, it seems most unlikely that the amount of the oxidoreductase changes significantly at adrenarche. P450 oxidoreductase also donates electrons to P450c21, yet 21-hydroxylase activity, as evidenced by production of aldosterone, corticosterone, and cortisol, does not increase at adrenarche. Therefore, because it seemed impossible to regulate 17,20 lyase activity by regulating the abundance of P450c17 mRNA or protein or by regulating P450 oxidoreductase, we hypothesized that the regulation of 17,20 lyase activity might be regulated by posttranslational modification of the P450c17 protein *(36)*.

Posttranslational modification had not been sought previously in P450c17 because western blotting of P450c17 produced by human adrenal cells or from transfected expression vectors reveals only a single molecular weight species of P450c17 *(20,28,36–38)*. However, we initially found charge isoforms of P450c17 by two-dimensional gel electrophoresis and western blotting of proteins extracted from human fetal adrenals, suggesting that P450c17 might indeed undergo posttranslational modification.

We then used human adrenal NCI-H295 cells and transfected COS-1 cells to study the posttranslational modifications of P450c17. NCI-H295 cells make C19 sex steroids and 17-hydroxylated C21 steroids *(39)*, and expresses abundant P450c17 mRNA *(40)* and immunodetectable protein. When NCI-H295 cells were labeled with either ^{32}P orthophosphate or [^{35}S]methionine for 2.5 h then treated for 2 h with or without cAMP, incorporation of [^{35}S]methionine into immunodetectable P450c17, an index of total P450c17 protein, increased by only one-third, but incorporation of ^{32}Pi, an index of phosphorylation, increased fourfold (Fig. 4A).

When the same experiment was done in nonsteroidogenic COS-1 cells transfected with a P450c17 expression vector, treatment with 200 µM 8Br-cAMP for 2 h did not increase immunoprecipitable [^{35}S]P450c17, but did increase ^{32}P labeling of P450c17 threefold. Similarly, cotransfection with a vector expressing the catalytic subunit of Protein Kinase A (RSV-Catβ) *(41)*, increased incorporation of ^{32}P orthophosphate about twofold. By contrast, incubation with phorbol ester (20 ng PMA/mL) had no effect. Thus the phosphorylation of P450c17 appeared to be catalyzed by a cAMP-dependent protein kinase. Two-dimensional phosphoamino acid analysis showed that about 70–80% of the incorporated ^{32}P was associated with serine and the remainder was associated with threonine, but none of the radioactivity was associated with tyrosine (Fig. 4B). Thus, P450c17 is posttranslationally modified by serine/threonine phosphorylation in response to a cAMP-dependent mechanism.

We examined the enzymatic consequences of this phosphorylation by transfecting COS-1 cells with P450c17 and incubating them with [^{14}C] pregnenolone. Cotransfecting the vector that expresses the catalytic subunit of protein kinase A or the vector that expresses P450 oxidoreductase increased the 17,20 lyase activity of P450c17, but cotransfecting the two together did not increase the lyase activity further. This suggests that P450c17 phosphorylation increases the efficiency of electron transfer, possibly by increasing the affinity of P450c17 for electron donors, such as P450 oxidoreductase. However, the induction of 17,20 lyase activity by cAMP was difficult to assess because of high background 17,20 lyase activity and high P450c17 phosphorylation in the untreated cells. Therefore, we performed the opposite experiment, assessing the effect of removing the phosphate from P450c17 in human fetal adrenal microsomes using alkaline phosphatase. We found that untreated microsomes incubated with [^{3}H]pregnenolone or [^{3}H]17-hydroxypregnenolone had both 17α-hydroxylase and 17,20 lyase activity, but microsomes that were dephosphorylated with alkaline phosphatase lost 17,20 lyase activity but retained 17α-hydroxylase activity. Furthermore, the amount of 17,20 lyase activity lost was strictly dependent on how long microsomes had been incubated with the alkaline phosphatase (Fig. 5). However, the alkaline phosphatase treatment had no effect on P450 oxidoreductase activity. The persistence of 17α-hydroxylase and P450 oxidoreductase activities indicated that the selective loss of 17,20 lyase activity was

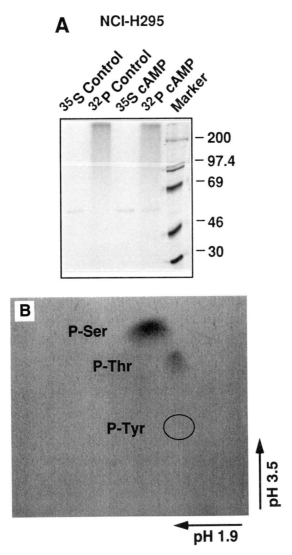

Fig. 4. Serine phosphorylation of P450c17. **(A)** Human adrenal NCI-H295 cells were labeled for 2.5 h with [^{35}S]methionine or ^{32}P orthophosphate, and then incubated another 2 h with or without 200 μ*M* 8Br-cAMP. P450c17 protein was collected with antiserum to P450c17 and staphylococcal protein A and displayed on an SDS gel. Note that the cAMP treatment does not increase the total amount of P450c17 protein (^{35}S) lanes, but does increase phosphorylation (^{32}P) lanes. **(B)** Immuno-isolated ^{32}P-labeled P450c17 was prepared from transfected COS-1 cells, and digested with trypsin and HCl. The hydrolyzed amino acids were electrophoresed along two axes, autoradiographed, and then the individual amino acids were identified by ninhydrin staining. About 80% of the ^{32}P is associated with serine and the remainder with threonine, but tyrosine is not phosphorylated.

not a result of proteolysis or disruption of the microsomes, and the persistence of 17α-hydroxylase activity, which requires NADPH, showed that the loss of 17,20 lyase activity was not caused by dephosphorylation of NADPH. Dephosphorylation of P450c17 with alkaline phosphatase treatment did not alter the substrate-induced difference spectrum of total microsomal P450 incubated with either pregnenolone or 17α-hydroxy-

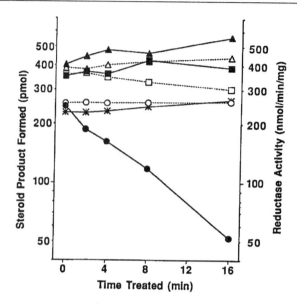

Fig. 5. Dephosphorylated microsomes loose 17,20 lyase activity. Human fetal adrenal microsomes were treated for 0–16 min with alkaline phosphatase (closed symbols) or control vehicle (open symbols), then incubated for 2 h with radiolabeled pregnenolone (△,▲). The resulting steroids were separated by chromatography and quantitated. Increasing the length of time the microsomes were dephosphorylated did not diminish the amount of 17α-hydroxypregnenolone (□,■) produced, but greatly diminished the amount of DHEA produced (○,●). The ability to reduce cytochrome c (*) right hand scale, was not affected by alkaline phosphatase.

pregnenolone, showing that the 17α-hydroxy pregnenolone could still bind to the active site of the enzyme. Thus, dephosphorylation did not affect substrate binding but did diminish 17,20 lyase activity.

MODELING OF P450c17 THREE-DIMENSIONAL STRUCTURE

Knowing the precise three-dimensional structure of P450c17 would provide substantial information about the enzymology of this enzyme. Unfortunately, none of the membrane-bound P450 enzymes, such as P450c17, has been able to be crystallized. However, several soluble P450 enzymes from bacteria have been crystallized; the best studied of these is the camphor-metabolizing enzyme P450cam from *Pseudomonas putida (42,43)*. Even though the amino acid sequences of P450c17 and P450cam are only 14–15% identical, we hypothesized in 1987 that the secondary structures of all the P450s, i.e., their array of α-helices and β-sheets, would be similar *(15,16)*; and mathematical predictions of protein secondary structures subsequently predicted that all P450 enzymes would have a similar architectural plan *(44,45)*.

Therefore, when sophisticated computer-graphic techniques became available we built first-generation models of P450c17 and P450c21 based on the crystallographically determined structure of P450cam using the MIDAS (Molecular Interactive Display and Simulation) system *(46,47)* at the Computer Graphics Laboratory at UCSF, and concentrated our efforts on the residues that appeared to define the steroid-binding pocket *(37)*. The model predicted that Leu102, Gly301, Met369, Ile371, and Gly111 should be involved in catalyzing the 17α-hydroxylase activity. To test this, we used site-directed mutagenesis to change these residues, singly or in combination, to the corresponding residues of P450c21 and we examined the 17α-hydroxylase and 21-hydroxylase activities of the resulting mutants *(37)*. The mutations Leu102Tyr and Met369Leu + Ile371Leu retained nearly full 17α-hydroxylase and 17,20 lyase activity, and the combination of all three mutations still retained 40–50% of activity, but the Gly301Ile and Gly111Asp mutations (and all multiple mutants that contained either of these mutations) lacked detectable 17α-hydroxylase and 17,20 lyase activity. The model also suggested that mutation of Asp298 should affect lyase and not hydroxylase activity, but the mutants Asp298Val and Asp298Ser were completely inactive. Thus, we could not confirm that the residues predicted to catalyze 17α-hydroxylase activity or 17,20 lyase activity actually played that role in the enzyme. However, the mutation Arg347Ala, analogous to the rat Arg346Ala mutation that selectively destroyed 17,20 lyase activity *(48)* also caused selective loss of 17,20 lyase activity in the human enzyme. The nearby residues Asn348 and Leu351 could be changed to the corresponding residues in P450c21 without affecting either 17α-hydroxylase or 17,20 activities. However, these Asn348Ala and Leu351Pro mutations changed the substrate-binding pockets of these mutants to resemble the binding pocket of P450c21. 11-Deoxycortisol, the predominant product produced by P450c21, had little effect on 17α-hydroxylase activity of wild type P450c17, but substantially inhibited the 17α-hydroxylase activities of both the Leu102Tyr and Met369Leu + Ile371Leu mutants. Thus, the mutagenesis experiments confirmed some features of the model and hence the utility of the approach *(37)*.

The principal limitation of our first model *(37)* was the structure of P450cam itself, which is a Type I enzyme analogous to a mitochondrial P450, as it receives electrons from NADPH via a flavoprotein and an iron/sulfur protein. By contrast, P450c17 is a Type II P450, which receives electrons directly from a flavoprotein and is substantially larger than P450cam. Three additional bacterial P450 enzymes have had their structures solved crystallographically since 1993 *(49–51)*, including P450BM-P *(49)*, which is the Type II P450 moiety of the 109 kDa P450BM-3 fusion protein found in *Bacillus megaterium* *(52)*. P450BM-P is 471 amino acids long (compared to 508 for P450c17 and 414 for P450cam) and shares 20% amino acid sequence identity with P450c17. We have constructed a new P450c17 model that incorporates structural information from the crystal structures of all four P450 enzymes, which share a common set of core α-helical and β-sheet elements *(53)*. We have identified the amino acids of P450c17 that probably comprise each of these structures by aligning the amino acid sequences using criteria that favor conformational similarity rather than simple amino acid identity *(54)*. Our data show that most mutations that cause 17α-hydroxylase deficiency lie on external helices of the model, away from the substrate binding pocket. The consensus sequence previously thought to be a substrate binding region *(55)* is in the region that corresponds to the presumed redox-partner interaction site in P450BM-P *(56)*. Thus, computer-graphic modeling of P450c17 also suggests that the interaction of P450c17 with its redox partner(s) may be involved in regulating 17,20 lyase activity.

17,20 LYASE DEFICIENCY

Consistent with the early presumption that 17α-hydroxylase and 17,20 lyase were separate enzymes, reports of isolated 17,20 lyase deficiency appeared in the early 1970s

(57–60), and by 1991, 10 reports describing 14 such patients had appeared *(61)*. These patients were typically 46,XY genetic males with ambiguous external genitalia, poor testosterone responses to gonadotropins, poor DHEA and androstenedione responses to ACTH, and normal cortisol secretion. Molecular genetic analysis of one of these patients revealed compound heterozygosity for a stop codon (Gln461Stop) and for a missense mutation (Arg496Lys) *(62)*. When the Arg496Lys mutation was recreated and expressed in transfected cells it had insignificant amounts of 17α-hydroxylase activity and 17,20 lyase activity *(62)*. Thus, this patient had combined 17α-hydroxylase and 17,20 lyase deficiency, so that it has not been clear if *bonafide* cases of isolated 17,20 lyase deficiency with normal 17α-hydroxylase activity exist.

Individual amino acid residues that appear to be crucial for 17,20 lyase activity have been identified. Based on the observation of conserved sequences in steroidogenic enzymes and steroid receptors *(55)*, Dufau's group mutagenized the arginine residues at positions 346, 357, 361, and 363 in rat P450c17 to either alanine or lysine *(48)*. The mutant Arg357Ala retained 35% of its 17α-hydroxylase activity but only 14% of its lyase activity, and the mutant Arg357Ala retained 80% of its 17α-hydroxylase activity but only 7% of its lyase activity. Thus, in rat P450c17, Arg346, and to a lesser degree Arg357, are specifically crucial for 17,20 lyase activity. We have made the corresponding human mutation (Arg357Ala) and shown that it severely reduced 17,20 lyase activity but not 17α-hydroxylase activity *(37)*. Thus, even though there have been no definitive clinical reports of human mutations specifically ablating 17,20 lyase activity whereas sparing 17α-hydroxylase activity, in vitro mutagenesis studies predict that such mutations can exist.

MOLECULAR BASIS OF 17,20 LYASE DEFICIENCY

Patients with true isolated 17,20 lyase deficiency could be considered as important site-directed mutagenesis experiments of nature, which should identify the specific P450c17 residues that are uniquely required for 17,20 lyase activity. We recently had the opportunity to study the DNA of two 46,XY individuals from rural Brazil who had the clinical phenotype predicted for isolated 17,20 lyase deficiency: female external genitalia, hypergonadotropic hypogonadism, sexual infantilism, and normal glucocorticoid and mineralocorticoid function *(63)*. At the time their intra-abdominal gonads were removed, their physicians in Brazil obtained testicular tissue and RNA, which we then used for reverse transcription, PCR, and direct sequencing to study their P450c17 sequences. We found that each patient was homozygous for a different missense mutation; one had Arg347His, whereas the other had Arg358Gln *(63)*. Both of these mutations lie within the conserved region previously thought to represent a steroid hormone binding site *(55)*, but which is now revealed by our molecular modeling as lying in the redox partner binding site. Furthermore, these two arginine residues correspond precisely to those identified by site-directed mutagenesis experiments in the rat as being specifically required for 17,20 lyase activity *(48)*. Expression of these mutations in transfected cells showed that they retained about 65% of 17α-hydroxylase activity but <5% of 17,20 lyase activity *(63)*. Thus, these two patients represent the first proven cases of 17,20 lyase deficiency, and are the first in which the precise location of a mutation had been previously predicted by mutagenesis studies in vitro.

A UNIFIED VIEW OF 17,20 LYASE ACTIVITY

All currently available observations are consistent with the hypothesis that the ratio of 17α-hydroxylase to 17,20 lyase activity of P450c17 is determined by the rate of flow of electrons to the enzyme. The enzyme will bind pregnenolone whether or not reducing equivalents are available. When electron donors are scarce, only the first reaction, 17α-hydroxylase activity, is catalyzed. The resulting 17α-hydroxypregnenolone is then released and a high ratio of 17α-hydroxylase to 17,20 lyase activity is observed. When electron donors are abundant, a second redox partner can interact with a P450c17 molecule that still retains 17α-hydroxypregnenolone, thus catalyzing the 17,20 lyase reaction, or 17α-hydroxyprogesterone may be released by one molecule of P450c17 and be rebound by another P450c17 molecule before the catalysis of 17,20 lyase activity.

The effective availability of electron-donating redox partners can be regulated by the relative molar abundance of P450 oxidoreductase, the availability of cytochrome b_5 or some other redox partner that may preferentially catalyze 17,20 lyase activity *(24–26)*, and Ser/Thr phosphorylation, which may either increase the enzyme's affinity for redox partners in general and/or participate in forming a modified redox partner site needed for binding of b_5. The selective disruption of 17,20 lyase activity by the artificial mutation Arg347Ala and by the natural mutations Arg347His and Arg358Gln supports the view that electrostatic interactions dictate the geometry, binding affinity and/or population of redox partners that can bind to P450c17. Thus, the relative 17,20 lyase activity is regulated by the availability of reducing equivalents.

ACKNOWLEDGMENTS

The author would like to thank Dong Lin, Steven Black, Eric Chiao, Lin-Hua Zhang, Henry Rodriguez, Shuji Ohno, David Geller, and Richard Auchus for their contributions to this work. This work was supported by the NIH under Grants DK37922 and DK42154 and by a grant from the March of Dimes.

REFERENCES

1. Miller WL. Molecular biology of steroid hormone synthesis. Endocr Rev 1988;9:295–318.
2. Fardella CE, Miller WL. Molecular biology of mineralocorticoid metabolism. Ann Rev Nutr 1996; 16:443–470.
3. Hum DW, Miller WL. Transcriptional regulation of human genes for steroidogenic enzymes. Clin Chem 1993;39:333–340.
4. Clark BJ, Wells J, King SR, Stocco DM. The purification, cloning and expression of a novel luteinizing hormone-induced mitochondrial protein in MA-10 cells mouse Leydig tumor cells. Characterization of the steroidogenic acute regulatory protein (StAR). J Biol Chem 1994;269:28,314–28,322.
5. Lin D, Sugawara T, Strauss JF III, Clark BJ, Stocco DM, Saenger P, et al. Role of steroidogenic acute regulatory protein in adrenal and gonadal steroidogenesis. Science 1995;267:1828–1831.
6. Clark BJ, Stocco DM. Regulation of the acute production of steroids in steroidogenic cells. Endocr Rev 1996;27:221–244.
7. Bose HS, Sugawara T, Strauss JF, III, Miller WL. The pathophysiology and genetics of congenital lipoid adrenal hyperplasia. N Engl J Med 1996;335:1870–1878.
8. Nakajin S, Hall PF. Microsomal cytochrome P450 from neonatal pig testis Purification and properties of a C_{21} steroid side-chain cleavage system (17α-hydroxylase-$C_{17,20}$ lyase). J Biol Chem 1981; 256:3871–3876.
9. Nakajin S, Shively JE, Yuan P, Hall PF. Microsomal cytochrome P450 from neonatal pig testis: Two enzymatic activities (17α-hydroxylase and C17,20-lyase) associated with one protein. Biochemistry 1981;20:4037–4042.

10. Kominami S, Shinzawa S, Takemori S. Purification and some properties of cytochrome P-450 for steroid 17α-hydroxylation and $C_{17,20}$ bond cleavage from guinea pig adrenal microsomes. Biochem Biophys Res Commun 1982;109:916–921.

11. Nakajin S, Shinoda M, Haniu M, Shively JE, Hall PF. C_{21} steroid side-chain cleavage enzyme from porcine adrenal microsomes. Purification and characterization of the 17α-hydroxylase/$C_{17,20}$ lyase cytochrome P450. J Biol Chem 1984;259:3971–3976.

12. Suhara K, Fujimura Y, Shiroo M, Katagiri M. Multiple catalytic properties of the purified and reconstituted cytochrome P-450 (P-450sccII) system of pig testis microsomes. J Biol Chem 1984;259: 8729–8736.

13. Zuber MX, John ME, Okamura T, Simpson ER, Waterman MR. Bovine adrenal cytochrome P45017: Regulation of gene expression by ACTH and eludication of primary sequence. J Biol Chem 1986;261:2475–2482.

14. Lin D, Harikrishna JA, Moore CCD, Jones KL, Miller WL. Missense mutation Ser[106]→ Pro causes 17α-hydroxylase deficiency. J Biol Chem 1991;266:15,992–15,998.

15. Chung B, Picado-Leonard J, Haniu M, Bienkowski M, Hall PF, Shivley JE, Miller WL. Cytochrome P450c17 (steroid 17α-hydroxylase/17,20 lyase): Cloning of human adrenal and testis cDNAs indicates the same gene is expressed in both tissues. Proc Natl Acad Sci USA 1987;84:407–411.

16. Picado-Leonard J, Miller WL. Cloning and sequence of the human gene encoding P450c17 (steroid 17α-hydroxylase/17,20 lyase): Similarity to the gene for P450c21. DNA 1987;6:439–448.

17. Matteson KJ, Picado-Leonard J, Chung B, Mohandas TK, Miller WL. Assignment of the gene for adrenal P450c17 (17α-hydroxylase/17,20 lyase) to human chromosome 10. J Clin Endocrinol Metab 1986;63:789–791.

18. Sparkes RS, Klisak I, Miller WL. Regional mapping of genes encoding human steroidogenic enzymes: P450scc to 15q23-q24, adrenodoxin to 11q22;adrenodoxin reductase to 17q24-q25;and P450c17 to 10q24-q25. DNA Cell Biol 1991;10:359–365.

19. Fan YS, Sasi R, Lee C, Winter JSD, Waterman MR, Lin CC. Localization of the human CYP17 gene (cytochrome P450 17α to 10q24.3) by fluorescence *in situ* hybridization and simultaneous chromosome banding. Genomics 1992;14:1110,1111.

20. Fardella CE, Hum DW, Homoki J, Miller WL. Point mutation Arg440 to His in cytochrome P450c17 causes severe 17α-hydroxylase deficiency. J Clin Endocrinol Metab 1994;79:160–164.

21. Yanase T. 17α-Hydroxylase/17,20 lyase defects. J Steroid Biochem 1995;53:153–157.

22. LaFlamme N, Leblanc J-F, Mailloux J, Faure N, Labrie F, Simard J. Mutation R96W in cytochrome P450c17 gene causes combined 17α-hydroxylase/17,20 lyase deficiency in two French Canadian patients. J Clin Endocrinol Metab 1996;81:264–268.

23. Yanagibashi K, Hall PF. Role of electron transport in the regulation of the lyase activity of C-21 side-chain cleavage P450 from porcine adrenal and testicular microsomes. J Biol Chem 1986;261: 8429–8433.

24. Onoda M, Hall PF. Cytochrome b_5 stimulates purified testicular microsomal cytochrome P450 (C_{21} side-chain cleavage). Biochem Biophys Res Commun 1982;108:454–460.

25. Kominami S, Ogawa N, Morimune R, Huang DY, Takemori S. The role of cytochrome b5 in adrenal microsomal steroidogenesis. J Steroid Biochem Mol Biol 1992;42:57–64.

26. Katagiri M, Kagawa N, Waterman MR. The role of cytochrome b_5 in the biosynthesis of androgens by human P450c17. Arch Biochem Biophys 1995;317:343–347.

27. Auchus RJ, Lee TC, Miller WL. Cytochrome b_5 augments the 17,20 lyase activity of human P450c17 without direct electron transfer. J Biol Chem 1998;273:3158–3165.

28. Lin D, Black SM, Nagahama Y, Miller WL. Steroid 17α-hydroxylase and 17,20 lyase activities of P450c17: Contributions of serine[106] and P450 reductase. Endocrinology 1993;132:2498–2506.

29. Cutler GB, Glenn M, Bush M, Hodgen GD, Graham CE, Loriaux DL. Adrenarche: a survey of rodents, domestic animals and primates. Endocrinology 1978;103: 2112–2118.

30. Apter D, Pakarinen A, Hammond GL, Vihko R. Adrenocortical function in puberty. Acta Paediatr Scand 1979;68:599–604.

31. Parker LN, Odell WD. Control of adrenal androgen secretion. Endocr Rev 1980;1:397–410.

32. Sklar CA, Kaplan SL, Grumbach MM. Evidence for dissociation between adrenarche and gonadarche: Studies in patients with idiopathic precocious puberty, gonadal dysgenesis, isolated gonadotropin deficiency, and constitutionally delayed growth and adolescence. J Clin Endocrinol Metab 1980; 51:548–556.

33. Orentreich N, Brind JL, Rizer RL, Vogelman JH. Age changes and sex differences in serum dehydroepiandrosterone sulfate concentrations throughout adulthood. J Clin Endocrinol Metab 1984;59:551–555.

34. Couch RM, Muller J, Winter JSD. Regulation of the activities of 17α-hydroxylase and 17,20-desmolase in the human adrenal cortex: Kinetic analysis and inhibition by endogenous steroids. J Clin Endocrinol Metab 1986;63:613–618.

35. Liu C, Laughlin GA, Fischer VG, Yen SSC. Marked attenuation of ultradian and circadian rhythms of dehydroepiandrosterone in postmenopausal women: Evidence for a reduced 17,20-demolase enzymatic activity. J Clin Endocrinol Metab 1990;71:900–906.

36. Zhang L, Rodriguez H, Ohno S, Miller WL. Serine phosphorylation of human P450c17 increases 17,20 lyase activity: Implications for adrenarche and for the polycystic ovary syndrome. Proc Natl Acad Sci USA 1995;92:10,619–10,623.

37. Lin D, Zhang L, Chiao E, Miller WL. Modeling and mutagenesis of the active site of human P450c17. Mol Endocrinol 1994;8:392–402.

38. Fardella CE, Zhang LH, Mahachoklertwattana P, Lin D, Miller WL. Deletion of amino acids Asp[487]-Ser[488]-Phe[489] in human cytochrome P450c17 causes severe 17α-hydroxylase deficiency. J Clin Endocrinol Metab 1993;77:489–493.

39. Gazdar AF, Oie HK, Shackleton CH, Chen TR, Triche TJ, Myers CE, et al. Establishment and characterization of a human adrenocortical carcinoma cell line that expresses multiple pathways of steroid biosynthesis. Cancer Res 1990;50:5488–5496.

40. Staels B, Hum DW, Miller WL. Regulation of steroidogenesis in NCI-H295 cells: A cellular model of the human fetal adrenal. Mol Endocrinol 1993;7:423–433.

41. Maurer RA. Both isoforms of the cAMP-dependent protein kinase catalytic subunit can activate transcription of the prolactin gene. J Biol Chem 1989;264:6870–6873.

42. Poulos TL, Finzel BC, Howard AJ. High-resolution crystal structure of cytochrome P450cam. J Mol Biol 1987;195:687–700.

43. Raag R, Poulos TL. Crystal structure of the carbon monoxide-substrate cytochrome P-450$_{CAM}$ ternary complex. Biochemistry 1989;28:7586–7592.

44. Nelson DR, Strobel HW. On the membrane topology of vertebrate cytochrome P450 proteins. J Biol Chem 1988;263:6038–6050.

45. Edwards RJ, Murray BP, Boobis AR, Davies DS. Identification and location of a-helices in mammalian cytochromes P450. Biochemistry 1989;28:3762–3770.

46. Ferrin TE, Huang CC, Jarvis LE, Langridge R. The MIDAS database system. J Mol Graphics 1988; 6:2–12.

47. Ferrin TE, Huang CC, Jarvis LE, Langridge R. The MIDAS display system. J Mol Graphics 1988; 6:13–27.

48. Kitamura M, Buczko E, Dufau ML. Dissociation of hydroxylase and lyase activities by site-directed mutagenesis of the rat P450-17α. Mol Endocrinol 1991;5:1373–1380.

49. Ravichandran KG, Boddupalli SS, Hasemann CA, Peterson JA, Deisenhofer J. Crystal structure of hemoprotein domain of P450BM-3, a prototype for microsomal P450's. Science 1993;261:731–736.

50. Hasemann CA, Ravichandran KG, Peterson JA, Deisenhofer J. Crystal structure and refinement of cytochrome P450terp at 2.3 Å resolution. J Mol Biol 1994;236:1169–1185.

51. Cupp-Vickery JR, Poulos TL. Structure of cytochrome P450eryF involved in erythromycin biosynthesis. Structural Biol 1995;2:144–153.

52. Fulco AJ. P450BM-3 and other inducible bacterial P450 cytochromes: biochemistry and regulation. Ann Rev Pharmacol Toxicol 1991;31:177–203.

53. Hasemann CA, Kurumbail RG, Boddupalli SS, Peterson JA, Deisenhofer J. Structure and function of cytochromes P450: A comparative analysis of three crystal structures. Structure 1995;3:41–62.

54. Graham-Lorence S, Amarneh B, White RE, Peterson JA, Simpson ER. A three-dimensional model of aromatase cytochrome P450. Prot Sci 1995;4:1065–1080.

55. Picado-Leonard J, Miller WL. Homologous sequences in steroidogenic enzymes, steroid receptors and a steroid binding protein suggest a consensus steroid-binding sequence. Mol Endocrinol 1988;2: 1145–1150.

56. Auchus RJ, Graham-Lorence S, Peterson JB, Miller WL. A second-generation molecular graphics model of human P450c17 based on assembly of core structures. 2nd Int Symp Molec Steroidogen 1996; Abs. P-36, Monterey, CA.

57. Zachman M, Vollmin JA, Hamilton W, Prader A. Steroid 17,20 desmolase deficiency: A new cause of male pseudohermaphroditism. Clin Endocrinol 1972;1:369–385.
58. Zachman M, Werder EA, Prader A. Two types of male pseudohermaphroditism due to 17,20 desmolase deficiency. J Clin Endocrinol Metab 1982;55:487–490.
59. Goebelsmann U, Zachmann M, Davajan V, Israel R, Mestman JH, Mishell DR. Male pseudohermaphroditism consistent with 17,20-desmolase deficiency. Gynecol Invest 1976;7:138–156.
60. Campo S, Stivel M, Nicolau G, Monteagudo C, Rivarola M. Testicular function in post-pubertal male pseudohermaphroditism. Clin Endocrinol 1979;11:481–490.
61. Yanase T, Simpson ER, Waterman MR. 17α-hydroxylase/17,20 lyase deficiency: From clinical investigation to molecular definition. Endocr Rev 1991;12:91–108.
62. Yanase T, Waterman MR, Zachmann M, Winter JSD, Simpson ER, Kagimoto M. Molecular basis of apparent isolated 17,20-lyase deficiency: Compound heterozygous mutations in the C-terminal region (Arg(496)$\rightarrow$Cys, Gln(461)$\rightarrow$Stop) actually cause combined 17α-hydroxylase/17,20-lyase deficiency. Biochem Biophys Acta 1992;1139:275–279.
63. Geller DH, Auchus RJ, Mendonça BB, Miller WL. The genetic and functional basis of isolated 17,20 lyase deficiency. Nat Genet 1997;17:201–205.

9

The Molecular Basis of Inherited Diabetes Insipidus

David R. Repaske, PhD, MD

CONTENTS

INTRODUCTION

Diabetes insipidus is a disease characterized by the excretion of an abnormally large amount of dilute urine that results from a failure of the water-conserving mechanism in the collecting ducts of the kidney. Inherited diabetes insipidus is a rare disorder, but the study of affected individuals and families has provided unique insights into the normal mechanisms involved in regulation of water balance. Water conservation in the kidney is regulated primarily by the hormone vasopressin. This hormone interacts with renal vasopressin receptors that cause intracellular water channels to be inserted into the luminal membrane of the cells lining the collecting duct to allow water resorption from the renal ultrafiltrate. Inherited forms of diabetes insipidus have been described that affect each of the key components in this water resorption system. Autosomal-dominant neurohypophyseal diabetes insipidus results from disruption of vasopressin production, X-linked diabetes insipidus results from abnormalities in the vasopressin receptor, and autosomal recessive diabetes insipidus results from defective water channels. A fourth inherited disease, Wolfram syndrome, involves inherited diabetes insipidus as one component of a cluster of abnormalities, and the molecular basis of this syndrome is being elucidated, but is not yet well understood. This article will explore the molecular biology of each of these inherited forms of diabetes insipidus and the current state of knowledge of the molecular mechanisms of production of vasopressin and action of vasopressin in the kidney.

From: *Molecular and Cellular Pediatric Endocrinology*
Edited by: S. Handwerger © Humana Press Inc., Totowa, NJ

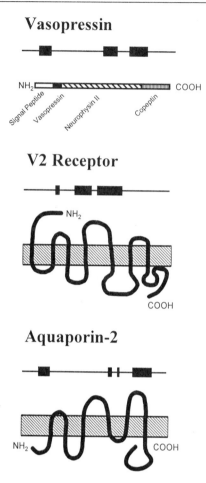

Fig. 1. Diagrams of the vasopressin, V2 receptor, and aquaporin-2 genes **(upper)** and proteins **(lower)**. The genes are represented by black rectangles (exons) connected by lines (introns and flanking regions). The vasopressin precursor protein is represented by a rectangle with signal peptide, vasopressin, neurophysin II, and copeptin domains indicated. The V2 receptor and aquaporin-2 proteins are represented as they appear in the plasma membrane with the extracellular surface superior.

PHYSIOLOGY

Vasopressin Production

Vasopressin is synthesized in the suprachiasmatic, supraoptic, and paraventricular nuclei of the hypothalamus of the brain. The vasopressin from the suprachiasmatic nucleus acts as a neurotransmitter within the brain, whereas the vasopressin from the large magnocellular neurons of the supraoptic and paraventricular nuclei acts as a hormone that is secreted into the bloodstream and regulates water resorption in the kidney. The human genome carries only one vasopressin gene (Fig. 1), and it encodes a precursor polypeptide that comprises vasopressin (9 amino acids), its carrier protein, neurophysin II (93 amino acids), and copeptin (39 amino acids). The gene is 2.5 kb in size and contains two introns *(1)*. It is highly homologous with the neighboring gene on human chromosome 20 that encodes oxytocin and its carrier protein, neurophysin I. The vasopressin gene is transcribed and translated into a preproprecursor polypeptide. The signal peptide is removed as the precursor enters the lumen of the endoplasmic reticulum, and then core glycosylation of the copeptin moiety is added. The proprecursor then folds with the first three amino acids (Cys-Tyr-Phe) of the vasopressin moiety entering into a binding pocket in neurophysin II *(2)*. One disulfide bond forms within the vasopressin moiety, and seven disulfides form within the neurophysin II domain *(3)*. One of these neurophysin disulfides (Cys^{10}-Cys^{54}) is critical for establishing and maintaining the proper secondary structure, but this bond is particularly unstable and only forms readily when the vasopressin portion of the proprecursor has bound within the neurophysin II binding pocket *(4)*. The first two amino acids of vasopressin (Cys-Tyr) are responsible for tight binding to neurophysin II, and therefore, for allowing disulfide bridge formation and stabilization of neurophysin II folding *(4)*. After folding, the precursor enters the Golgi complex where core glycosylation is modified and the intact proprecursor is packaged into neurosecretory granules. The granules are transported down the magnocellular neuron axons to the nerve terminals in the posterior pituitary. During transport, the three product peptides are cleaved from one another by dibasic-specific endoproteases. This processing releases a 10-amino acid peptide that is vasopressin with an additional C-terminal glycine. A peptidylglycine alpha-amidating monooxygenase removes a portion of this glycine but leaves the amino group attached to the nine amino acids of vasopressin creating an amidated peptide *(2)*. Even after vasopressin is proteolytically cleaved from neurophysin and amidated, it remains bound in the binding pocket of neurophysin II. This binding also promotes dimerization of neurophysin II, presumably allowing denser packaging of the hormone within the neurosecretory granules. Vasopressin is stored within the posterior pituitary until released into the circulation in response to serum hyperosmolality or hypovolemia/hypotension. In the circulation, vasopressin dissociates from neurophysin II and circulates freely.

Renal Vasopressin Receptors

There are at least three distinct membrane-bound G protein-linked vasopressin receptors expressed in mammals. The V2 class of receptors is linked to an increase in intracellular cAMP concentration via stimulation of adenylate cyclase. These receptors mediate increased free-water resorption via the principal cells of the collecting duct of the kidney, vasodilation in the peripheral vasculature, and release of coagulation factor VIII and von Willebrand factor from the endothelium and from the liver *(5–7)*. The V2 receptor is a 371-amino acid "serpentine" receptor encoded on chromosome Xq28 in a compact gene that contains only two small introns *(8)* and is similar to many other serpentine receptor genes. The protein has an extracellular N terminus, seven transmembrane domains, and an intracellular C terminus. There are, therefore, also three extracellular loops and three intracellular loops *(9)*. Investigation of the V2 receptor has been aided by the existence of a V2-specific agonist, 1-desamino[8-D-arginine]vasopressin, or dDAVP *(6)*. The V2 receptors are expressed on the basal aspect of the principal cells of the collecting ducts and bind vasopressin circulating in the bloodstream. Binding of vasopressin activates the receptor, and an intramolecular signal is transduced across the cell membrane that activates a G protein that in turn activates adenylate cyclase. The increased production of cAMP shifts the balance between production of cAMP by adenylate cyclase and degradation of cAMP by cyclic nucleotide phosphodiesterases, and the intracellular concentration of cAMP increases. An increase in cAMP can even be quantitated in the urine. The increased concentration of cAMP binds to and releases an inhibitory regulatory subunit from protein kinase A and therefore stimulates the catalytic activity of protein kinase A.

Renal Effector Molecules

The renal ultrafiltrate from the glomeruli is typically 125 mL/min/1.73m² or approx 180 L/day in an adult. Approximately 90% of this volume is resorbed in the proximal and distal tubules of the kidney, along with more than 90% of the solute. The collecting ducts are therefore presented with approx 18 L/d of dilute renal ultrafiltrate. In complete diabetes insipidus, or under conditions such as serum hypoosmolality when serum vasopressin is absent, almost this entire volume of fluid is excreted as dilute urine. However, in the normal kidney in the presence of vasopressin, protein kinase A is activated within the principal cells of the collecting duct via activation of V2 receptors. By an as yet unknown mechanism, protein kinase A allows intracellular clathrin-coated vesicles containing aquaporin-2 water channels to fuse with the apical cell membrane and to insert these water channels into the cell membrane. Water then flows down a concentration gradient out of the renal ultrafiltrate and into the principal cells of the collecting ducts. Water subsequently leaves the principal cells through aquaporin-3 channels in the basolateral membrane and flows into the relative hyperosmotic environment of the renal medullary interstitium. Aquaporin-2 is encoded on chromosome 12 and encodes a 271-amino acid protein that has six putative transmembrane domains with both the N and C termini within the intracellular compartment *(10)*. The first intracellular loop and the second extracellular loop have extended homology with analogous portions of five other known water channels and are relatively hydrophobic, suggesting that they extend into the membrane lipid bilayer to form the water pore. Aquaporin-3 channels that allow water to flow out of the principle cells seem to be constitutively present in the membrane and are not known to be regulated by vasopressin.

Summary

This discussion outlines the regulation of water balance in mammals. Regulation of the amount of vasopressin released from the posterior pituitary normally controls the amount of free water excreted by the kidneys. This system requires normal production of the hormone vasopressin, normal action of the renal V2 receptor, and the ability of the renal aquaporin-2 water channels to be inserted into the luminal membrane of the principle cells of the renal collecting duct. Four inherited disruptions of this process have been studied at the molecular level and will now be described to examine how each of these diseases produces diabetes insipidus.

AUTOSOMAL-DOMINANT
NEUROHYPOPHYSEAL DIABETES INSIPIDUS

Clinical

Autosomal-dominant neurohypophyseal diabetes insipidus, or ADNDI, is caused by deficiency of circulating vasopressin *(11)*. The disease is transmitted as an autosomal-dominant trait with essentially complete penetrance. Affected individuals are completely asymptotic at birth but develop polyuria and polydipsia at 1–6 yr of age *(12)* and have been shown to have a declining ability to produce vasopressin as symptoms progress *(13)*. Autopsy results have been reported on only four individuals with classic ADNDI, and each has shown degeneration of the supraoptic and paraventricular nuclei of the hypothalamus *(14–16)*. The degeneration involves specifically the hormone-producing magnocellular neurons and spares the medium and small neurons of the hypothalamus and the balance of the brain and anterior pituitary. Immunostaining *(16)* demonstrated almost complete loss of vasopressin-containing magnocellular neurons with preservation of some magnocellular neurons that do not stain for vasopressin. These observations have led to the hypothesis that ADNDI is a progressive neurodegenerative disorder that specifically involves vasopressinergic magnocellular neurons *(17,18)*. Interestingly, vasopressin also is produced in the adrenal glands *(19)* ovaries, testes *(20,21)*, and other areas of the brain, including the suprachiasmatic nucleus. Immunostaining does not show evidence of degeneration of these other vasopressinergic neurons *(16)* and there is no recognized adrenal or gonadal dysfunction in individuals affected with ADNDI.

Magnetic resonance imaging (MRI) studies of the posterior pituitary in normal individuals show a high-intensity "bright spot" on T1-weighted images in normal subjects *(22,23)*. Other retrospective reviews of MRI scans from patients with neurologic disorders but without DI reveal the presence of a bright spot in all subjects *(23–26)* or in most subjects *(27–29)*. However, individuals with acquired neurohypophyseal diabetes insipidus (caused by trauma, surgery, infiltrative disease, and so forth) are uniformly missing this bright spot *(24,26,29–35)*. The exact nature of the spot remains a subject of investigation *(33)*, but it seems to be associated with the presence of neurosecretory granules. In ADNDI the bright spot is absent in most patients with longstanding diabetes insipidus *(36,37)* but has been detected in individuals who have only been symptomatic for 1 or 2 yr *(25)*, in "mildly affected" individuals *(38)*, and in a patient with severe long-standing disease who had an attenuated bright spot *(39)*.

Treatment of ADNDI consists of administration of exogenous vasopressin or vasopressin analog. Usually the V2-specific analog dDAVP is administered once or twice a day intranasally or orally. Because this is a disease of diminished vasopressin production, the kidney remains responsive to exogenously administered V2 receptor agonist.

Animal Model

There is no animal model for autosomal-dominant diabetes insipidus. The Brattleboro rat has inherited vasopressin-deficient diabetes insipidus, but this disease is autosomal recessive, congenital, and involves hypertrophy of vasopressinergic magnocellular neurons in the hypothalamus *(40)*. The genetic locus of the murine disease is the vasopressin gene, and the mutation is a single base deletion within the coding sequence for neurophysin II *(41)*. The resulting frameshift mutation encodes a vasopressin/neurophysin/copeptin precursor with a completely novel C terminus. Furthermore, the frameshift mutation eliminates the normal stop codon, and no additional stop codon is created. Therefore the poly-A tail of the mRNA is translated and adds a highly positively charged polylysine tail to the already abnormal precursor polypeptide *(42)*. The mutant mRNA has been shown to be transcribed and translated *(42,43)*. The abnormal precursor is present in magnocellular neurons but accumulates abnormally in the endoplasmic reticulum, Golgi apparatus, and lysosomes, and little of the mutant precursor seems to be processed properly *(44,45)* so that essentially no mature vasopressin is produced in the homozygous mutant rat. In vitro and *Xenopus* oocyte expression studies indicate that the signal peptide of the mutant preproprecursor is removed by signal peptidase on the inner membrane of the endoplasmic reticulum, but the proprecursor is unable to be translated fully across the membrane for further glycosylation and processing. This processing blockage seems to be caused by the point mutation in the precursor and not by the presence of the polylysine tail or the loss of the glycosylation site because removal of the tail or introduction of an alternate glycosylation site does not allow the precursor to traverse the membrane *(46)*. However, murine magnocellular neurons are apparently not irreversibly harmed by this accumulation of precursor because intrahypothalamic injection of normal vasopressin gene mRNA *(47)* and gene conversion whereby recombination between the vasopressin and highly homologous oxytocin gene within the magnocellular neuron "repairs" the mutation *(48)* can both restore the ability to produce vasopressin in the homozygous Brattleboro rat. Similarly, the heterozygous rat shows no discernible dysfunction in anatomy or in production of vasopressin, suggesting that, although the mutant gene product is not processed correctly, it does not interfere with the production and processing of the normal allele *(40)*. This interpretation is complicated by the unexplained observation that in the heterozygote, the mutant mRNA is only detected at 5% of the level of the normal allele, and thus relatively decreased production of the mutant precursor may contribute to the normal phenotype of the heterozygote *(49)*.

Genetic Locus of Human ADNDI

Although the Brattleboro rat disease is different from human ADNDI in several significant ways, the vasopressin gene mutation in the Brattleboro rat suggested this gene as a candidate locus for ADNDI. Linkage analysis using restriction fragment length polymorphisms (RFLPs) as chromosomal markers to trace the inheritance of individual vasopressin alleles through three affected families was used *(50)*. In two families, the inheritance of one particular vasopressin allele was always associated with inheritance of ADNDI. The third family was uninformative using the identified RFLPs. The strength of the statistical association was such that the odds of this association between inheritance of one vasopressin allele and inheritance of ADNDI occurring by chance alone were <1:500. Thus, the genetic locus for ADNDI was established to be in, or very near, the vasopressin gene.

Identification of ADNDI Mutations

With the vasopressin gene identified as the genetic locus of ADNDI, the nucleotide sequence of this gene was examined in affected individuals from a number of different kindreds. A surprising heterogeneity of mutations that cause apparently identical disease was found. To date, 27 mutations that cause ADNDI have been described within the vasopressin gene and fall into one of four classes: signal peptide mutations, missense or deletion mutations within the neurophysin II-encoding portion of the gene, nonsense mutations within the neurophysin II-encoding portion of the gene, and one missense mutation within the vasopressin-encoding portion of the gene. These mutations are summarized in Table 1. In all cases, these mutations are found to be heterozygous, consistent with a dominant mode of inheritance. In all cases, the mutations detected by sequence analysis of genomic DNA have been confirmed by changes in restriction endonuclease recognition sites in genomic DNA.

Four mutations have been described that fall within the signal peptide. Each of these mutations is predicted to decrease the ability of signal peptidase to remove the signal

Table 1
Mutations That Cause Autosomal Dominant Neurohypophyseal Diabetes Insipidus

Mutation	Type	CpG dinucleotide	Amino acid alteration	Families reported	Reference
Signal peptide					
DelG227	Deletion		Del MPDT -19 - -16	1	37
C274T	Missense		Ser-3 Phe	1	53
G279A	Missense	CpG	Ala-1Thr	6	13,51,53,134
G280T	Missense	CpG	Ala-1 Val	4	12,53,62
Vasopressin					
T285C	Missense		Tyr2His	1	66
Neurophysin II					
G1730C	Missense		Gly14Arg	1	53
G1740T	Missense		Gly17Val	1	57
C1748T	Missense	CpG	Arg20Cys	1	53
G1757C	Missense		Gly23Arg	1	62
G1758T	Missense		Gly23Val	1	39
C1761T	Missense		Pro24Leu	2	59,134
DelAGG1827–1829	Deletion		Del Glu47	2	53,58
A1830G	Missense		Glu47Gly	1	53
T1839C	Missense		Leu50Pro	1	53
C1857T	Missense		Ser56Phe	1	61
G1859A	Missense	CpG	Gly57Ser	3	53,56,134
G1859C	Missense		Gly57Arg	1	53
G1872C	Missense		Cys61Ser	1	53
G1872A	Missense		Cys61Tyr	1	61
C1873A	Nonsense		Cys61X	1	53
G1874T	Missense		Gly62Trp	1	36
G1883T	Missense		Gly65Cys	1	53
G1884T	Missense		Gly65Val	2	60,135
C1891A	Nonsense		Cys67X	1	36
C2094A	Nonsense		Cys79X	1	53
CG2106/7GT	Nonsense		Pro83X	1	53
G2116T	Nonsense		Glu87X	1	53

peptide from the precursor. Two of the mutations change the last amino acid of the signal peptide (normally Ala) to amino acids [Thr *(13,51,52)* and Val *(12,53)*] that do not naturally occur in this position in signal peptides *(54)* and that do not support the proper targeting of signal peptidase *(55)*. One mutation disrupts the initiation methionine presumably forcing use of the subsequent methionine as the initiation amino acid *(37)*, and one mutation disrupts the codon for the −3 amino acid of the signal peptide substituting Phe for Ser *(53)*. These two mutations theoretically affect important recognition sites for signal peptidase and are expected to decrease the removal of signal peptide from the precursor *(37,53,54)*.

Sixteen missense mutations and one three-base deletion have been reported within the coding sequence of neurophysin II *(36,53,56–62)*. Almost all of the amino acids altered by these mutations can be hypothesized to affect the binding of vasopressin to neurophysin

II. Some mutations alter amino acids that are directly involved with vasopressin binding. For instance, Cys^1 of vasopressin forms a strong salt bridge with Glu^{47} of neurophysin II and has hydrogen bonds with Leu^{50} and Ser^{52} (63). Tyr^2 of vasopressin tightly binds neurophysin II with apolar and hydrogen bond interactions involving Cys^{10}, Cys^{21}, Phe^{22}, Gly^{23}, Pro^{24}, Cys^{44}, Glu^{47}, Asn^{48}, and Cys^{54} (63). Vasopressin has additional interactions with Leu^{50}, Pro^{51}, Ser^{52}, Pro^{53}, and Cys^{54}. Thus, the mutations that alter Gly^{14}, Gly^{17}, Arg^{20}, Gly^{23}, Pro^{24}, Glu^{47}, and Leu^{50} of neurophysin II could all reasonably be expected to alter directly binding of vasopressin to neurophysin II. Other mutations affect amino acids that are probably important for the three dimensional configuration of neurophysin II. Alteration of Cys^{61} will prevent formation of one disulfide bridge, and alterations of Gly^{57}, Gly^{62}, and Gly^{65} all place a bulky side chain in a position where no side chain normally exists. Proper folding of the precursor seems to be dependent on binding of the vasopressin moiety in the neurophysin II binding site, and thus each of these mutations might reasonably be expected to alter efficient folding and processing of the precursor polypeptide (2,4,64,65).

One missense mutation within the vasopressin coding sequence (66) has been reported to cause dominantly inherited diabetes insipidus. Consistent with the above hypotheses, the mutation alters Tyr^2 that is critically involved with the binding of vasopressin to neurophysin II (63). Therefore, this mutation, too, is hypothesized to disrupt intramolecular binding, folding, and processing of the precursor polypeptide.

Five nonsense mutations, within the coding sequence of the 93 amino acids of neurophysin II, have been described that cause ADNDI (36,53,56–60). These all fall within the C-terminal domain of neurophysin II, suggesting that nonsense mutations that might occur in the N-terminal or mid portion of the precursor do not cause ADNDI. In all five cases, a substantial portion of the proprecursor is produced before the polypeptide chain is prematurely terminated. These mutations, too, would significantly disrupt the ability of the precursor to fold and be processed, but the precursor peptide is large enough (approx 10–12 kDa for the known nonsense mutations) potentially to cause a significant accumulation of abnormal precursor.

Thus, the unifying hypothesis for each of these 27 different mutations all causing identical disease is that each in its own way disrupts proper processing of the precursor and leads to a toxic accumulation of misprocessed precursor.

Biochemical Studies

Several studies have examined the ability of a mutant precursor protein to be processed in vitro or in tissue culture systems. Two signal peptide mutations, $Ala^{-1}Thr$ and $Ala^{-1}Val$, both demonstrate decreased processing in in vitro transcription/translation/processing systems in which the initial steps of peptide precursor processing were accomplished by the presence of pancreatic microsomal membranes (51,67). The $Ala^{-1}Thr$ mutation supported a low rate of signal peptidase activity, whereas the $Ala^{-1}Val$ mutation did not support detectable signal peptidase activity. In both cases, core glycosylation proceeded normally.

Unfortunately, magnocellular neuron tissue culture is not feasible, and so expression of mutant precursor protein must be performed in heterologous tissue culture systems. The wild-type vasopressin gene and the mutation encoding the $Gly^{17}Val$ substitution were stably expressed in the AtT20 anterior pituitary cell line (68). Normal processing and regulated secretion of neurophysin II were detected in the presence of the normal gene, but the mutation dramatically decreased the amount of neurophysin II that was secreted. The intracellular mutant precursor was glycosylated in the endoplasmic reticulum but remained endoglycosidase H sensitive, indicating that glycoprotein did not transit to the Golgi where further modifications render glycoproteins endoglycosidase H resistant. Another recent study (69) used the Neuro2A neuroblastoma cell line stably expressing wild-type and mutant vasopressin genes. In this system the wild-type vasopressin gene was expressed, and vasopressin secretion was measured. Four different mutant vasopressin genes ($Arg^{-1}Thr$, $delGlu^{47}$, $Gly^{57}Ser$, and $Cys^{67}Ter$) each supported production of the predicted mRNA and precursor polypeptide, but all had significantly reduced secretion of vasopressin. Again, the precursor was shown to arrest in the endoplasmic reticulum because each remained endoglycosidase H sensitive. Additionally, when Neuro2A cell division was arrested with valproic acid, cells expressing the wild-type vasopressin gene remained viable, whereas cells expressing each of the mutant vasopressin genes had significantly decreased viability over a 6-wk time period. Although these studies do not use hypothalamic neural tissues, they suggest that a variety of vasopressin gene mutations cause accumulation of abnormal precursor in the endoplasmic reticulum and may lead to premature cell death.

Discussion

Individuals affected with ADNDI are not symptomatic at birth. They lose the ability to produce an adequate amount of vasopressin and develop symptoms of diabetes insipidus typically over the first 1–6 yr of life. ADNDI is inherited in an autosomal dominant manner, and sequence analysis has confirmed heterozygosity for mutations within the vasopressin gene. Thus, diabetes insipidus develops even in the presence of one normal vasopressin gene. Autopsy studies have shown degeneration of the vasopressinergic magnocellular neurons of the supraoptic and paraventricular nuclei of the hypothalamus. Taken together, these observations suggest that ADNDI is caused by progressive neurodegeneration of vasopressinergic magnocellular neurons. This hypothesis explains both the delayed onset (the normal gene can produce vasopressin at birth) and the dominant nature of the disease (the normal gene can no longer be expressed after the mutant gene triggers degeneration of magnocellular neurons). The diverse range of mutations that all cause clinically identical ADNDI has been surprising. The postulate that each mutation somehow alters processing of the precursor and causes accumulation of misprocessed precursor within the magnocellular neuron is now beginning to gain experimental support, although in heterologous systems.

Although this model for ADNDI accounts for many of the known features of the disease, there are some assumptions that have been made. The neurodegeneration that has been detected in autopsy studies has been examined in only four individuals, and none of these individuals has had a molecular diagnosis that confirms the presence of a vasopressin gene mutation or demonstrates which mutation is involved. It is unlikely, but possible, that only a small class of the vasopressin gene mutations that cause ADNDI are actually associated with neurodegeneration.

The model for ADNDI also creates several unanswered questions. The foremost question is how do these diverse mutations all cause abnormal precursor processing and accumulation? A related question is why can the abnormally processed precursor not be effectively handled by the proteasome pathway that is designed to degrade such misprocessed protein? A corollary question is why is this mechanism of dominant disease not recognized to occur in other cells that secrete peptide hormones? It is possible that toxic accumulation of misprocessed protein precursors actually does underlie dominantly inherited forms of other human diseases, including neurodegenerative diseases such as dominantly inherited forms of Alzheimer's or Parkinson's disease, but this is not recognized. These neurologic diseases, similar to ADNDI, involve degeneration of one specific population of neurons, perhaps because they express a mutant neuron-type specific peptide that cannot be processed properly. Neurons would be particularly susceptible to accumulation of misprocessed precursor because these are nondividing cells and, at least in the case of vasopressin, a relatively small number of cells are called on to produce a large amount of the hormone. Neurons may have an absence of or a relative deficiency in a critical class of chaperone protein that assists in proper folding of precursor peptides, making neurons particularly susceptible to accumulation of misprocessed precursor. Notably, neurons in other tissues, such as parvocellular neurons in the suprachiasmatic nucleus, the adrenals, and the gonads, that also express the mutant vasopressin gene, but express the gene in smaller quantities are apparently not troubled by accumulation of misprocessed precursor. In these tissues, the production of aberrant precursor may be slow enough to allow the cells to dispose of it, these cells may have additional capacity to handle misprocessed precursor, or continued cell division may dilute any accumulation of misprocessed precursor.

Finally, there remain the intriguing differences between the diabetes insipidus of the Brattleboro rat and human ADNDI. Many different human vasopressin gene mutations uniformly produce dominant diabetes insipidus, yet the one known mutation in the rat gene produces recessive disease and does not seem to kill these magnocellular neurons. The human and rat diseases could be different because of a truly unique feature of the Brattleboro rat mutation or of the Brattleboro rat mutation specifically in the context of the rat vasopressin gene. Alternatively, the difference in disease might be attributable to a difference between the human and the rat magnocellular neurons, such as a more active proteasome pathway or different expression of chaperone proteins. Another possibility is that the rat disease is identical to the early stages of the human disease, but the rat never lives long enough to manifest neurodegeneration and dominant disease. Perhaps a homozygous human would have congenital disease, initially with hypertrophy of the magnocellular neurons as seen in the homozygous rat. Further investigation of the mechanism of accumulation of the mutant precursor polypeptides and experiments introducing human and rat vasopressin transgenes into heterologous animals will be required to answer these questions fully.

One of the most striking features of ADNDI is the similarity of disease caused by a diverse range of mutations. However, there are also instances of the same mutation causing different manifestations that suggest that there are additional genetic or environmental influences on the presentation of the disease. Two families have been described with ADNDI that is caused by precisely the same mutation, encoding Thr^{-1}Val *(12)*. In one family from the United States, affected members have onset of symptoms at a typical age of one to two years. In the other family from Lebanon, there is an unusually delayed onset with a median age of onset of 12 yr. The delayed onset may reflect an ethnic or familial genetic difference either in some aspect of the vasopressin production pathway such as a more efficient proteasome system or in the vasopressin response in the kidney such as greater sensitivity to a low concentration of vasopressin. The different age of onset might also reflect an environmental influence such as more frequent water consumption that would lead to less production of vasopressin and therefore slower damage to magnocellular neurons.

Another variation among individuals with ADNDI is in the presentation of the posterior pituitary bright spot on MRI. In individuals with vasopressin deficiency caused by trauma or infiltrative disease, the posterior bright spot is uniformly absent. However, in individuals with ADNDI, the presence, absence, or attenuation of the bright spot has been reported. These results may indicate that some vasopressin-containing neurosecretory granules persist in the posterior pituitary for a variable period of time after onset of significant symptoms in affected individuals. These findings may also be explained by the presence of a variable amount of another substance that could generate a posterior pituitary bright signal, such as oxytocin-containing neurosecretory granules. In acquired diabetes insipidus caused by trauma, tumor, or inflammation, both oxytocin- and vaso-pressin-containing neurosecretory granules are expected to be absent from the posterior pituitary because of generalized damage to the hypothalamus and/or pituitary. In these individuals the posterior bright spot is completely absent. On the other hand, in ADNDI, only the vasopressin-containing granules are expected to be absent, and the persistence of a bright spot may reflect persistence of a normal signal from oxytocin-containing neurosecretory granules.

Another striking feature of ADNDI is the recurrence in multiple, unrelated families of a few specific mutations. The explanation may be that each of the mutations that has been reported in more than two families falls at a CpG mutational hot spot. In mammalian cells, there is an enzyme that methylates cytosine that occurs 5' of guanosine. Spontaneous demethylation of methylcytosine (which can occur either on the sense or antisense strand) creates a mutation (70), and this type of mutation is up to four orders of magnitude more frequent than other spontaneous mutations (71). The recurrent Ala^{-1}Thr, Ala^{-1}Val, and Gly^{57}Ser substitutions are all explained by mutations that occur at CpG mutational hot spots. The Arg^{20}Cys substitution is also caused by mutation at a CpG hot spot, but recurrences have not yet been reported.

X-LINKED NEPHROGENIC DIABETES INSIPIDUS

Clinical

X-linked nephrogenic diabetes insipidus is caused by abnormal functioning of the V2 vasopressin receptors. The gene for the V2 receptor is located at Xq28 on the distal tip of the long arm of the X chromosome. There is high penetrance in males who inherit a defective gene, and heterozygous females occasionally are symptomatic, presumably because of extreme lyonization of the X chromosome carrying the normal allele (72–74) or increased vasopressinase activity during pregnancy (75). Affected individuals are symptomatic from birth. Nephrogenic diabetes insipidus is frequently associated with growth failure, mental retardation and megacystis, megaureter, and hydronephrosis (76). The mental retardation is probably secondary to bouts of severe neonatal dehydration, perhaps complicated by overvigorous rehydration (77), and the dilated urinary tract is likely secondary to the elevated urine output. Presenting symptoms in a neonate are frequently irritability, intermittent fever, poor feeding, and poor weight gain, because the polyuria and polydipsia is often unrecognized (78). Definitive diagnosis of nephrogenic diabetes insipidus is made by demonstration of development of hyperosmolality with inappropriately dilute urine without an adequate urine-concentrating response to vasopressin or vasopressin analog. Additionally, an elevated serum vasopressin concentration is present because the normal neural sensing system for hyperosmolality is intact and vasopressin is secreted into the circulation in an attempt to communicate the need for increased free water resorption to the kidney. Individuals with nephrogenic diabetes insipidus have been reported to have a diminished or absent posterior bright spot by MRI in spite of their normal ability to produce vasopressin-containing granules *(25,26,29)*. This finding seems to be paradoxical, but is attributed to chronic vasopressin secretion with depletion of neurosecretory granules from the posterior pituitary, as demonstrated in an animal model *(79)*. Normally vasopressin signaling at vasopressin receptors increases cAMP production and therefore increases urinary cAMP concentration. In X-linked nephrogenic diabetes insipidus, the defective receptor abolishes this increase in urinary cAMP. V2 receptors are also located in the vascular endothelium and, when triggered, cause release of coagulation factor VIII, von Willebrand factor antigen, and tissue-type plasminogen activator, and cause vascular smooth muscle relaxation that is manifest as a decrease in blood pressure *(80)*. In patients with X-linked nephrogenic diabetes insipidus, all of these V2 receptor-mediated responses are deficient *(7,81)*.

Treatment of X-linked nephrogenic diabetes insipidus is less straightforward than the hormone replacement therapy for central diabetes insipidus. Sodium depletion induced by sodium restriction and thiazide natriuresis is a form of indirect therapy that is somewhat successful *(82)*. Sodium depletion results in vigorous sodium resorption in the proximal tubules of the kidney, and water follows passively resulting in decreased fluid delivery to the collecting duct. The presence of elevated urinary prostaglandins in nephrogenic diabetes insipidus prompted therapeutic trials of prostaglandin synthesis inhibitors alone or in combination with thiazide diuretics *(83,84)*. Some patients show significant responses, but side effects are frequent. Therapy with thiazide plus amelioride (which contributes to natriuresis by blocking sodium/potassium exchange in the collecting duct) augments the therapeutic effect of thiazide alone and prevents the hypokalemia frequently associated with prolonged thiazide therapy *(85,86)* and is perhaps the best therapeutic option.

An autosomal recessive form of nephrogenic diabetes that also involves the receptors or an early postreceptor defect has been reported *(87)* in sisters of consanguineous parents. They had a nonaffected father, inherited different X chromosomes from their mother, and did not increase urinary cAMP in response to vasopressin. Thus the disease does not seem to be X-linked but, similar to X-linked diabetes insipidus, involves defective coupling of vasopressin receptors to cAMP production.

Gene Structure and Mutations

The human V2 receptor was cloned in 1992 and found to belong to the family of seven transmembrane-spanning domain G protein-coupled receptors *(8,9)*. The cDNA encodes a 371-amino acid polypeptide with a molecular weight of 40,285 Daltons. The N terminus is predicted to be extracellular, and the C terminus is intracellular. With seven transmembrane spans, there are three intracellular and three extracellular loops formed. The gene contains two small introns and three coding exons. The first exon encodes the first nine amino acids that are all in the extracellular domain. The second exon encodes six transmembrane domains, and the third encodes the seventh transmembrane domain. Expression of the cDNA in G9 cells produced vasopressin-specific binding activity and vasopressin-stimulated cAMP production *(9)*. The rat V2 receptor was cloned by homology with the rat V1 receptor and was found to be structurally and functionally similar to the human V2 receptor *(88)* and to have numerous phosphorylation consensus sites that were identified in the C-terminal domain. Many mutations in the V2 receptor gene in individuals with nephrogenic diabetes insipidus were thereafter reported in rapid succession. The first two were a frameshift mutation that created a premature stop codon in the third intracellular loop and a missense mutation that predicted substitution of Asp for Ala^{132} in the third transmembrane domain *(89)*. Other mutations included deletion, insertion, missense, and nonsense mutations throughout the receptor *(90–100)*. Approximately 70 mutations have been reported, and a recent summary of mutations has been published *(101)*. Nonsense mutations occur throughout the cDNA, including one that encodes Arg^{337}X and truncates the C terminal of the receptor by only 35 amino acids. Missense mutations are likewise scattered throughout the cDNA and create amino acid substitutions in the extracellular, transmembrane, and intracellular domains. There is a particularly high density of missense mutations that fall within the transmembrane domains. A 28-base-pair deletion flanked by a 9-base-pair direct repeat was reported in one family *(98)*, and a duplication of these same nucleotides is reported in several families *(98,99)*. This duplication and deletion fall within the N-terminal extracellular domain of the receptor. Several unexpected findings have been reported in otherwise typical X-linked nephrogenic diabetes insipidus. There are occasionally patients with no mutation identified in the V2 receptor gene, suggesting a defect in an accessory protein or in a regulatory sequence of the V2 receptor gene. In one case, two affected brothers inherited different V2 receptor genes from their mother, demonstrating that the V2 gene is not the genetic locus of diabetes insipidus in this family *(91)*. Another case report revealed an unexpected silent polymorphism, reported as Val^{108}Met, that was present in unaffected male relatives of a patient *(91)*.

Functional Studies

Numerous mutations have been described in the V2 receptor gene, but proof that these mutations cause receptor dysfunction is not presented in most reports. For normal functioning, V2 receptors require proper gene transcription, translation, processing, and insertion into the membrane, as well as normal vasopressin binding activity, transmembrane signal transduction, and coupling to G proteins. Truncated receptors are reasonably presumed to have lost at least their capacity for coupling, which is a property of the third intracellular loop and C terminus of the other seven transmembrane domain receptors. Depending on the location of the premature stop codon, transmembrane signaling and vasopressin binding activity may be presumed to be lost, as well. However, the effect of missense mutations on the receptor is harder to predict. The first mutation to be studied functionally was the Arg^{137}His substitution that falls just at the boundary of the membrane and the second intracellular loop. This mutation is highly conserved in G protein-coupled receptors. The mutation was recreated in cDNA, cloned into the expression vector pKNH, and transfected transiently into COS.M6 cells and stably into Ltk$^-$ cells *(102)*. The wild-type and mutant receptors bound vasopressin with equal affinity, but surprisingly the amount of expression of the mutant protein was only 7% that of the wild-type in the transient transfections. Furthermore, the mutant receptor, in contrast to the wild-type, did not mediate stimulation of cAMP production in the presence of vasopressin. Even in a stably transfected cell line selected for a high level of expression of the mutant cDNA, no vasopressin-stimulated increase in cAMP could be detected. Thus, this mutation does not affect the binding of ligand but does demonstrate reduced expression of protein on the membrane, perhaps as a consequence of protein misfolding, and furthermore does not support coupling of ligand binding to stimulated cAMP production. In contrast, when the mutation encoding Tyr^{205}Cys at the interface between the transmembrane domain and the second extracellular loop was transiently expressed in COS cells, equivalent numbers of receptors were expressed on the cell surface. However, the affinity of the mutant receptor for vasopressin was reduced 10-fold, and there was a reduced maximum accumulation of cAMP in response to vasopressin, raising the question of reduced transmembrane signaling or coupling to G protein *(103)*. The deletion of Val^{278} in the sixth transmembrane domain did not support any vasopressin binding, but it was not determined whether this is because of reduced expression or reduced binding of vasopressin *(101)*. Another mutation encoding Arg^{143}Pro in the second intracellular loop was stably expressed in CHO cells and showed a 10-fold decrease in cell-surface expression but normal affinity and the ability to stimulate cAMP production to up to 50% of the level of the wild-type construct *(101)*. The mutation encoding Arg^{113}Trp has been shown to have a combination of partial defects including binding capacity, affinity, and coupling *(104)*. Arg^{202}Cys in the third extracellular domain was demonstrated by transient transfection in COS-7 to have binding affinity for vasopressin reduced to 15% of normal and to have the maximal capacity to stimulate cAMP production reduced to 30% of normal *(105)*. This same study found that the Arg^{202}Cys mutation produced no binding at all in stable transfections in CHO cells, and this binding deficit could be explained by reduced binding affinity or, more likely, by absence of cell surface expression of the protein. Similarly, the insG^{804} that produces a premature stop in the third intracellular loop abolished all vasopressin binding *(105)*. One elegant study *(106)* confirmed the observation that many mutations disrupt cell surface expression of the receptor protein and in addition examined the total amount of mutant receptor protein produced. The V2 receptor cDNA was engineered to encode an epitope tag of 10 amino acids from the influenza hemagglutinin protein at the N terminus of the V2 receptor. The cDNA was cloned into a mammalian expression vector, and four mutations that cause X-linked nephrogenic diabetes insipidus were individually recreated in this construct. The epitope tag allowed immunologic localization of the expressed protein in stably transfected CHO cells. This study defined four classes of mutations: those that express protein normally on the cell surface but are defective in binding vasopressin (such as Arg^{202}Cys), those that express protein normally on the cell surface and bind vasopressin but have defective signal transduction or coupling to G proteins (such as Arg^{137}His), those that make V2 receptor protein but do not express the protein on the cell surface (such as Arg^{143}Pro or delVal^{278}), and those that do not produce detectable protein at all (such as InsG^{804}).

Surprisingly, the loss of vasopressin-stimulated increases in cAMP caused by V2 receptor mutations in the third intracellular loop or in the sixth or seventh transmembrane domains could be reversed by coexpression with a cDNA encoding the mutation-free C-terminal domain of the V2 receptor *(107)*. This rescuing V2 receptor tail includes a portion of the third intracellular loop and the sixth and seventh transmembrane domains *(107)*. Nine mutations were all shown to be partially to fully functionally rescued and included missense, nonsense, frameshift, and deletion mutations. The rescued abnormal receptors included some that were not expressed on the cell surface as determined by the epitope tag approach. In these coexpression studies, vasopressin was able to stimulate almost normal amounts of cAMP production. However, the study did not report the effect on cAMP generation of expressing the V2 receptor tail alone and did not explore the surprising finding that the response to vasopressin was restored without significant restoration of cell surface expression of the mutant V2 receptors. The report suggests that the V2 receptor has several domains that fold independently and that the presence of a normal C-terminal domain may facilitate the folding of a receptor with a mutation in this domain, suggesting a potential approach to gene therapy.

Discussion

Classical X-linked nephrogenic diabetes insipidus is caused by mutations in the V2 receptor gene, but there are reports of apparent X-linked nephrogenic diabetes insipidus that do not involve this gene. As seen for ADNDI, a wide range of mutations in different portions of the V2 receptor have been described that each cause a clinically indistinguishable disease phenotype. Each mutation seems to prevent coupling between the presence of vasopressin and the generation of cAMP within the principle cell of the collecting duct. However, four different mechanisms have been identified that block this coupling, including decreased production of the receptor, decreased expression of the receptor on the cell surface, decreased binding of vasopressin, and decreased transmembrane signal transduction or coupling to G protein. Thus as seen for ADNDI, clinical homogeneity results even though there is diverse molecular heterogeneity.

The fact that X-linked nephrogenic diabetes insipidus results from receptor dysfunction makes effective treatment challenging. Current therapy does not address the underlying misfunction but instead only partially compensates for it. With the molecular mechanisms of various forms of X-linked nephrogenic diabetes insipidus beginning to be understood, alternative therapies could be explored such as maximizing a small signal from a receptor with subnormal signaling ability by use of a cyclic nucleotide phosphodiesterase inhibitor to slow the degradation of cAMP, overcoming the defect in a receptor with a lowered affinity for vasopressin by use of a high dose of dDAVP, and perhaps some day rescuing poorly expressed protein by use of gene therapy.

AUTOSOMAL-RECESSIVE NEPHROGENIC DIABETES INSIPIDUS

Clinical

Autosomal-recessive nephrogenic diabetes insipidus is caused by abnormality in the aquaporin-2 water channels. The gene for this protein was assigned to chromosome 12q13 by *in situ* hybridization *(108)*. Heterozygotes are clinically unaffected, and thus one functional allele of this gene is sufficient to mediate water resorption in the collecting duct of the kidney. Clinically, this disorder is indistinguishable from X-linked nephrogenic diabetes insipidus, but biochemical testing demonstrates an intact increase in urinary cAMP in response to vasopressin challenge. The disease is distinguished from X-linked nephrogenic diabetes insipidus by its unique inheritance pattern, by intact urinary cAMP response to vasopressin, and by intact nonrenal V2 receptor-mediated responses, such as release of coagulation factor VIII. Treatment of autosomal recessive nephrogenic diabetes insipidus is the same as that described for the X-linked form.

Biochemistry and Molecular Genetics

There is a family of at least six homologous proteins that confer water permeability to lipid bilayer membranes *(109)*. Aquaporin-1 was the first to be described as a component of the red blood cell membrane and in fact was later shown to be responsible for the Colton blood group antigen. Aquaporin-1 is a 28 kDa protein, and examination of the amino acid sequence encoded by the cDNA reveals six membrane-spanning domains *(110)*. The ability of aquaporins to allow water flow across a biological membrane has been most elegantly demonstrated by expression of aquaporin mRNA in *Xenopus* oocytes. The oocytes acquire a 10-fold increased water permeability measured as a dramatic increase in the rate of osmotic swelling *(111,112)*. Reconstitution of purified aquaporin-1 in artificially created phospholipid liposomes demonstrated that this protein does not need accessory proteins to confer increased water permeability. Aquaporin-1 was subsequently identified as an abundant protein in the proximal tubule and the descending thin limb of the loop of Henle where the initial 90% of the volume of the renal ultrafiltrate is resorbed *(113)*. Amazingly, individuals found to be missing aquaporin-1 (identified by absence of Colton antigen) appear to be clinically normal *(114)*. A rat homolog of aquaporin-1 was cloned *(115)* and found to be expressed exclusively in the renal collecting duct and was called WCH-CD for water channel collecting duct. This clone was used to screen a human kidney cDNA library, and a human cDNA clone was isolated and called aquaporin-2. This clone encodes a 291 amino acid protein that has 90% sequence identity with rat WCH-CD and was assigned to human chromosome 12q13 by *in situ* hybridization *(108,112,116)*. The gene comprises four exons and spans five kilobases of genomic DNA *(117)*. It is expressed in principal cells of the collecting duct of the kidney both in intracellular vesicles and on the apical membrane in contact with the renal ultrafiltrate *(118)*. Vasopressin causes both the translocation of aquaporin-2-containing vesicles to the apical membrane and an increase in aquaporin-2 expression *(119)*. Lithium, which can cause drug-induced nephrogenic diabetes insipidus, produces decreased expression of aquaporin-2 *(120)*. Aquaporin-3 is constitutively expressed on the basolateral aspects of the principal cell of the collecting duct and allows water resorbed from the ultrafiltrate to exit the principal cell and enter the renal interstitium. Aquaporin-3 is also widely expressed in other tissues. Aquaporin-4 is widely expressed in the brain, including in the supraoptic and paraventricular nuclei of the hypothalamus, and may, therefore, allow the stretch and shrinking of hypothalamic neurons that mediate measurement of plasma osmolality and release of vasopressin. Other members of the aquaporin family include aquaporin-0 found in the lens of the eye and aquaporin-5 found in salivary and lacrimal glands.

The aquaporins all have six putative membrane-spanning domains with the first half of the protein, containing three of these domains, homologous with the second half, but with opposite intracellular/extracellular orientation in the two halves. Both the N and C termini are intracellular, and therefore, there are three extracellular loops and two intracellular loops. The protein seems to insert into the membrane as a tetramer, but each polypeptide chain is an independently functioning water channel.

Mutations and Functional Studies

The initial patient with autosomal recessive nephrogenic diabetes insipidus, whose aquaporin-2 genes were analyzed *(112)*, was found to be a compound heterozygote with a mutation in one aquaporin-2 gene encoding $Arg^{187}Cys$ in the third extracellular loop and a mutation in the other aquaporin-2 gene encoding $Ser^{216}Pro$ in the sixth transmembrane domain. Each mutation was recreated in cDNA and expressed in *Xenopus* oocytes; neither facilitated osmotic swelling *(112)*. Three patients with consanguineous parents were studied, and one was found to be homozygous for the mutation encoding Arg[187]Cys, one was homozygous for a novel mutation encoding Gly[64]Arg, and the third was homozygous for a single-base mutation, delC369, that results in a premature termination in the second extracellular loop *(121)*. Again, expression studies in *Xenopus* oocytes produced no functional water channels with any of the mutants. The molecular basis for the reduced activity in *Xenopus* oocytes was studied for Gly[64]Arg, Arg[187]Cys, and Ser[216]Pro *(122)*. In each case, the protein was translated into precursor polypeptide but abnormally processed and retained in the endoplasmic reticulum, suggesting that the molecular basis for the dysfunction of these mutant proteins is impaired routing to the intracellular vesicles and plasma membrane *(122)*. Similarly, Ala[147]Thr and Thr[126]Met confer a small increase in water permeability to *Xenopus* oocyte membranes, whereas Asn[68]Ser does not, and none of these is significantly routed to the cell membrane *(123)*. Recently, mutations encoding Trp[202]Cys in the third extracellular loop *(124)* and Gly[100]Ter in the third transmembrane domain *(125)* were also identified but not functionally characterized.

Discussion

Autosomal recessive nephrogenic diabetes insipidus is caused by mutation in the aquaporin-2 gene. Only nine mutations have been found in association with this disease, and studies in a model system suggest that at least some of these mutations prevent proper processing and impair routing of the water channel protein.

DIDMOAD OR WOLFRAM SYNDROME

Clinical

The DIDMOAD syndrome is an autosomal recessive disorder named as an acronym for its principle clinical features: acquired Diabetes Insipidus, Diabetes Mellitus, Optic Atrophy, and Deafness. It is also variably associated with other neurodegenerative features including progressive ataxia, peripheral neuropathy, dementia, depression, and other psychiatric illnesses. The syndrome was first described by Wolfram and Wagener *(126)* and is frequently referred to as Wolfram syndrome. Symptoms typically develop over the first three decades of life with diabetes mellitus as the most frequent initial presenting feature. The diabetes mellitus was not associated with antiislet cell antibodies in one patient *(127)*. The diabetes insipidus was demonstrated to be caused by vasopressin deficiency in one 14-yr-old patient who also had diabetes mellitus and optic atrophy but normal hearing *(128)*. She, along with many other DIDMOAD patients, also had hydronephrosis and dilation of the urinary bladder, and these resolved after vasopressin analog therapy for her diabetes insipidus, suggesting that these features may be secondary to polyuria alone. There is some evidence of an increased incidence of psychiatric illness in heterozygotes as well as in homozygotes *(129)*. MRI studies of two unrelated patients demonstrated widespread atrophic changes throughout the brain *(130)*.

Molecular Genetics

The mutation that is responsible for DIDMOAD was demonstrated by linkage analysis to map to chromosomal locus 4p16.1 *(131)* and there is some evidence of a second locus in a minority of families. The gene that is responsible has not been identified. Biochemical investigation of a 13-yr-old girl with DIDMOAD revealed a generalized deficiency of mitochondrial respiratory chain enzymes in lymphocytes and in skeletal muscle *(127)*. Further investigation revealed that the patient had two populations of mitochondrial DNA (mtDNA): normal 16.5 kb circular mtDNA and partially deleted, approx 9 kb circular mtDNA. Mitochondrial DNA normally contains 15 genes that encode 2 rRNAs and 13 respiratory chain enzyme components. Nuclear DNA encodes the remainder of the respiratory chain components. This patient had a specific 7.7 kb mtDNA deletion that involved deletion of 11 respiratory chain protein genes. The deletion was flanked by 11 base-pair direct repeats that presumably targeted this segment for deletion via homologous recombination or slippage mispairing. The autosomal recessive inheritance of DIDMOAD is not consistent with inheritance of a mtDNA deletion, because mtDNA is maternally inherited. In addition, neither parent of the index patient had detectable mtDNA deletions. In another study *(132)*, a 20-yr-old female with DIDMOAD was found to have mild mitochondrial enzyme deficiencies and a subpopulation of 8 kb mtDNA that was present in 23% of lymphocyte mtDNA molecules. The 8.5 kb deletion almost coincided with the 7.7 kb deletion described previously and was flanked by imperfect 7 base-pair direct repeats. This deletion was not detected in lymphocyte mtDNA from 40 control individuals but was present in 4–6% of lymphocyte mtDNA from each parent and a sister unaffected by DIDMOAD. The fact that the father's mtDNA was also abnormal demonstrates that the mtDNA mutations are not inherited but presumably arise as a result of the chromosome 4p16.1 mutation, which in fact must be semidominant. One additional study *(133)* reported two affected families. In one, lymphocyte mitochondrial enzyme studies were performed and confirmed a deficit in activity. In both, mtDNA deletions were identified that involved the same region of the mtDNA described in the other studies, but there was heterogeneity in the endpoints of the deletions identified from each affected individual. In each case, the deletions involved mtDNA segments flanked by direct repeats. Family members who were shown to be carriers of the 4p16.1 mutation also had a low frequency of mtDNA deletions. Of particular interest in this study was the finding that the brain contained a much higher percentage of deleted mtDNA (85–90%) compared with lymphocytes, liver, or skeletal muscle (5%) in the one affected patient studied. Thus, the predominant clinical picture of neurodegenerative defects correlates with the higher level of defective mtDNA in the brain.

Discussion

DIDMOAD is an autosomal recessive syndrome that includes vasopressin-deficient diabetes insipidus and seems to involve mutations that increase the incidence of mtDNA deletions. The precise sites of mtDNA deletions varies in different families (and perhaps within affected individuals). These deletions cause a generalized deficiency in mitochondrial respiratory chain enzyme activity, presumably causing a deficiency in ATP production. The mitochondrial enzyme deficiency is most severe in brain tissues and corresponds with the anatomic site of greatest general functional defect. However, the mechanism by which a generalized deficiency in energy production causes specific loss of insulin and vasopressin secretion is not clear. One potential explanation is that the autosomal mutation has independent parallel effects on mitochondria and on insulin and vasopressin production. One hypothetical possibility would be a defect in a precursor protein-processing enzyme that leads to defective production of insulin, vasopressin, and a mitochondrial DNA repair protein.

SUMMARY AND CONCLUSIONS

Four different inherited forms of diabetes insipidus have been described. Three involve specific defects in the hypothalamic/posterior pituitary/renal water conservation axis, and one is a syndrome that includes vasopressin-deficient diabetes insipidus along with other hormone and neurologic deficits. Specific mutations have been described that cause abnormality of vasopressin production, of renal vasopressin receptors, and of the ultimate renal effector molecule, aquaporin-2. Each can be distinguished biochemically, and fortuitously, each has a distinct pattern of inheritance. Surprisingly, there is a large and diverse group of mutations that produce each specific form of diabetes insipidus, and each mutant gene seems to produce a protein that is dysfunctional in large part because of abnormality in processing and intracellular trafficking of the precursor protein. However, only ADNDI seems to cause a defect significant enough to compromise the viability of the cell in which it is produced.

Many other proteins are presumably involved in the water resorption axis, including G proteins, adenylyl cyclase, protein kinase A, a phosphorylation acceptor protein responsible for translocation of aquaporin-2 vesicles to the apical membrane, and others. Thus, it is likely that additional mutations that produce inherited diabetes insipidus will be identified in the future.

REFERENCES

1. Sausville E, Carney D, Battey J. The human vasopressin gene is linked to the oxytocin gene and is selectively expressed in a cultured lung cancer cell line. J Biol Chem 1985;260:10,236–10,241.
2. Breslow E, Burman S. Molecular, thermodynamic, and biological aspects of recognition and function in neurophysin-hormone systems: a model system for the analysis of protein-peptide interactions. Adv Enzymol Relat Areas Mol Biol 1990;63:1–67.
3. Burman S, Wellner D, Chait B, Chaudhary T, Breslow E. Complete assignment of neurophysin disulfides indicates pairing in two separate domains. Proc Natl Acad Sci USA 1989;86:429–433.
4. Huang HB, Breslow E. Identification of the unstable neurophysin disulfide and localization to the hormone-binding site. Relationship to folding-unfolding pathways. J Biol Chem 1992;267:6750–6756.
5. Orloff J, Handler J. The role of adenosine 3',5'-phosphate in the action of antidiuretic hormone. Amer J Med 1967;42:757–768.
6. Richardson DW. Desmopressin. Ann Int Med 1985;103:228–239.
7. Bichet DG, Razi M, Lonergan M, Arthus M-F, Papukna V, Kortas C, Barjon J-N. Hemodynamic and coagulation responses to 1-desamino[8-D-arginine]vasopressin in patients with congenital nephrogenic diabetes insipidus. N Engl J Med 1988;318:881–886.
8. Seibold A, Brabet P, Rosenthal W, Birnbaumer M. Structure and chromosomal localization of the human antidiuretic hormone receptor gene. Am J Hum Genet 1997;51:1078–1083.
9. Birnbaumer M, Seibold A, Gilbert S, Ishido M, Barberis C, Antaramian A, Rosenthal W. Molecular cloning of the receptor for human antidiuretic hormone. Nature 1992;357:333–335.
10. van Lieburg AF, Knoers NVAM, Deen PMT. Discovery of aquaporins: a breakthrough in research on renal water transport. Pediatr Nephrol 1995;9:228–234.
11. Kaplowitz PB, D'Ercole AJ, Robertson GL. Radioimmunoassay of vasopressin in familial central diabetes insipidus. J Pediatr 1982;100:76–81.
12. Repaske DR, Medlej R, Gultekin EK, Krishnamani MRS, Halaby G, Findling JW, Phillips JA III. Heterogeneity in clinical manifestation of autosomal dominant neurohypophyseal diabetes insipidus caused by a mutation encoding Ala -1 -> Val in the signal peptide of the arginine vasopressin/neurophysin II/copeptin precursor. J Clin Endocrinol Metab 1997;82:51–56.
13. McLeod JF, Kovacs L, Gaskill MB, Rittig S, Bradley GS, Robertson GL. Familial neurohypophyseal diabetes insipidus associated with a signal peptide mutation. J Clin Endocrinol Metab 1993;77:599A–599G.

14. Braverman LE, Mancini JP, McGoldrich DM. Hereditary idiopathic diabetes insipidus. A case report with autopsy findings. Ann Int Med 1965;63:503–508.
15. Green JR, Buchan GC, Alvord EC Jr, Swanson AG. Hereditary and idiopathic types of diabetes insipidus. Brain 1967;90:707–714.
16. Bergeron C, Kovacs K, Ezrin C, Mizzen C. Hereditary diabetes insipidus: an immunohistochemical study of the hypothalamus and pituitary gland. Acta Neuropathol 1991;81:345–248.
17. Repaske DR, Phillips JA, III. The molecular biology of human hereditary central diabetes insipidus. In: Swaab DF, Hofman MA, Mirmiran M, Ravid R, Van Leeuwen FW, eds., The Human Hypothalamus in Health and Disease. Elsevier, Amsterdam, 1992, pp. 295–308.
18. Miller WL. Editorial: Molecular genetics of familial central diabetes insipidus. J Clin Endocrinol Metab 1993;77:592–595.
19. Nussey SS, Ang VTY, Jenkins JS, Chowdrey HS, Bisset GW. Brattleboro rat adrenal contains vasopressin. Nature 1984;310:64–66.
20. Lim ATW, Lolait SJ, Barlow JW, Autelitano DJ, Toh BH, Boublik J, et al. Immunoreactive arginine-vasopressin in Brattleboro rat ovary. Nature 1984;310:61–64.
21. Kasson BG, Hsueh AJW. Arginine vasopressin as an intragonadal hormone in Brattleboro rats: presence of a testicular vasopressin-like peptide and functional vasopressin receptors. Endocrinology 1986;118:23–31.
22. Fujisawa I, Asato R, Nishimura K, Togashi K, Itoh K, Nakano Y, Itoh H, et al. Anterior and posterior lobes of the pituitary gland: assessment by 1.5 T Imaging. J Comput Assist Tomogr 1987;11:214–220.
23. Mark LP, Haughton VM, Hendrix LE, Daniels DL, Williams AL, Czervionke LF, Asleson RJ. High-intensity signals within the posterior pituitary fossa: a study with fat-suppression MR techniques. Am J Neuroradiol 1991;12:529–532.
24. Gudinchet F, Brunelle F, Barth MO, Taviere V, Brauner R, Rappaport R, Lallemand D. MR imaging of the posterior hypophysis in children. Am J Neuroradiol 1989;10:511–514.
25. Maghnie M, Villa A, Arico M, Larizza D, Pezzotta S, Beluffi G, et al. Correlation between magnetic resonance imaging of posterior pituitary and neurohypophyseal function in children with diabetes insipidus. J Clin Endocrinol Metab 1992;74:795–800.
26. Sato N, Ishizaka H, Yagi H, Matsumoto M, Endo K. Posterior lobe of the pituitary in diabetes insipidus: dynamic MR imaging. Radiology 1993;186:357–360.
27. Colombo N, Berry I, Kucharczyk J, Kucharczyk W, de Groot J, Larson T, et al. Posterior pituitary gland: appearance on MR images in normal and pathologic states. Neuroradiology 1987;165:481–485.
28. Brooks BS, El Gammal T, Allison JD, Hoffman WH. Frequency and variation of the posterior pituitary bright signal on MR images. Am J Neuroradiol 1989;10:943–948.
29. Moses AM. Use of T1-weighted MR imaging to differentiate between primary polydipsia and central diabetes insipidus. Am J Neuroradiol 1992;13:1273–1277.
30. Fujisawa I, Nishimura K, Asato R, Togashi K, Itoh K, Noma S, et al. Posterior lobe of the pituitary in diabetes insipidus: MR findings. J Comput Assist Tomogr 1987;11:221–225.
31. Chiumello G, Di Natale B, Pellini C, Beneggi A, Scotti G, Triulzi F. Magnetic resonance imaging in diabetes insipidus. Lancet 1989;i:901.
32. Cacciari E, Zucchini S, Carla G, Pirazzoli P, Cicognani A, Mandini M, et al. Endocrine function and morphological findings in patients with disorders of the hypothalamo-pituitary area: a study with magnetic resonance. Arch Dis Child 1990;65:1199–1202.
33. Tien R, Kucharczyk J, Kucharczyk W. MR imaging of the brain in patients with diabetes insipidus. Am J Neuroradiol 1991;12:533–542.
34. Imura H, Nakao K, Shimatsu A, Ogawa Y, Sando T, Fujisawa I, Yamabe H. Lymphocytic infundibulo-neurohypophysitis as a cause of central diabetes insipidus. N Engl J Med 1993;329: 683–689.
35. Appignani B, Landy H, Barnes P. MR in idiopathic central diabetes insipidus of childhood. Am J Neuroradiol 1993;14:1406,1407.
36. Nagasaki H, Ito M, Yuasa H, Saito H, Fukase M, Hanada K, et al. Two novel mutations in the coding region for neurophysin-II associated with familial central diabetes insipidus. J Clin Endocrinol Metab 1995;80:1352–1356.
37. Rutishauser J, Boni-Schnetzler M, Boni J, Wichmann W, Huisman T, Vallotton MB, Froesch ER. A novel point mutation in the translation initiation codon of the pre-pro-vasopressin-neurophysin II gene: cosegregation with morphological abnormalities and clinical symptoms in autosomal dominant neurohypophyseal diabetes insipidus. J Clin Endocrinol Metab 1996;81:192–198.
38. Lacombe LU. De la polydipsie. J Med Chir 1841;7:305–339.

39. Gagliardi PC, Bernasconi S, Repaske DR. Autosomal dominant neurohypophyseal diabetes insipidus associated with a missense mutation encoding Gly23 -> Val in neurophysin II. J Clin Endocrinol Metab 1997;82:3643–3646.

40. Ivell R, Burbach PH, Van Leeuwen FW. The molecular biology of the Brattleboro rat. Frontiers in Neuroendocrinology 1990;11:313–338.

41. Schmale H, Richter D. Single base deletion in the vasopressin gene is the cause of diabetes insipidus in Brattleboro rats. Nature 1984;308:705–709.

42. Ivell R, Schmale H, Krisch B, Nahke P, Richter D. Expression of a mutant vasopressin gene: differential polyadenylation and read-through of the mRNA 3' end in a frameshift mutant. EMBO J 1986;5:971–977.

43. McCabe JT, Morrell JI, Ivell R, Schmale H, Richter D, Pfaff DW. Brattleboro rat hypothalamic neurons transcribe vasopressin gene: Evidence from in situ hybridization. Neuroendocrinology 1986;44:361–364.

44. Krisch B, Nahke P, Richter D. Immunocytochemical staining of supraoptic neurons from homozygous Brattleboro rats by use of antibodies against two domains of the mutated vasopressin precursor. Cell Tissue Res 1986;244:351–358.

45. Van Leeuwen FW, van der Beek EM. The amount of mutant vasopressin precursor in the supraoptic and paraventricular nucleus of Brattleboro rats increases with age. Brain Res 1991;542:163–166.

46. Schmale H, Borowiak B, Holtgreve-Grez H, Richter D. Impact of altered protein structures on the intracellular traffic of a mutated vasopressin precursor from Brattleboro rats. Eur J Biochem 1989;182:621–627.

47. Jirikowski GF, Sanna PP, Maciejewski-Lenoir D, Bloom FE. Reversal of diabetes insipidus in Brattleboro rats: Intrahypothalamic injection of vasopressin mRNA. Science 1992;255:996–998.

48. van Leeuwen F, van der Beek E, Seger M, Burbach P, Ivell R. Age-related development of a heterozygous phenotype in solitary neurons of the homozygous Brattleboro rat. Proc Natl Acad Sci USA 1989;86:6417–6420.

49. Sherman TG, Watson SJ. Differential expression of vasopressin alleles in the Brattleboro heterozygote. J Neurosci 1988;8:3797–3811.

50. Repaske DR, Phillips JA, III, Kirby LT, Tze WJ, D'Ercole AJ, Battey J. Molecular analysis of autosomal dominant neurohypophyseal diabetes insipidus. J Clin Endocrinol Metab 1990;70:752–757.

51. Ito M, Oiso Y, Murase T, Kondo K, Saito H, Chinzei T, Racchi M, Lively MO. Possible involvement of inefficient cleavage of preprovasopressin by signal peptidase as a cause for familial central diabetes insipidus. J Clin Invest 1993;91:2565–2571.

52. Krishnamani MRS, Phillips JA, III, Copeland KC. Detection of a novel arginine vasopressin defect by dideoxy fingerprinting. J Clin Endocrinol Metab 1993;77:596–598.

53. Rittig S, Robertson GL, Siggaard C, Kovacs L, Gregersen N, Nyborg J, Pedersen EB. Identification of 13 new mutations in the vasopressin-neurophysin II gene in 17 kindreds with familial autosomal dominant neurohypophyseal diabetes insipidus. Am J Hum Genet 1996;58:107–117.

54. von Heijne G. A new method for predicting signal sequence cleavage sites. Nucleic Acids Res 1986;14:4683–4691.

55. Folz RJ, Nothwehr SF, Gordon JI. Substrate specificity of eukaryotic signal peptidase. Site-saturation mutagenesis at position-1 regulates cleavage between multiple sites in human pre(delta-pro)apolipoprotein A-II. J Biol Chem 1988;263:2070–2078.

56. Ito M, Mori Y, Oiso Y, Saito H. A single base substitution in the coding region for neurophysin II associated with familial central diabetes insipidus. J Clin Invest 1991;87:725–728.

57. Bahnsen U, Oosting P, Swaab DF, Nahke P, Richter D, Schmale H. A missense mutation in the vasopressin-neurophysin precursor gene cosegregates with human autosomal dominant neurohypophyseal diabetes insipidus. EMBO J 1992;11:19–23.

58. Yuasa H, Ito M, Nagasake H, Oiso Y, Miyamoto S, Sasake N, Saito H. Glu-47, which forms a salt bridge between neurophysin-II and arginine vasopressin, is deleted in patients with familial central diabetes insipidus. J Clin Endocrinol Metab 1993;77:600–604.

59. Repaske DR, Browning JE. A de novo mutation in the coding sequence for neurophysin II (Pro24->Leu) is associated with onset and transmission of autosomal dominant neurohypophyseal diabetes insipidus. J Clin Endocrinol Metab 1994;79:421–427.

60. Rauch F, Lenzner C, Nurnberg P, Frommel C, Vetter U. A novel mutation in the coding region of neurophysin-II is associated with autosomal dominant neurohypophyseal diabetes insipidus. Clin Endocrinol 1996;44:45–51.

61. Grant FD, Ahmadi A, Majzoub J. Identification of novel vasopressin mutations in two familial diabetes insipidus kindreds. Endocrine Soc 1997; P1–481 (abstract).

62. Heppner C, Kotzka J, Bullman C, Crone W, Muller-Wieland D. Identification of mutations of the arginine vasopressin-neurophysin II gene in two kindreds with familial central diabetes insipidus. Endocrine Soc 1997; P3–472 (abstract).

63. Chen LQ, Rose JP, Breslow E, Yang D, Chang WR, Furey WF, Jr., Sax M, Wang BC. Crystal structure of a bovine neurophysin II dipeptide complex at 2.8 A determined from the single-wavelength anomalous scattering signal of an incorporated iodine atom. Proc Natl Acad Sci USA 1991;88:4240–4244.

64. Breslow EMG. The conformation and functional domains of neurophysins. In: Gross P, Richter D, Robertson GL, eds. Vasopressin John Libbey Eurotext, Paris, 1993; pp. 143–157.

65. Huang H-B, Breslow E. Identification of the unstable neurophysin disulfide and localization to the hormone-binding site. Relationship to folding-unfolding pathways. J Biol Chem 1996;267: 6750–6756.

66. Rittig S, Siggaard C, Ozata M, Yetkin I, Gundetrgorn MA, Robertson GL, Pedersen EB. Familial neurohypophyseal diabetes insipidus due to mutation that substitutes histidine for tyrosine 2 in the antidiuretic hormone. J Invest Med 1996;44:387A (abstract).

67. Srivuthana K, Gultekin EK, Browning JE, Repaske DR. Misprocessing of preprovasopressin associated with familial central diabetes insipidus. Endocrine Soc 1997; P1–482 (abstract).

68. Olias G, Richter D, Schmale H. Heterologous expression of human vasopressin-neurophysin precursors in a pituitary cell line: defective transport of a mutant protein from patients with familial diabetes insipidus. DNA Cell Biol 1996;15:929–935.

69. Ito M, Jameson JL, Ito MA. Molecular basis of autosomal dominant neurohypophyseal diabetes insipidus. Cellular toxicity caused by the accumulation of mutant vasopressin precursors within the endoplasmic reticulum. J Clin Invest 1997;99:1897–1905.

70. Cooper DN, Youssoufian H. The CpG dinucleotide and human genetic disease. Hum Genet 1988;78:151–155.

71. Bellus GA, Hefferon TW, Ortiz de Luna RI, Hecht JT, Horton WA, Machado M, Kaitila I, McIntosh I, Francomano CA. Achondroplasia is defined by recurrent G380R mutations of FGFR3. Am J Hum Genet 1995;56:368–373.

72. Knoers N, Monnens LAH. Nephrogenic diabetes insipidus: clinical symptoms, pathogenesis, genetics and treatment. Pediatr Nephrol 1992;6:476–482.

73. Moses AM, Sangani G, Miller JL. Proposed cause of marked vasopressin resistance in a female with an X-linked recessive V2 receptor abnormality. J Clin Endocrinol Metab 1995;80:1184–1186.

74. van Lieburg AF, Verdijk MAJ, Schoute F, Ligtenbery MJL, van Oost BA, Waldhauser F, Dobner M, Monnens LAH, Knoers NVAM. Clinical phenotype of nephrogenic diabetes insipidus in females heterozygous for a vasopressin type 2 receptor mutation. Hum Genet 1995;96:70–78.

75. Lightman SL. Molecular insights into diabetes insipidus. N Engl J Med 1993;328:1562,1563.

76. Uribarri J, Kaskas M. Hereditary nephrogenic diabetes insipidus and bilateral nonobstructive hydronephrosis. Nephron 1993;65:346–349.

77. Niaudet P, Dechaux M, Trivin C. Nephrogenic diabetes insipidus; clinical and pathophysiological aspects. In: Grunfeld JP, Maxwell MH, eds., Advances in Nephrology. Yearbook Medical, Chicago, 1984; pp. 247–260.

78. Niaudet P, Dechaux M, Leroy D, Broyer M. Nephrogenic diabetes insipidus in children. Front Horm Res 1985;13:224–231.

79. Fujisawa I, Asato R, Kawata M, Sano Y, Nakao K, Yamada T, Imura H, Naito Y, Hoshino K, Noma S, Nakano Y, Konishi J. Hyperintense signal of the posterior pituitary on T1-weighted MR images: an experimental study. J Comput Assist Tomogr 1989;13:371–377.

80. Knoers N, van der Ouweland A, Dreesen J, Verdijk M, Monnens LAH, van Oost BA. Nephrogenic diabetes insipidus: identification of the genetic defect. Pediatr Nephrol 1993;7:685–688.

81. Kobrinsky NL, Doyle JJ, Israels ED, Winter JSD, Cheang MS, Walker RD, Bishop AJ. Absent factor VIII response to synthetic vasopressin analogue (DDAVP) in nephrogenic diabetes insipidus. Lancet 1985;i:1293,1294.

82. Earley LE, Orloff J. The mechanism of antidiuresis associated with the administration of hydrochlorothiazide to patients with vasopressin-resistant diabetes insipidus. J Clin Invest 1962;41:1988–1997.

83. Blachar Y, Zadik Z, Shemesh M, Kaplan BS, Levin S. The effect of inhibition of prostaglandin synthesis on free water and osmolar clearances in patients with hereditary nephrogenic diabetes insipidus. Int J Pediatr Nephrol 1980;1:48–52.

84. Rascher W, Rosendahl W, Henrichs IA, Maier R, Seyberth HW. Congenital nephrogenic diabetes insipidus—vasopressin and prostaglandins in response to treatment with hydrochlorothiazide and indomethacin. Pediatr Nephrol 1987;1:485–490.

85. Alon U, Chan JCM. Hydrochlorothiazide-amiloride in the treatment of congenital nephrogenic diabetes insipidus. Am J Nephrol 1985;5:9–13.

86. Knoers N, Monnens LAH. Amiloride-hydrochlorothiazide versus indomethacin-hydrochlorothiazide in the treatment of nephrogenic diabetes insipidus. J Pediatr 1989;117:499–502.

87. Langley JM, Balfe JW, Selander T, Ray PN, Clarke JTR. Autosomal recessive inheritance of vasopressin-resistant diabetes insipidus. Am J Med Genet 1991;38:90–94.

88. Lolait SJ, O'Corroll A-M, McBride OW, Konig M, Morel A, Brownstein MJ. Cloning and characterization of a vasopressin V2 receptor and possible link to nephrogenic diabetes insipidus. Nature 1992;357:336–339.

89. Rosenthal W, Seibold A, Antaramian A, Lonergan M, Arthus M-F, Hendy GN, Birnbaumer M, Bichet DG. Molecular identification of the gene responsible for congenital nephrogenic diabetes insipidus. Nature 1992;359:233–235.

90. van den Ouweland AMW, Dreesen JCFM, Verdijk M, Knoers NVAM, Monnens LAH, Rocchi M, van Oost BA. Mutations in the vasopressin type 2 receptor gene (AVPR2) associated with nephrogenic diabetes insipidus. Nature Genet 1992;2:99–102.

91. Pan Y, Metzenberg A, Das S, Jing B, Gitschier J. Mutations in the V2 vasopressin receptor gene are associated with X-linked nephrogenic diabetes insipidus. Nature Genet 1992;2:103–106.

92. Holtzman EJ, Harris HW, Jr., Kolakowski LF, Jr., Guay-Woodford LM, Botelho B, Ausiello DA. Brief report: a molecular defect in the vasopressin V_2-receptor gene causing nephrogenic diabetes insipidus. N Engl J Med 1993;328:1534–1537.

93. Merendino JJ, Jr., Spiegel AM, Crawford JD, O'Carroll A-M, Brownstein MJ, Lolait SJ. Brief report: a mutation in the vasopressin V2-receptor gene in a kindred with X-linked nephrogenic diabetes insipidus. N Engl J Med 1993;328:1538–1541.

94. Bichet DG, Arthus M-F, Lonergan M, Hendy GN, Paradis AJ, Fuuiwara TM, Morgan K, Gregory MC, Rosenthal W, Didwania A, Antaramian A, Birnbaumer M. X-linked nephrogenic diabetes insipidus mutations in North America and the Hopewell hypothesis. J Clin Invest 1993;92:1262–1268.

95. Holtzman EJ, Kolakowski LF, O'Brian D, Crawford JD, Ausiello DA. A Null mutation in the vasopressin V2 receptor gene (AVPR2) associated with nephrogenic diabetes insipidus in the Hopewell kindred. Hum Mol Genet 1993;2:1201–1204.

96. Faa V, Ventruto ML, Loche S, Bozzola M, Podda R, Cao A, Rosatelli MC. Mutation in the vasopressin V2-receptor gene in three families of Italian descent with nephrogenic diabetes insipidus. Hum Mol Genet 1994;3:1685–1686.

97. Tsukaguchi H, Matsubara H, Aritaki S, Kimura T, Abe S, Inada M. Two novel mutations in the vasopressin V2 receptor gene in unrelated Japanese kindreds with nephrogenic diabetes insipidus. Biochem Biophys Res Commun 1993;197:1000–1010.

98. Wildin RS, Antush MJ, Bennett RL, Schoof JM, Scott CR. Heterogeneous AVPR2 gene mutations in congenital nephrogenic diabetes insipidus. Am J Hum Genet 1994;55:266–277.

99. Holtzman EJ, Kolakowski LF, Geifman-Holtzman O, O'Brian DG, Rasoulpour M, Guillot AP, Ausiello DA. Mutations in the vasopressin V2 receptor gene in two families with nephrogenic diabetes insipidus. J Am Soc Nephrol 1994;5:169–176.

100. Oksche A, Dickson J, Schulein R, Seyberth HW, Muller M, Rascher W, Birnbaumer M, Rosenthal W. Two novel mutations in the vasopressin V2 receptor gene in patients with congenital nephrogenic diabetes insipidus. Biochem Biophys Res Commun 1994;205:552–557.

101. Tsukaguchi H, Matsubara H, Mori Y, Yoshimasa Y, Yoshimasa T, Nakao K, Inada M. Two vasopressin type 2 receptor mutations R143P and delV278 in patients with nephrogenic diabetes insipidus impair ligand binding of the receptor. Biochem Biophys Res Commun 1995;211:967–977.

102. Rosenthal W, Antaramian A, Gilbert S, Birnbaumer M. Nephrogenic diabetes insipidus. A V2 vasopressin receptor unable to stimulate adenylyl cyclase. J Biol Chem 1993;268:13,030–13,033.

103. Yokoyama K, Yamauchi A, Izumi M, Itoh T, Imai E, Kamada T. A low-affinity vasopressin V2-receptor gene in a kindred with X-linked nephrogenic diabetes insipidus. J Am Soc Nephrol 1995;7:410–414.

104. Birnbaumer M, Gilbert S, Rosenthal W. An extracellular congenital nephrogenic diabetes insipidus mutation of the vasopressin receptor reduces cell surface expression, affinity for ligand, and coupling to the Gs/adenylyl cyclase system. Mol Endocrinol 1994;8:886–894.

105. Tsukaguchi H, Matsubara H, Inada M. Expression studies of two vasopressin V2 receptor gene mutations, R202C and 804insG, in nephrogenic diabetes insipidus. Kidney Int 1995;48:554–562.

106. Tsukaguchi H, Matsubara H, Taketani S, Mori Y, Seido T, Inada M. Binding-, intracellular transport-, and biosynthesis-defective mutants of vasopressin type 2 receptor in patients with X-linked nephrogenic diabetes insipidus. J Clin Invest 1995;96:2043–2050.

107. Schoneberg T, Yun J, Wenkert D, Wess J. Functional rescue of mutant V2 vasopressin receptors causing nephrogenic diabetes insipidus by a co-expressed receptor polypeptide. EMBO J 1996; 15:1283–1291.

108. Sasaki S, Fushimi K, Saito H, Saito F, Uchida S, Ishibashi K, et al. Cloning, characterization, and chromosomal mapping of human aquaporin of collecting duct. J Clin Invest 1994;93:1250–1256.

109. King LS, Agre P. Pathophysiology of the aquaporin water channels. Annu Rev Physiol 1996;58: 619–648.

110. Preston GM, Agre P. Molecular cloning of the red cell integral protein of Mr 28,000: a member of an ancient channel family. Proc Natl Acad Sci USA 1991;88:11,110–11,114.

111. Preston GM, Carroll TP, Guggino WB, Agre P. Appearance of water channels in Xenopus oocytes expressing red cell CHIO28 protein. Science 1992;256:385–387.

112. Deen PMT, Verdijk MAJ, Knoers NVAM, Wieringa B, Monnens LAH, van Oost BA. Requirement of human renal water channel aquaporin-2 for vasopressin-dependent concentration of urine. Science 1994;264:92–95.

113. Nielsen S, Pallone T, Smith BL, Christensen EI, Agre P. Aquaporin-1 water channels in short and long loop descending thin limbs and in descending vasa recta in rat kidney. Amer J Physiol 1995;268: F1023–F1037.

114. Preston GM, Smith BL, Zeidel ML, Moulds JJ, Agre P. Mutations in aquaporin-1 in phenotypically normal humans without functional CHIP water channels. Science 1994;265:1585–1587.

115. Fushimi K, Uchida S, Hara Y, Hirata Y, Marumo F, Sasaki S. Cloning and expression of apical membrane water channel of rat kidney collecting tubule. Nature 1993;361:549–552.

116. Deen PM, Weghuis DO, Sinke RJ, Geurts van Kessel A, Wieringa B, van Os CH. Assignment of the human gene for the water channel of renal collecting duct aquaporin 2 (AQP2) to chromosome 12 region q12->q13. Cytogenet Cell Genet 1994;66:260–262.

117. Uchida S, Sasaki S, Fushimi K, Marumo F. Isolation of human aquaporin-CD gene. J Biol Chem 1994;269:23,451–23,455.

118. Nielsen S, DiGiovanni SR, Christensen EI, Knepper MA, Harris HW. Cellular and subcellular immunolocalization of vasopressin-regulated water channel in rat kidney. Proc Natl Acad Sci USA 1993;90:11,663–11,667.

119. Neilsen S, Chou CL, Marples D, Christensen EI, Kishore BK, Knepper MA. Vasopressin increases water permeability of kidney collecting duct by inducing translocation of aquaporin-CD water channels to plasma membrane. Proc Natl Acad Sci USA 1995;92:1013–1017.

120. Marples D, Christensen S, Christensen EI, Ottesen PD, Nielsen S. Lithium-induced down-regulation of aquaporin-2 water channel expression in rat kidney medulla. J Clin Invest 1995; 95:1838–1845.

121. van Lieburg AF, Verdijk MAJ, Knoers VVAM, van Essen AJ, Proesmans W, Mallmann R, et al. Patients with autosomal nephrogenic diabetes insipidus homozygous for mutations in the aquaporin 2 water-channel gene. Amer J Hum Genet 1994;55:648–652.

122. Deen PMT, Croes H, van Aubel RAMH, Ginsel LA, van Os CH. Water channels encoded by mutant aquaporin-2 genes in nephrogenic diabetes insipidus are impaired in their cellular routing. J Clin Invest 1995;95:2291–2296.

123. Mulders SM, Knoers NVAM, van Lieburg AF, Monnens LAH, Leumann E, Wuhl E, et al. New mutations in the AQP2 gene in nephrogenic diabetes insipidus resulting in functional but misrouted water channels. J Am Soc Nephrol 1997;8:242–248.

124. Oksche A, Moller A, Dickson J, Rosendahl W, Rascher W, Bichet DG, Rosenthal W. Two novel mutations in the aquaporin-2 and the vasopressin V2 receptor genes in patients with congenital nephrogenic diabetes insipidus. Human Genetics 1996;98:587–589.

125. Hochberg Z, Van Lieburg A, Even L, Brenner B, Lanir N, van Oost BA, Knoers NV. Autosomal recessive nephrogenic diabetes insipidus caused by an aquaporin-2 mutation. J Clin Endocrinol Metab 1997;82:686–689.

126. Wolfram DJ, Wagener HP. Diabetes mellitus and simple optic atrophy among siblings: report of four cases. Mayo Clin Proc 1938;13:715–718.

127. Rotig A, Cormier V, Chatelain P, Francois R, Saudubray J-M, Rustin P, Munnich A. Deletion of mitochondrial DNA in a case of early-onset diabetes mellitus, optic atrophy, and deafness (Wolfran Syndrome, MIM 222300). J Clin Invest 1993;91:1095–1098.
128. Wit JM, Donckerwolcke RAMG, Schulpen TWJ, Deutman AF. Documented vasopressin deficiency in a child with Wolfram syndrome. J Pediatr 1986;109:493,494.
129. Swift RG, Perkins DO, Chase CL, Sadler DB, Swift M. Psychiatric disorders in 36 families with Wolfram syndrome. Amer J Psychiat 1991;148:775–779.
130. Rando TA, Horton JC, Layzer RB. Wolfram syndrome: evidence of a diffuse neurodegenerative disease by magnetic resonance imaging. Neurology 1992;42:1220–1224.
131. Collier DA, Barrett TG, Curtis D, Maclead A, Arranz MJ, Maassen JA, Bundy S. Linkage of Wolfram syndrome to chromosome 4p16.1 and evidence for heterogeneity. Amer J Hum Genet 1996;59: 855–863.
132. Barrientos A, Casademont J, Saiz A, Cardellach F, Volpini V, Solans A, et al. Autosomal recessive Wolfram syndrome associated with a 8.5-kb mtDNA single deletion. Amer J Hum Genet 1995; 58:963–970.
133. Barrientos A, Volpini V, Casademont J, Genis D, Manzanares J-M, Ferrer I, et al. A nuclear defect in the 4p16 region predisposes to multiple mitochondrial DNA deletions in families with Wolfram syndrome. J Clin Invest 1996;97:1570–1576.
134. Repaske DR, Summar ML, Krishnamani MRS, Gultekin EK, Arriazu MC, Roubicek ME, et al. Recurrent mutations in the vasopressin-neurophysin II gene cause autosomal dominant neurohypophyseal diabetes insipidus. J Clin Endocrinol Metab 1996;81:2328–2334.
135. Ueta Y, Taniguchi S, Yoshida A, Murakami I, Mitani Y, Hisatome I, et al. A new type of familial central diabetes insipidus caused by a single base substitution in the neurophysin II coding region of the vasopressin gene. J Clin Endocrinol Metab 1996;81:1787–1790.

10

Molecular Biology of Gonadotropin-Releasing Hormone and the Gonadotropin-Releasing Hormone Receptor

Dorothy I. Shulman, MD and Barry B. Bercu, MD

CONTENTS

INTRODUCTION

Gonadotropin-releasing hormone (GnRH) is a hypothalamic decapeptide that plays a fundamental role in the reproductive events of all mammalian species. GnRH was first isolated in the early 1970s by Schally *(1)* and Guillemin *(2)*. Since that time there has been an explosion of knowledge regarding the physiology and genetic structure of GnRH and its membrane receptor, leading to the development of synthetic analogs with clinical utility in the treatment of GnRH deficient states, infertility, hormone-dependent cancers, precocious puberty, and a variety of gynecologic conditions.

GONADOTROPIN-RELEASING HORMONE

General Anatomy and Physiology

GnRH neurons migrate during early fetal life from the olfactory placode to their ultimate primary location, the arcuate nuclei of the hypothalamus. Nerve terminals extend into the median eminence, releasing GnRH into the hypophyseal portal circulation. GnRH neuronal cells express abundant GnRH receptors indicating that autocrine regulation of GnRH release can occur within the brain. GnRH axons terminating on other GnRH cell bodies or dendrites are speculated to be involved in the pulsatile release of GnRH *(3)*. Defects in the migration of these neurons may account for some cases of GnRH deficiency

From: *Molecular and Cellular Pediatric Endocrinology*
Edited by: S. Handwerger © Humana Press Inc., Totowa, NJ

associated with absence of the olfactory bulb and tract in humans, an entity called Kallmann's syndrome. GnRH occurs in the brain in locations other than the arcuate nucleus and may act as a neurotransmitter, neuromodulator or local hormone (4). The presence of GnRH in the midbrain, hindbrain and spinal cord of some mammals suggests that GnRH may directly regulate sexual behavior. GnRH has also been isolated in breast and prostate tumor cells, in human placenta, gonads, the immune system, pituitary gland, and in pancreatic tumor cells (3). In the placenta GnRH acts as a local hormone releasing human chorionic gonadotropin (5). There is evidence that GnRH directly affects steroidogenesis in the ovary (6,7). The role of GnRH production in most peripheral tissues is not yet known.

GnRH is synthesized and stored primarily in neurons of the medial basal hypothalamus. In response to neural signals, pulses of GnRH are released into the hypophyseal portal circulation. GnRH then travels to the anterior pituitary where it selectively stimulates *de novo* synthesis and release of luteinizing hormone (LH) and follicle stimulating hormone (FSH) from the gonadotroph cells. These glycoproteins consist of a common α and unique β subunits. LH and FSH, in turn, stimulate the gonadal production of sex steroids and gametogenesis. The amount of LH and FSH released by the pituitary is a function of both the concentration of GnRH applied to the pituitary gonadotroph cell and the pattern of its application. Physiologic secretion of gonadotropins requires intermittent GnRH secretion (8). The frequency of GnRH stimulation can differentially control FSH and LH secretion; slower pulse frequency favors the secretion of FSH (9). Continuous stimulation of the pituitary by either GnRH or long-acting GnRH agonists results in "desensitization" of gonadotropin secretion and gonadal suppression (10).

The distribution of hypothalamic GnRH is restricted to the hypothalamic hypophyseal portal system due to lack of plasma protein binding and rapid dilution of portal blood into the general circulation. Exogenous GnRH is distributed widely into the extracellular fluid space and is metabolized by enzymatic degradation and renal excretion (11).

The hypothalamic-pituitary-gonadal axis is active during the neonatal period, quiescent during childhood, and reemerges during puberty (12,13). Pubertal secretion of GnRH is initially nocturnal and sleep-entrained. As puberty progresses, daytime and nighttime patterns become similar. In adult men, pulse frequency is approximately every 2 h; in women, pulse frequency varies considerably during the menstrual cycle. As GnRH has a very short plasma half-life (2–4 min), and its location in the hypophyseal portal circulation is inaccessible for sampling, most of the information regarding the physiologic secretion of GnRH in humans has been learned indirectly from intensive peripheral sampling of LH and FSH concentrations (10).

Structure of GnRH Peptide and Its Precursor

The linear sequence the GnRH decapeptide is Glu[1]-His[2]-Trp[3]-Ser[4]-Tyr[5]-Gly[6]-Leu[7]-Arg[8]-Pro[9]-Gly[10]-amide. The GnRH molecule has existed for at least 500 million years, the human form 400 million years. Only one form of GnRH has been identified in most placental mammals, and this is still considered to be the sole neuropeptide causing the release of LH and FSH. Most nonmammalian vertebrates possess at least two forms of GnRH which may have functions separate from gonadotropin release (3,4).

GnRH exists as part of a larger precursor protein, a prepropeptide 92 amino acids in length (14). The human GnRH precursor molecule is produced throughout life in the

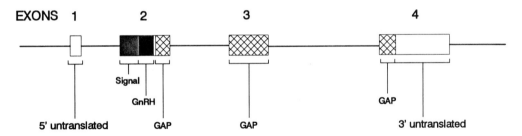

Fig. 1. The human GnRH gene consists of four exons separated by three introns. Exon 2 contains the signal peptide, the decapeptide GnRH, a processing site following GnRH, and the amino terminal portion of the GAP.

human hypothalamus, including the earliest stages of development of the peptidergic neurons (9 wk gestation) prior to organization of the hypophyseal portal circulation *(15)*. This prepropeptide is identical in the placenta and hypothalamus. Within the precursor protein, GnRH decapeptide is preceded by a 23-amino acid signal peptide containing a hydrophobic middle section, a feature characteristic of many secreted proteins. At the C-terminus end is a Gly-Lys-Arg sequence, characteristic of an enzymatic amidation and precursor processing site. Following this, in mammals, is a GnRH-associated propeptide (GAP) that is 56 amino acids long and has an unknown function *(3)*. The C-terminus of this peptide consists of the sequence Lys-Lys-Ile, which represents an enzymatic cleavage site for further processing *(14)*. GAP has been shown to coexist with GnRH in hypothalamic neurons and was initially thought to inhibit the secretion of prolactin (PRL). The relationship between GnRH, GAP, and PRL in vivo is not clear. GAP and GAP-related peptides have been shown to stimulate gonadotropin release from rat anterior pituitary cells in culture, but these peptides did not affect the secretion of gonadotrophs or of PRL in vivo in ewes. It is possible that GAP, in common with some other cryptic peptides associated with neurohormones, is involved in the correct processing and packaging of the hormone *(3)*. In the GAP peptides from mammals and fish the conservation of the leucine and arginine residues may be an indication that secondary structure is being maintained, similar to the retention of cysteine residues in the neurophysin portion of the vasotocin precursor. An endocrine disorder resulting from the loss of part of the GnRH gene in mammals provides some evidence that GAP is acting as a conformational assistant. In "hypogonadal" mice, the third and fourth exons, which encode most of GAP, have been deleted from the GnRH gene. Although exon 2, which encodes GnRH, remains intact, these mice do not appear to release GnRH, circulating gonadotropins are undetectable, and the animals are sexually immature *(16)*. Full-length transcripts, in the correct reading frame, may be required for effective processing of the GnRH peptide.

GnRH Gene

The GnRH gene in mammals consists of four exons and three introns *(17)* (Fig. 1). The first exon encodes the 5'-untranslated region. The second exon encodes the signal peptide, mGnRH, the enzymatic amidation and precursor processing site, and the first 11 amino acids of GAP. The third exon encodes GAP amino acids and the 3'-untranslated region.

GnRH Gene Regulation

The mammalian GnRH gene appears to have a different transcriptional start site depending on the species. The 5'-untranslated region (exon 1) from brain tissue in rats is 145 nucleotide bases, which is longer than the same region in the human (61 bases) or mouse (58 bases) (3). The transcriptional start site for GnRH in the placenta is reported to be upstream from that in the hypothalamus (17). Evidence suggests that the first intron is not removed from the GnRH mRNA in the placenta resulting in a 5'-untranslated region of about 900 kbases. As a result the first exon in the placenta is much longer than that in the hypothalamus reflecting tissue-specific gene processing (3,17). Different regions of the promoters are likely to be activated for the expression of the GnRH gene in neural and nonneural tissues.

In the 5'-flanking region of the mammalian GnRH genes, the TATA and CAAT boxes, which are important in the efficient transcription of genes by RNA polymerase II, have been identified for the gene in the hypothalamus. Deletion experiments for the 5'-flanking region in the rat GnRH gene have revealed both activating and inhibiting regions (17). Consensus sequences for putative DNA binding sites exist in the rat GnRH promoter region for transcription factors similar to oct-1, tst-1, and pit-1 (18). These factors are associated with regulation of gene expression in different tissues and during development.

Peptide hormones that bind to GnRH neurons via their membrane receptors activate the protein kinase C pathway and may trigger fos-mediated acute release of GnRH as well as rapid repression of GnRH gene transcription. This process may be important during normal physiologic processes, such as a mechanism to limit the LH surge at ovulation (17).

Direct steroid hormone regulation of GnRH gene expression is suggested by the presence of retinoic acid elements in the 5'-flanking region in the rat (18); a region with high homology to known palindromic estrogen response elements in humans (19); and by half-sites for estrogen and thyroid hormone receptors (18). Additional evidence that estrogen directly regulates GnRH gene expression was provided by experiments in which the estrogen receptor was shown to bind to the 5'-flanking region of the GnRH gene (19).

GNRH RECEPTOR

Location of GnRH Binding Sites

The action of GnRH in pituitary gonadotrophs is initiated by its interaction with a specific membrane receptor. In the anterior pituitary, GnRH high affinity binding activity resides in the gonadotrophs, which make up <20% of anterior pituitary cells (20). High-affinity binding also occurs in hypothalamic neurons in a dose, time, and temperature dependent manner (5). Specific GnRH binding occurs in other parts of the brain including the hippocampus, lateral septal nucleus, anterior cingulate cortex, subiculum, and entorhinal cortex. In the gonads, GnRH binding activity is specific to the Leydig cells of the testis and the granulosa cells of the ovary. Human placenta contains low-affinity GnRH binding sites that interact with GnRH agonist and antagonist analogs. They may be a variant of the GnRH receptor. The current hypothesis suggests that GnRH produced locally in these peripheral tissues acts on the receptors in an autocrine-paracrine mechanism.

GnRH Receptor Gene and Protein Structure

The mouse GnRH receptor was cloned in 1992 (21) in a mouse transgene gonadotroph cell line. Shortly thereafter the human GnRH receptor was cloned (22,23). The human

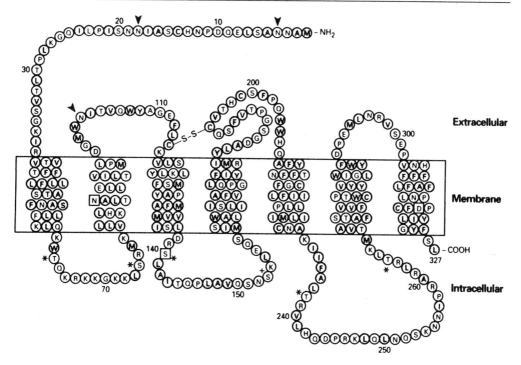

Fig. 2. Amino acid sequence of the murine GnRH receptor shown in its proposed configuration in the membrane. Hydrophobic residues are shaded, and potential N-linked glycosylation sites are marked with arrowheads. Possible phosphorylation sites are marked with asterisks. The casein kinase II phosphorylation site is marked with a cross. (Reproduced with permission from ref. *24a*.)

GnRH receptor gene has been localized to chromosome 4q13.2–13.3 and has been shown to comprise three exons spanning 18.9 kbases. To date, only the mouse GnRH receptor gene has been mapped *(24)*. The mouse and human receptors share 89% homology. The murine receptor is a 327-amino acid single polypeptide chain which has the heptahelical structure of a member of the family of G protein-coupled receptors (Fig. 2). The human receptor has one more amino acid, a lysine residue in the second extracellular loop. The GnRH receptor contains seven transmembrane regions similar to other G protein receptors. However, it differs most notably in that it terminates after the seventh transmembrane domain and does not have a cytoplasmic C-terminal tail *(5,24)*. In other seven-transmembrane receptors this region has been implicated in coupling to G proteins and in desensitization and internalization. The GnRH receptor is an exception in that these functions must be dependent on parts of the receptor other than the C-terminal cytoplasmic domain. Other unique features of the GnRH receptor include an unusually long first intracellular loop with a high content of basic amino acids, and its phenylalanine-rich seventh transmembrane domain. Three consensus sequences for N-linked glycosylation are present in the extracellular domains of the cloned receptor. Potential sites for phosphorylation by cAMP-dependent protein kinase and protein kinase C are located in the first cytoplasmic domain. A potential casein kinase II phosphorylation site is in the second cytoplasmic domain, and a potential protein kinase C site is present in the third cytoplasmic domain. Other possible phosphorylation sites are at tyrosine[238] and serine[140]. The binding site of the neurotransmitter receptors is believed to reside within the transmembrane helical bundle. The extracellular domains may serve critical roles in binding peptide hormones. GnRH receptors have relatively little sequence homology with other G protein-coupled receptors, apart from those for the oxytocin-vasopressin family of peptides with which they share approx 25% homology. The human receptor clone has a dissociation constant of 2.8 nM with GnRH *(5)*.

Location of GnRH Receptor mRNA

Results of in vivo studies indicate that mRNA levels of the GnRH receptor correlate closely with GnRH binding activity. Human GnRH receptor mRNA was detected by poly-merase chain amplification but not Northern blot analysis of ovary, testes, breast, prostate, and a breast tumor cell line and in epithelial ovarian carcinomas *(5)*. GnRH receptor mRNA has not been identified in the placenta by Northern analysis although previous binding studies have identified a low-affinity receptor in this tissue. *In situ* hybridization has revealed GnRH receptor mRNA in the rat hippocampus and hypothalamus.

Regulation of GnRH Receptors

GnRH receptor expression may be an important control point in the reproductive pathway. Marked changes in receptor number, but not in binding affinity, occur in a number of different endocrine states including development, estrous cycle, lactation, castration, hormone replacement, and aging *(5)*. Inhibin decreases upregulation of GnRH receptor mRNA after exposure to GnRH *(25)*. Treatment of rats with estrogen and tes-tosterone decreased receptor mRNA. Suckling causes significant suppression of receptor mRNA expression and consequently of GnRH receptors in the gonadotrophs of lactating female rats. Hypothalamic lesions, GnRH antibodies, and GnRH agonists also influence GnRH receptor number. GnRH regulates the expression of its own receptor; pulsatility, frequency, and amplitude of GnRH delivery are important factors in this regulation. Low concentrations or pulsatile administration of GnRH increases GnRH receptor mRNA levels. Conversely, high concentration or continuous GnRH treatment results in desen-sitization of the receptor. If GnRH is administered continuously to pituitary cell cultures a biphasic pattern of receptor regulation can be seen. Initially receptor number is decreased, however, later receptor numbers return to normal and then to supranormal *(26)*. Ca^{2+} mobilization is required for recovery of receptor number but not for receptor loss. Reduction of receptor number after GnRH treatment has also been observed in testicular and hippocampal GnRH receptors *(5)*. A GnRH antagonist alone had no effect on GnRH receptor synthesis in rat gonadotroph cell cultures *(25)*.

Recent isolation and characterization of the 5'-flanking region of the mouse GnRH receptor has identified an initiation transcription site 62 nucleotides upstream of the translational start site *(27)*. In addition, several minor transcription start sites occur fur-ther upstream. Within this promoter region the TATA box, which is important for deter-mining the accurate start site of transcription, appears to be absent as is true of other G protein-coupled receptors (LH, FSH, TSH). Transient expression of the promoter-reporter construct was greater in pituitary cells of gonadotroph origin (aT3 cells) than in those of somatomammotropic origin (GH3 cells) or in those of nonpituitary origin (JEG-3 cells), suggesting that in this promoter region are regulatory elements for tissue specific gene expression. Also in this 5' region is a site homologous to the gonadotroph-specific ele-ment (GSE). The GSE is a highly conserved 30 base-pair sequence that has been proposed to dictate the expression of the gonadotropin α-subunit in gonadotroph cells *(28)*. A tissue-specific 54-kDa nuclear protein, steroidogenic factor-1, has been shown to bind to an 8 base-pair stretch of nucleotides (TGTCCTTG) within the GSE *(29)*. An identical 8 base-pair sequence is present in the 5'-untranslated region of the GnRH receptor gene (+48/+55) promoter region. Consensus sequences similar to the GnRH response elements found in the α-subunit promoter have also been identified *(30)*. These sequences may be important in the autoregulatory role of GnRH on its receptor expression.

Activation of GnRH Receptors

The GnRH receptor is initially distributed uniformly on the surface of the cell. When activated it internalizes via receptor mediated endocytosis. The internalized complex then undergoes dissociation, followed by degradation of the ligand and partial recycling of the receptors. High-resolution electron micrographs reveal that GnRH agonists coupled to colloidal gold or ferritin are internalized and routed to the lysosome *(26)*.

Activation of GnRH receptors during agonist stimulation initiates a series of steps that lead to a cascade of intracellular responses *(5,25)*. Mobilization of calcium ions resulting in a net increase of intracellular calcium is required for GnRH-induced gonadotropin release. In vivo human studies also show that serum gonadotropins are lowered by infusion of calcium channel blockers *(10)*. The first step after agonist binding of the GnRH receptor is G protein-mediated activation of phospholipase C, leading to hydrolysis of phosphoinositides and the formation of inositol phosphates and diacylglycerol. These initial changes determine the second step in signaling; inositol phosphates induce oscillatory or biphasic elevations in cytoplasmic Ca^{2+}, depending on the cell type expressing the receptor, and Ca^{2+} and diacylglycerol activate protein kinase C. Cytoplasmic Ca^{2+} and protein kinase C subsequently serve as interacting signals in the regulation of several cellular responses, including the control of Ca^{2+} signaling and secretion, as well as the control of primary and secondary gene responses (c-fos, c-jun, junB) *(5)*. Calmodulin is also a potential intracellular mediator of the Ca^{2+} signal *(25)*. The signaling molecules of the phospholipase C-dependent pathway also exert positive and negative control on the signal transduction mechanism. These feedback mechanisms provide complexity in signaling that is important in the amplification, maintenance, and termination of specific aspects of the activation pathways. They may also contribute to the termination of signaling as observed during desensitization of gonadotrophs by continuous exposure to high agonist concentrations. A similar signaling pathway has been demonstrated for GnRH receptors in other tissues including gonads, placenta, and GT1 neuronal cells *(5)*.

The cellular mechanism of desensitization of the GnRH receptor is still unknown. Conn et al. *(25)* have suggested that desensitization of the receptor occurs in two phases. Initially, loss of responsiveness is due to receptor loss. As receptor number returns to normal and then supranormal, desensitization is maintained because receptors are uncoupled from their effector system resulting in loss of functional activity of the Ca^{2+} ion channel.

CLINICAL AND THERAPEUTIC USES OF GNRH AND ITS ANALOGS

GnRH

In the human, disorders of GnRH secretion, as in patients with Kallmann's syndrome, have long been known to cause hypogonadism. Quantifiable abnormalities of GnRH secretion are discernible in both males and females with hypogonadotropic hypogonadism, including total absence of GnRH secretion, defects of the amplitude and frequency of its secretion, and altered bioactivity of gonadotropins. Physiological regimens of hypothalamic replacement therapy with exogenous GnRH, which mimic the normal frequency of endogenous GnRH secretion, result in normalization of reproductive function and fertility in hypogonadotropic subjects of both sexes. Crowley *(31)* reported replacement of hypogonadotropic men with exogenous GnRH delivered subcutaneously via an infusion pump. Twenty-five to 200 ng/kg boluses every 2 h restored normal pituitary and gonadal responses. Growth of the testes and induction of spermatogenesis was achieved in several months of therapy and is an alternative to therapy with exogenous gonadotropins. In women pulsatile GnRH, 25–100 ng/kg given intravenously hourly, induced ovulatory cycles. This therapy was associated with a lower incidence of pregnancies complicated by multiple gestations compared to therapy with exogenous gonadotropins *(10)*.

Intravenous bolus injection of GnRH is also used as a diagnostic tool to assess gonadotropin secretion in suspected disorders of pituitary function (precocious puberty, hypogonadotropic hypogonadism).

GnRH Agonists

Since the determination of the primary structure of GnRH, over 2000 analogs of GnRH have been synthesized *(32)*. The original incentive for the development of more potent GnRH agonists was the hope of providing treatment for male and female infertility. Because of the short half-life of GnRH, there was a need for development of GnRH analogs with greater potency and longer activity thought to be necessary for practical clinical utility. Various methods were used to increase the potency of native GnRH, including but not limited to the following structural modifications: D-amino acid substitution at position 6, modification of position 10 incorporating a Pro^9-ethyl amide or an α-aza-Gly^{10} replacement, and a N-Me-Leu^7 substitution. These substitutions inhibit enzymatic degradation and enhance receptor binding affinity. Agonist activity requires conservation of the N- and C-terminus residues, whereas antagonist activity requires conservation of only C-terminal residues *(24)*. The residues most critical for agonist binding and/or activity are the lactam ring of $pGlu^1$, the aromatic side chain of Trp^3, and the carboxy-terminal amide of Gly-amide[10]. The basic Arg^8 of GnRH is critical for high-affinity agonist and antagonist binding. Appreciation of an ionic interaction between Arg^8 of GnRH and the third extracellular loop of the GnRH receptor, and the proximity of helix 2 and helix 7 of the receptor have provided a foundation on which to develop a predictive model of the interaction of GnRH and its analogs with the receptor *(24)*.

Early in the development of long-acting GnRH agonists, their gonadal suppressive effects, owing to pituitary receptor desensitization, became apparent. When administered in a pulsatile fashion, similar to the pattern of release of endogenous GnRH, the analogs stimulate LH and FSH secretion. With continuous administration, however, these agonists produce a fully reversible inhibition of the pituitary-gonadal axis. Initial stimulation of gonadotropins occurs within the first 7–14 d of therapy; within 4 wk after initiation, circulating gonadal sex steroid levels fall to the castrate range. GnRH agonists are inactivated by gastric peptidases, therefore they must be administered by either injection or nasal spray. Single daily subcutaneous injections or depot formulations of GnRH agonists (given intramuscularly lasting 28 d) have been introduced for the treatment of disorders which require sustained suppression of gonadotropin and gonadal steroid secretion.

GnRH agonists are now recognized as powerful pharmacologic tools for treating various diseases mediated by gonadal hormones. Use in endometriosis, advanced prostate cancer, and precocious puberty has been approved by the Food and Drug Administration in the United States. GnRH analogs have also proven useful in the treatment of uterine leiomyomas, polycystic ovary disease, fibrocystic breast disease, premenstrual syndrome, dysfunctional uterine bleeding, and for ovulation induction in vitro fertilization protocols. They have also been reported to be of benefit in the treatment of benign prostatic hyperplasia, estrogen receptor positive breast cancer and irritable bowel syndrome *(33)*. A direct antiproliferative effect of GnRH analogs on ovarian tumor cells has been observed as well as on prostate cancers *(5,34)*.

GnRH agonists are generally well tolerated because of their selective ability to downregulate GnRH receptors in the pituitary gland and the absence of inherent steroidal activity. Their principal side effects are attributable to the reduction in plasma concentrations of estrogens and testosterone, including decreased libido, hot flashes, emotional lability, and headache *(33)*. Decreased bone mineral density has been observed in women treated with GnRH analogs for extended periods (> 6 mo) *(35)*. Therefore, in gynecologic conditions, such as endometriosis, in which there appears to be no adverse affect on the primary disease, the addition of estrogen and progesterone may prevent excessive bone loss *(35,36)*. An adverse effect of GnRH analogs on plasma lipid profile has not been demonstrated. GnRH analog treatment abruptly halts the progression of puberty and appears to increase final adult stature in children with central precocious puberty with onset before age 6 yr *(37,38)*. Ovulatory menstrual cycles are restored within 2 yr of stopping analog therapy *(39)*. Long-term effects on bone mineral density in treated children are not yet available.

GnRH Antagonists

The initial rational for the GnRH antagonist was for its potential antireproductive effects. Also, an antagonist would avoid the initial stimulatory effect on gonadotropin and sex steroid secretion observed with agonists, particularly in the treatment of steroid-sensitive cancers. Pituitary suppression in response to the administration of a GnRH antagonist is based on its ability to induce competitive blockade of the receptor, precluding substantial occupation by endogenous GnRH *(10,32)*. Suppression is immediate and there is no initial increase in gonadal steroid secretion, which is seen in the first 2 wk of agonist therapy *(32,40)*. With the development of more potent antagonists, and the introduction of D-Arg and other basic side-chains into position 6, came the unexpected finding that they triggered edema by means of histamine release. Current structural modifications of GnRH antagonists have been undertaken to reduce the histamine releasing potential while increasing the GnRH antagonist potency. Most contain hydrophobic D-amino acids in positions 1, 2, and 3 and a D-Ala at position 10. GnRH antagonists are not yet approved for clinical use.

REFERENCES

1. Matsuo H, Bab Y, Nair RMG, et al. Structure of the porcine LH- and FSH- releasing hormone. I. The proposed amino acid sequence. Biochem Biophys Res Commun 1971;43:1334–1339.
2. Burgus R, Butcher M, Amoss M, et al. Primary structure of ovine hypothalamic luteinizing hormone-releasing factor (LRF). Proc Natl Acad Sci USA 1972;69:278–282.
3. Sherwood NM, Lovejoy DA, Coe IR. Origin of mammalian gonadotropin-releasing hormones. Endocr Rev 1993;14:241–254.

4. King JA, Millar RP. Evolutionary aspects of gonadotropin-releasing hormone and its receptor. Cell Mol Neurobiol 1995;15:5–23.

5. Stojilkovic SS, Catt KJ. Expression and signal transduction pathways of gonadotropin-releasing hormone receptors. Rec Prog Horm Res 1995;50:161–205.

6. Bussenot I, Azoulay-Barjonet C, Parinaud J. Modulation of the steroidogenesis of cultured human granulosa-lutein cells by gonadotropin-releasing hormone agonist. J Clin Endocrinol Metab 1993;76:1376–1379.

7. Srivastava K, Luu-The V, Marrone BL, et al. Suppression of luteal steroidogenesis by an LHRH antagonist (Nal-Lys antagonist:antide) in vitro during early pregnancy in the rat. J Mol Endocrinol 1994;13:87–94.

8. Belchetz PE, Plant TM, Nakai Y, et al. Hypophysial responses to continuous and intermittent delivery of hypothalamic gonadotropin-releasing hormone. Science 1978;202:631–633.

9. Gross KM, Matsumoto AM, Bremner SJ. Differential control of luteinizing hormone and follicle-stimulating hormone-releasing hormone pulse frequency in man. J Clin Endocrinol Metab 1987;64:675–680.

10. Conn PM, Crowley WF. Gonadotropin-releasing hormone and its analogues. N Engl J Med 1991;324:93–103.

11. Handelsman DJ, Swerdloff RS. Pharmacokinetics of gonadotropin-releasing hormone and its analogs. Endo Rev 1986;7:95–105.

12. Conte FA, Grumbach MM, Kaplan SL, et al. Correlation of luteinizing hormone-releasing factor-induced luteinizing hormone and follicle-stimulating hormone release from infancy to 19 years with the changing pattern of gonadotropin secretion in agonadal patients: relation to the restraint of puberty. J Clin Endocrinol Metab 1980;50:163–168.

13. Bercu BB, Lee, BC, Spiliotis BE, et al. Male sexual development in the monkey. II. Cross-sectional analysis of pulsatile hypothalamic-pituitary secretion in castrated males. J Clin Endocrinol Metab 1983;56:1227–1235.

14. Seeburg PH, Adelman JP. Characterization of cDNA for precursor of human luteinizing hormone releasing hormone. Nature 1984;311:666–668.

15. Bloch B, Gaillard RC, Culler MP, et al. Immunohistochemical detection of proluteinizing hormone-releasing hormone peptides in the neurons in the human hypothalamus. J Clin Endocrinol Metab 1992;74:135–138.

16. Seeburg PH, Mason AJ, Stewart TA, et al. The mammalian GnRH gene and its pivotal role in reproduction. Recent Prog Horm Res 1987;43:69–91.

17. Wierman ME, Bruder JM, Kepa JK. Regulation of gonadotropin-releasing hormone (GnRH) gene expression in hypothalamic neuronal cells. Cell Mol Neurobiol 1995;15:79–88.

18. Kepa JK, Wang C, Neeley CI, et al. Structure of the rat gonadotropin releasing hormone (rGnRH) gene promoter and functional analysis in hypothalamic cells. Nucleic Acid Res 1992;20:1393–1399.

19. Radovick S, Ticknor CM, Nakayama Y, et al. Evidence for direct estrogen regulation of the human gonadotropin-releasing hormone gene. J Clin Invest 1991;88:1649–1655.

20. Childs GV, Unabia G, Tibolt R, et al. Cytological factors that support nonparallel secretion of luteinizing hormone and follicle-stimulating hormone during the estrous cycle. Endocrinology 1987;121:1801–1813.

21. Tsutsumi M, Zhou W, Millar RP, et al. Cloning and functional expression of a mouse gonadotropin-releasing hormone receptor. Mol Endocrinol 1992;6:1163–1169.

22. Kakar SS, Musgrove LC, Devor DC, et al. Cloning, sequencing, and expression of human gonadotropin releasing hormone (GnRH) receptor. Biochem Biophys Res Commun 1992;189:289–295.

23. Chi L, Zhou, W, Prikhozhan A, et al. Cloning and characterization of the human GnRH receptor. Mol Cell Endocrinol 1993;91:R1–R6.

24. Sealfon SC, Millar RP. Functional domains of the gonadotropin-releasing hormone receptor. Cell Mol Neurobiol 1995;15:25–42.

24a. Stojikovic SS, Reinhart J, Catt KJ. Gonadotropin-releasing hormone receptors: structure and signal transduction pathways. Endocr Rev 1994;15:462–499.

25. Conn PM, Janovick JA, Stanislaus D, et al. Molecular and cellular bases of gonadotropin-releasing hormone action in the pituitary and central nervous system. Vitamins Hormones 1995;50:151–214.

26. Conn PM. The molecular basis of gonadotropin-releasing hormone action. Endocr Rev 1986;7:3–10.

27. Albarracin CT, Kaiser UB, Chin WW. Isolation and characterization of the 5'-flanking region of the mouse gonadotropin-releasing receptor gene. Endocrinology 1994;135:2300–2306.

28. Horn F, Windle JJ, Barnhart KM, et al. Tissue-specific gene expression in the pituitary: the glycoprotein hormone α-subunit gene is regulated by a gonadotrope-specific protein. Mol Cell Biol 1992;12: 2143–2153.
29. Barnhart KM, Mellon PL. The orphan nuclear receptor, steroidogenic factor-1, regulates the glycoprotein hormone α-subunit gene in pituitary gonadotrophs. Mol Endocrinol 1994;8:878–885.
30. Schoderbek W, Roberson, M, Maurer R. Two different DNA elements mediate gonadotropin-releasing hormone effects on expression of the glycoprotein hormone α-subunit gene. J Biol Chem 1993;268: 3903–3910.
31. Crowley WF, Jr., Filicori M, Spratt DI, et al. The physiology of gonadotropin-releasing hormone (GnRH) secretion in men and women. Rec Prog Horm Res 1985;41:473–526.
32. Karten MJ, Rivier JE. Gonadotropin-releasing hormone analog design. Structure-function studies toward the development of agonist and antagonists: rationale and perspective. Endocr Rev 1986;7:44–66.
33. Winkel CA. Gonadotropin-releasing hormone agonists. Current uses for these increasingly important drugs. Post Grad Med 1994;95:111–118.
34. Limonta P, Dondi D, Moretti RM, et al. Antiproliferative effects of luteinizing hormone-releasing hormone agonists on the human prostatic cancer cell line LNCaP. J Clin Endocrinol Metab 1992;75: 207–212.
35. Lemay A, Surrey ES, Friedman AJ. Extending the use of gonadotropin-releasing hormone agonists: the emerging role of steroidal and nonsteroidal agents. Fertil Steril 1994;61:21–34.
36. Kiilholma P, Tuimala R, Kivinen S, et al. Comparison of the gonadotropin-releasing hormone agonist goserelin acetate alone versus goserelin combined with estrogen-progestogen add-back therapy in the treatment of endometriosis. Fertil Steril 1995;64:903–908.
37. Kletter GB, Kelch RP. Effects of gonadotropin-releasing hormone analog therapy on adult stature in precocious puberty. J Clin Endocrinol Metab 1994;79:331–339.
38. Paul D, Conte FA, Grumbach MM, et al. Long term effect of gonadotropin-releasing hormone agonist therapy on final and near-final height in 26 children with true precocious puberty treated at a median age of less than 5 years. J Clin Endocrinol Metab 1995;80:546–551.
39. Jay N, Mansfield MJ, Blizzard RM, et al. Ovulation and menstrual function of adolescent girls with central precocious puberty after therapy with gonadotropin-releasing hormone agonists. J Clin Endocrinol Metab 1992;75:890–894.
40. Pineda J, Lee BC, Spiliotis BE, et al. Effect of a potent GnRH antagonist, [Ac-Δ^3 Pro^1, pFDPhe^2, DTrp3,6] GnRH, on pulsatile secretion of gonadotropin secretion in the castrate male primate. J Clin Endocrinol Metab 1983;56:420–422.

11   Estrogen Biology
Evolving New Concepts

Eric P. Smith, MD

CONTENTS

INTRODUCTION

Understanding of the biology of estrogen has progressed markedly over the past decade. The definition of what constitutes an estrogen has expanded, the mechanism of action is increasingly understood and the full scope of physiologic actions in both sexes is now better appreciated. This chapter will summarize well-known basic concepts of estrogen biology while incorporating in more detail specific advances that have particular implications for pediatric endocrinology.

ESTROGEN BIOSYNTHESIS AND METABOLISM

Estrogen Biosynthesis

Estrone (E1) and estradiol (E2) enzymatically derived from androstenedione and testosterone respectively under the control of p450 aromatase enzyme are traditionally perceived to be the primary active estrogens *(1)*. Estradiol is significantly more potent than estrone. The principle source of estrogen in the female is the ovary with some contribution from the adrenal gland and peripheral aromatization of androgen *(2)*. In the male, most estrogen is derived from peripheral aromatization of androgen with some direct synthesis from the testis and adrenal. In the ovary, under the primary control of the gonadotropin hormones, FSH and LH, the granulosa cell expresses aromatase activity. Peripheral conversion of androstenedione and testosterone to estrone and estradiol, respectively, is in both sexes under the complex tissue-specific extragonadal expression of the CYP19 gene *(3)*.

From: *Molecular and Cellular Pediatric Endocrinology*
Edited by: S. Handwerger © Humana Press Inc., Totowa, NJ

Estrogen Metabolism

Similar to other classes of steroid hormones, E1 and E2 are subject to complex further metabolism. There is considerable speculation regarding what constitutes the activity of these metabolites. E1 and E2, which can themselves be interconverted, are oxidized at the C2 position to form 2–3 and 3–4 catechols that retain significant estrogenic activity *(4,5)*. The catechol estrogens are inactivated by O-methylation, glucuronidation, and sulfation but also can be converted to semiquinones implicated in carcinogenesis in part because of their capacity to covalently bind to DNA and generate reactive oxygen intermediates that can cause oxidative DNA damage *(4,6)*. Catechol estrogens, however, are thought to be, in general, rapidly metabolized reducing the possibility of significant actions. Interestingly, catechol *O*-methyl transferase levels vary from target tissues and defects in the activity of this neutralizing pathway may have important implications *(4)*.

Two novel case reports have served to clarify some physiologically important aspects of estrogen synthesis; specifically, the physiologic role of the p450 aromatase enzyme. It is instructive to review them in some detail.

The first is a case of ambiguous sex differentiation secondary to altered aromatase function in the placenta. Specifically, in 1990, Shozu *(7)* described a woman with maternal virilization secondary to apparent placental aromatase deficiency. In this individual, there were low levels of maternal estrogen and 7–10-fold increase in maternal androgen. The androgen excess led to progressive maternal virilization and to fetal masculinization. Direct in vitro analysis of placental steroidogenesis demonstrated markedly impaired aromatization strongly suggesting that the absence of placental aromatization resulted in large quantities of androstenedione and testosterone transferred to the maternal and fetal circulation. The specific lesion was determined by Harada and coworkers in 1992 to be a homozygous point mutation (GT-GC) in the 5'-splice acceptor sequence in the CYP19 gene *(8)*. Figure 1 shows the fetoplacental unit and the impact of p450 aromatase deficiency on steroidogenesis.

The second case reported in 1994 involved a karyotypic female with pseudohermaphroditism secondary to a disruptive mutation of the CYP19 aromatase gene *(9)*. This individual, who initially presented as a newborn with ambiguous genitalia of undetermined origin, was reevaluated at 14 yr of age because of marked virilization without breast development. Deficient aromatase activity resulted in elevated serum androgen and undetectable circulating estrogen concentrations. Despite persistent androgen excess, which would have been expected to rapidly advance skeletal maturation, bone age was strikingly delayed at 10 yr. Estrogen treatment resulted in suppression of elevated gonadotropins, normalization of androgen production, breast enlargement, a growth spurt, and bone-age advancement. DNA analysis revealed two discrete point mutations in the heme binding domain of the aromatase enzyme gene accounting for the impaired aromatase activity. Treatment with estrogen led to suppression of elevated gonadotropins, normalization of androgen production, breast enlargement, a growth spurt, and bone-age advancement.

These cases reveal the importance of aromatase in limiting the androgen exposure in the fetus and establish a new etiology for female pseudohemaphroditism. It is interesting to compare these observations to some studies in animals where the regulation of estrogen production appears particularly critical. For example, the female spotted hyena is born with masculinized appearance secondary to low aromatase activity *(10)*. The female

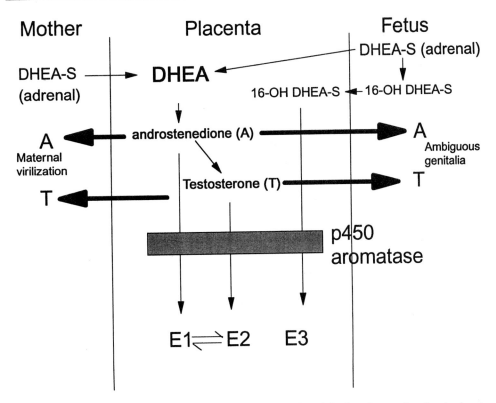

Fig. 1. Effect of p450 aromatase deficiency on maternal and fetal androgen levels. Androstene-dione and testosterone in the placental compartment are not aromatizable to E1 and E2, respectively, leading to transfer of excess androgen to maternal and fetal circulations.

reproductive structures develop normally but external genitalia display a male-like phallus with a urogenital sinus. In addition, the augmented androgen levels appear to serve a behavioral function as the females are bigger than males and are more dominant and aggressive. Even more striking are studies in poultry. Administration of an aromatase inhibitor to a female hen on d 5 of egg development will result in a testis forming instead of an ovary; estrogen rescue therapy will result in ovarian formation *(11)*. In contrast, estrogen does not appear to be required in humans for normal ovarian development. It is likely that further functions for the aromatase enzyme will be appreciated as mice with disruptions of this enzyme are characterized in detail. One prediction would be that alterations in ovarian aromatase activity may explain such human conditions as "polycystic ovary disease" *(12)*.

ESTROGEN-LIKE COMPOUNDS

A key feature of the basic estrogen structure is the aromatic ring; therefore, any compound that possesses this molecular feature has a potential for being an estrogen agonist or antagonist *(12,13)*. For example, diethylstilbestrol (DES) is a nonsteriodal analog with affinity for estrogen receptor (ER) greater than estradiol (Fig. 2). Tamoxifen and clomifene represent examples of a class of substituted triphenylethylene antiestrogens that have variable tissue and specific actions (Fig. 2). Tamoxifen antagonizes breast

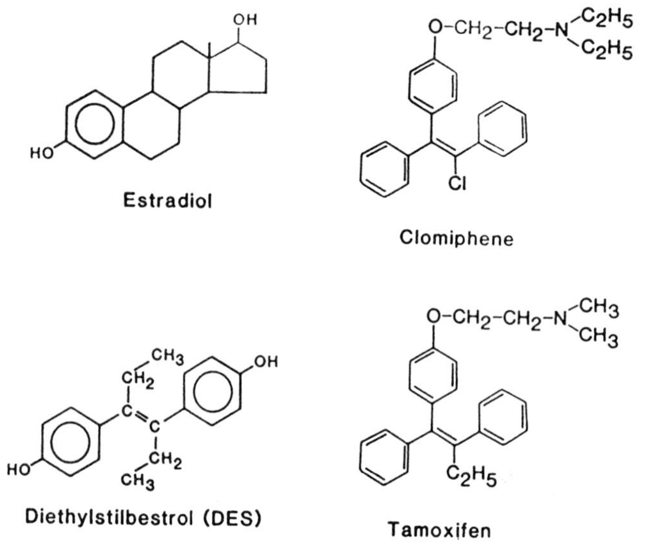

Fig. 2. Chemical structures of estradiol, diethylstilbestrol (DES), and the triphenylethylene type estrogen-like compounds, tamoxifen and clomiphene.

epithelial growth, stimulates bone mineralization and has a mixed agonist-antagonist action on the uterus *(13,14)*. More complete or pure antiestrogens include such agents as the 7-α alkylamide analog of estrogen, ICI 164384; this compound possesses little or no agonist properties, and, therefore, has harmful effects on the skeleton when used as an adjuvant in breast cancer therapy *(13,15)*.

In addition, compounds with estrogen biological activity have been identified in the environment along with plant estrogens termed "phytoestrogens" *(16,17)*. Examples include the bioflavonoids in foods and synthetic environmental contaminants, such as polychlorinated biphenyls (PCBs), DDT being a particularly familiar one. Recent evidence has accrued that these compounds can synergize with each other to generate much more potent estrogenic activity than any component individually *(18)*. The presence of these ubiquitous estrogen mimetics, contaminating synthetic estrogens, multiple naturally synthesized estrogen and the interconversion of androgen and estrogen presents an challenge to understanding the full impact of estrogen biologic activity in a given organism. For example, is the reduced incidence of heart disease in Asian cultures where diets are high in soy products secondary to a protective effect of plant estrogens on the cardiovascular system *(16,17)*? Are the declining sperm counts observed in humans secondary to environmental estrogens *(19)*?

ESTROGEN MECHANISM OF ACTION

Estrogen Receptors

The estrogen receptor is a member of a superfamily of nuclear receptors that includes those for steroids, thyroid hormone, certain vitamins, and orphan receptors for which no known ligand has been identified *(20)*. Members of the nuclear steroid family receptor contain a highly conserved DNA binding domain, a less well-conserved C-terminal ligand binding domain and a variable N-terminal domain *(22,23)*. Estrogen binds to the estrogen receptor residing predominantly in the cell nucleus regardless of ligand occupancy. Contained with the receptor protein are three basic domains signaling nuclear localization. There is evidence that the receptor is, in fact, constantly diffusing into the cytoplasm, but is then rapidly transported back into the nucleus in an energy-dependent process. Without ligand, the receptor exists as an inactive oligomeric complex that contains other proteins, including heat shock protein. Upon ligand binding, the heat shock protein dissociates allowing DNA interaction and/or interaction with a number of possible proteins involved in transcription.

Lubahn et al. in 1993 helped to clarify the function of the estrogen receptor by the development of the estrogen receptor deficient ERKO mouse by insertional disruption of the estrogen-receptor gene *(23)*. Also, these studies were performed in part to confirm the importance of estrogen in early development. Exon 2 of the mouse gene was targeted downstream of the translation start site in order to block expression of the estrogen receptor gene and protein. Homologous recombination resulted in replacement of a portion of the endogenous ER gene sequence of exon 2 with the engineered DNA sequence.

Significantly, all animals were viable suggesting that the estrogen receptor is not required for early development events that ensure survival. The female animals displayed intact differentiation of the Müllerian structures and ovaries as would be anticipated and the breast analgem was differentiated. However, there was no endometrial response to estrogen and the ovaries, reminiscent of the aromatase patient, were polycystic in appearance. The males appeared unaffected initially, but displayed infertility ultimately secondary to progressive primary testicular failure possibly secondary to seminiferous tubule fluid production/absorption abnormality *(24)*.

These observations on the murine model were insightful regarding the true physiologic role of estrogen and ongoing studies continue to reveal expected and unexpected results. For example, the behavior of the adult animals is not normal. Male animals display normal motivation to mount females but exhibit decreased intromission and ejaculation. Even more striking is substantially less aggressive behaviors and male-typical offensive attacks *(25)*. Another behavior particularly linked in prior studies to estrogen exposure in the newborn period is open-field behaviors. ERKO male mice display demasculinized open-field behaviors manifested as fewer defecations and urinations and increased rearings and leanings. Interestingly, testosterone levels are normal in these ERKO males. Female animals are less affected and appear to primarily have decreased receptivity *(26)*. These results suggest that, at least in the rodent, estrogen is important for intact reproductive behavior.

Coincident to the development of the mouse model a human karyotypic male was identified in 1994 with a disruptive mutation of the estrogen receptor gene *(27)*. Similar to the aromatase cases described earlier, a detailed review is revealing. A 28-yr-old man presented with tall stature (204 cm) and incomplete closure of the epiphyses (bone age of left wrist and hand, 15 yr) with a history of continued linear height was growth into adulthood despite otherwise normal pubertal development and apparently normal gender identification. Serum FSH, LH, estradiol, and estrone concentrations were elevated but serum testosterone concentrations were normal. The bone mineral density of the lumbar spine measured by dual-energy X-ray absorptiometry was low. To test the hypothesis of estrogen resistance, the man was treated with high-dose transdermal estrogen for 6 mo, but there was no physical or biochemical response despite a 10-fold elevation in serum

Table 1
Expected Phenotypic Findings

	Estrogen resistance Male	Aromatase deficiency Male	Female
Fetal life	Normal	Maternal virilization	Maternal virilization
Genital formation	Normal	Normal	Ambiguous genitalia
Pubertal changes	Normal	Normal	Virilization cystic ovaries amenorrhea
Pubertal growth	Attenuated	Attenuated	Attenuated
Postpubertal growth	Persistant tall stature	Persistant tall stature	?
Bone age	Delayed	Delayed	Delayed
Androgen levels	Normal	Elevated	Elevated
Estrogen levels	Elevated	Low	Low
Bone density	Low	Low	Low

estradiol concentration. DNA analysis performed by Korach and colleagues revealed a homozygous mutation of his estrogen-receptor.

Finally, in 1996 a 24-yr-old male with aromatase deficiency secondary to a CYP19 mutation was reported revealing incomplete epiphyseal closure of the left wrist and hand, (14 yr), decreased bone mass and tall stature (204 cm) (28). The mineral density of the lumbar spine low and biochemical markers for bone turnover were elevated. Serum androgen levels were elevated and serum estrogen was undetectable. Parental target achieved at the normal age of 16–17 yr followed by continued growth into his early twenties.

These two cases, consistent with the aromatase-deficient females, reveal that estrogen is particularly critical for the final phases epiphyseal maturation and normal bone mineral accretion. Another inference is that androgen alone is relatively ineffective in promoting epiphyseal fusion. Table 1 shows a comparison of the phenotype of the cases described.

However, another level of complexity was the discovery in 1996 of an additional estrogen receptor, ER-β (29). The rat ER β, encoding a protein of 485 amino acids, displays >90% homology to ER α in the DNA binding domain and approx 55% amino acid identity in the carboxyterminal ligand binding domain. Analogous to what has been known for other classes of steroid receptors is the observation that ER β is expressed differently than ER α. For example, mRNA levels as determined by reverse transcriptase PCR in the rat demonstrates that ER α expression to be predominant in the uterus, testis, pituitary, ovary, kidney, epididymus, and adrenal (30). In contrast, ER β displays preferential abundance in bladder, prostate, lung, brain, uterus, ovary, and testis. Furthermore, though most known ligands bind with similar affinity, some display markedly different affinity. For example, RU 2858 or moxestrol possess approx 10-fold different affinity for ER α vs ER β. Two plant-derived nonsteroidal compounds, coumestrol, and genistein, displayed significantly higher affinity for ER β. This may have clinical implications because ER β is particularly highly expressed in the prostate and these compounds have been associated with prostate cancer protection. By the time of publication of this textbook, the role for this new receptor will certainly be more apparent than is appreciated at this very preliminary phase (31).

Estrogen Response Elements

The ligand receptor complex interacts with cognate DNA sequences referred to as estrogen response elements *(21,22)*. There is considerable similarity among the REs for the different steroids suggesting that the specificity of response is likely to include many other factors *(21,22)*. Of recent interest, with respect to mechanisms of estrogen action, is the possibility of actions of estrogen via alternative EREs. Evidence for alternative estrogen action pathway include recent studies by Yang and colleagues *(32)*. Employing the estrogen analog, raloxifene, which similar to tamoxifen appears to antagonize estrogen action in breast while mimicking it in bone, these investigators asked the question why this analog could convey these different specificities. Estrogen, as previously mentioned, binds to the estrogen receptor inducing interaction with DNA through the classic ERE. In a MG63 osteosarcoma cell line in vitro model system employing activation of the TGF beta gene, activation involved a sequence distinct from the classic ERE. Evidence suggested that an "adapter protein" after interaction with the estrogen receptor was responsible for DNA interaction. This coupled with evidence that estrogen, but not roloxifene, may mediate some of its actions on uterine tissue through AP-1 sites on DNA may begin to explain how estrogen analogs display a myriad of tissue selective effects.

Alternate Receptors

Another intriguing aspect of estrogen mechanism of action with major implication for the physiological role for estrogen is evidence that estrogen may act independently of the classical DNA binding estrogen receptor. There is evidence for a lower affinity binding species within the nucleus termed the "Type II" receptor; its function is not known *(14,33)*. In addition, there is evidence that specific estrogen receptor(s) may be present in the plasma membrane similar to classic peptide hormone receptors *(14)*. Immunologic methods show localization of estrogen to putative binding location on the plasma membrane *(14,34)*. These studies coupled with the observation that estrogen effects are often measurable with in minutes of exposure suggest that some actions of estrogen are "nongenomic" and do not require DNA interaction *(14)*. A particularly convincing study showed, for example, that the ability of estrogen to stimulate the release of prolactin from a GH3 pituitary tumor cell line within one minute of exposure can be blocked by external trypsin exposure. The inhibition correlates with the absence of immunological localization of estrogen to the plasma membrane of these cells *(34)*.

In this context, it is of interest to include studies exploring the actions of estrogen on the vasculature *(35)*. Estrogen, which is well known to exert cardiovascular protection, may act through direct actions on the vasculature in addition to effects on lipid metabolism. The vascular wall contains estrogen receptors, vascular tone is affected by estrogen and endothelial cells in culture proliferate in response to estrogen *(36,37)*. Intriguingly, E2 in vivo and in vitro can induce an acute vasodilatory effect suggesting that membrane localized receptors distinct from the ER alpha and beta exist with signal transduction capability. However, the pharmocologic amounts raise questions about the specificity of the response. Signal transduction pathways mediating the actions of estrogen are not precisely described but calcium fluxes and changes in nitric oxide appear to be involved *(38)*.

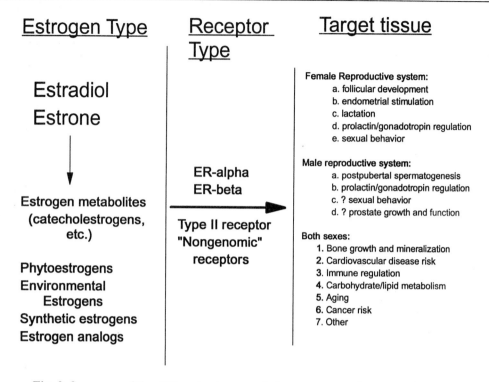

Fig. 3. Summary of the different estrogens, their receptors, and targets of action.

SUMMARY

Estrogen biology has entered a particularly complex and intriguing phase based on the combined efforts of basic science and clinical investigations *(39–42)*. Figure 3 summarizes the status of estrogen biology in terms of estrogen classification, receptor types, and targets of action. Previous notions suggested that estrogen deficiency states would be embryonically lethal *(43)*, but the validity of the lethality hypothesis is now in question. Estrogen is responsible in both males and females for the final phase of epiphyseal maturation leading to fusion and for normal bone mineralization. Indeed, estrogen can be viewed as a primary determinant of the final height of a child in the sense that estrogen initiates and completes epiphyseal closure. Clinical conditions in pediatrics such as premature thelarche, obesity-associated early puberty in girls, delayed puberty in obese boys, gynecomastia in boys, polycystic ovary disease, and decreased bone mineral density states need to be reassessed in light of these new insights *(44)*. Estrogen biological activity and the impact of estrogen in normal and pathologic conditions must be considered the sum total of estrogen biosynthesis, metabolism, and exogenous environmental compounds impacting on a array of possible receptors each modulated by the tissue specific subcellular milieu.

REFERENCES

1. Carr BR. Disorders of the ovary and female reproductive tract. In: Wilson JD, Foster DW, eds. Williams Textbook of Endocrinology, 8th ed, Saunders, Philadelphia, 1992, pp. 733–798.
2. MacDonald PC, Madden JD, Brenner PF, Wilson JD, Sitteri PK. Origin of estrogen in normal men and in women with testicular feminization. J Clin Endocrinol Metab 1979;49:905–916.

3. Simpson ER, Mahendroo MS, Means GD, Kilgore MW, Hinshelwood MM, Graham-Larence S, et al. Aromatase cytochrome p450, the enzyme responsible for estrogen biosynthesis. Endocrine Rev 1994;15:342–355.

4. Yager JD, Liehr JG. Molecular mechanisms of estrogen carcinogenesis. Annu Rev Pharmacol Toxicol 1996;36:203–232.

5. Schutze N, Vollmer G, Knuppen R. Catecholestrogens are agonists of estrogen receptor dependent gene expression in MCF-7 cells. J Steroid Biochem Mol Biol 1994;48:453–461.

6. Nutter LM, Ngo EO, Abul-Hajj YJ. Characterization of DNA damage induced by 3,4-estrone-o-quinone. J Biol Chem 1991;226:16,380–16,386.

7. Shozu M, Akasofu K, Harada T, Kubota Y. A new cause of female pseudohermaphroditism: placental aromatase deficiency. J Clin Endocrinol Metab 1991;72:560–566.

8. Harada N, Ogawa H, Shozu M, Yamada K, Sukara K, Nishida E, Takagi Y. Biochemical and molecular genetic analyses on placental aromatase (p-450 arom) deficiency. J Biol Chem 1992;267: 4781–4785.

9. Conte FA, Grumbach MM, Ito Y, Fisher CR, Simpson ER. A syndrome of female pseudo-hemaphroditism, hypergonadotropic hypogonadism, and multicystic ovaries associated with missense mutations in the gene encoding aromatase (p450). J Clin Endocrinol Metab 1994;78:1287–1292.

10. Yalcinkaya TM, Siiteri PK, Vigne J-L, Licht P, Pavgi S, Frank LG, Glickman SE. A mechanism for virilization of female hyenas in utero. Science 1993;260:1929–1931.

11. Elbrecht A, Smith RG. Aromatase enzyme activity and sex determination in chickens. Science 1992;255:467–470.

12. Bulun SE. Aromatase deficiency in women and men: would you have predicted the phenotypes? J Clin Endocrinol Metab 1996;81:867–871.

13. Evans GL, Turner RT. Tissue-selective actions of estrogen analogs. Bone 1995;17:181S–190S.

14. Clark JH, Schrader WT, O'Malley BW. Mechanisms of action of steroid hormones. In: Wilson JD, Foster DW, eds. Williams Textbook of Endocrinology, 8th ed, Saunders, Philadelphia, 1992, pp. 35–90.

15. Wiseman LR, Wakeling AE, May FE, Westley BR. Effects of the antioestrogen, ICI 164,384, on oestrogen induced RNAs in MCF-7 cells. J Steroid Biochem 1989;33:1/6.

16. Cooper RI, Kavlock RJ. Endocrine disrupters and reproductive development: a weight of the evidence overview. J Endocrinol 1997;152:159–166.

17. Safe SH. Environmental and dietary estrogens and human health: is there a problem? Environ Health Perspect 1995;103:346–351.

18. Arnold SF, Klotz DM, Collins BM, Vonier PM, Guillette LJ Jr., Mclachlan JA. Synergistic activation of estrogen receptor with combinations of environmental chemicals. Science 1996;272:1489–1492.

19. Toppari J, Larsen JC, Christiansen P, Giwercman A, Grandjean P, Guilletter LJ Jr., et al. Male reproductive health and environmental estrogens. Environ Health Perspect 1996;104(suppl 4):741–803.

20. Walter P, Green S, Greene G, Krust A, Bornert JM, Jeltsch JM, et al. Cloning of the human estrogen receptor cDNA. Proc Natl Acad Sci USA 1985;82:7889–7893.

21. Parker MG. Structure and function of estrogen receptors. Vitamins Hormones 1995;51:267–287.

22. Katzenellenbogen BS. Estrogen receptors: bioactivities and interactions with cell signaling pathways. Biol Reproduct 1996;54:287–293.

23. Lubahn DB, Moyer JS, Golding TS, Couse JF, Korach KS, Smithies O. Alteration of reproductive function but not prenatal sexual development after insertional disruption of the mouse estrogen receptor gene. Proc Natl Acad Sci USA 1993;90:11,162–11,166.

24. Eddy EM, Wahburn TF, Bunch DO, Goulding EH, Gladen BC, Lubahn DB, Korach KS. Targeted disruption of the estrogen receptor gene in the male mice causes alteration of spermatogenesis and infertility. Endocrinology 1996;137:4796–4805.

25. Ogawa S, Lubahn DB, Korach KS, Pfaff DW. Behavioral effects of estrogen receptor gene disruption in male mice. Proc Natl Acad Sci USA 1997;94:1476–1481.

26. Rissman EF, Early AH, Taylor JA, Korach KS, Lubahn DB. Estrogen receptors are essential for female sexual receptivity. Endocrinology 1997;138:507–510.

27. Smith EP, Boyd J, Frank GR, Takahashi H, Cohen RM, Specker B, et al. Estrogen resistance caused by a mutation in the estrogen-receptor gene in a man. N Engl J Med 1994;331:1056–1061.

28. Morishima A, Grumbach MM, Simpson ER, Fisher C, Qin K. Aromatase deficiency in male and female siblings caused by a novel mutation and the physiological role of estrogens. J Clin Endocrinol Metab 1995;80:3689–3698.

29. Kuiper GGJM, Enmark E, Pelto-Huikko M, Nilsson S, Gustafsson JA. Cloning of a novel estrogen receptor expressed in rat prostate and ovary. Proc Natl Acad Sci USA 1996;93:5925–5930.
30. Kuiper GGJM, Carlson B, Grandien K, Enmark E, Haggblad J, Nilsson S, Gustafsson JA. Comparison of the ligand binding specificity and transcript tissue distribution of estrogen receptors alpha and beta. Endocrinology 1997;138:863–870.
31. Katzenellenbogen BS, Korach KS. Editorial: a new actor in the estrogen receptor drama-enter ER-beta. Endocrinology 1997;138:861,862.
32. Yang NN, Venugopalan M, Hardikar S, Glasebrook A. Identification of an estrogen response element activated by metabolites of 17 beta-estradiol and roloxifene. Science 1996;273:1222–1225.
33. Markaverich BM, Clark JH. Two binding sites for estradiol in rat uterine nuclei: relationship to uterotropic response. Endocrinology 1979;105:1458–1462.
34. Watson CS, Pappas TC, Gametchu B. The other estrogen receptor in the plasma membrane: implication for the actions of environmental estrogens. Environ Health Perspect 1995;103:41–50.
35. Farhat MY, Lavigne MC, Ramwell PW. The vascular protective effects of estrogen. FASEB J 1996;10:615–624.
36. Kim-Schulze S, McGowan KA, Hubchak SC, Cid MC, Martin B, Kleinman HK, et al. Expression of an estrogen receptor by human coronary artery and umbilical vein endothelial cells. Circulation 1996;94:1402–1407.
37. Sudhir K, Chou TM, Mullen WL, Hausmann K, Collins P, Yock PG, Chatterjee K. Mechanisms of estrogen-induced vasodilitation: in vivo studies in canine coronary conductance and resistance arteries. J Am Coll Cardiol 1995;26:807–814.
38. Rosenfeld CR, Cox BE, Roy T, Mangess RR. Nitric oxide contributes to estrogen-induced vasodilitation of the ovine uterine circulation. J Clin Invest 1996;98:2158–2166.
39. Tonetti DA, Jordan VC. Targeted anti-estrogens to treat and prevent diseases in women. Mol Med Today 1996;2:218–223.
40. Frank GR. The role of estrogen in pubertal skeletal physiology: epiphyseal maturation and mineralization of the skeleton. Acta Paediatr 1995;84:627–630.
41. Federman DD. Life without estrogen. N Engl J Med 1994;331:1088,1089.
42. Korach KS. Insights from the study of animals lacking functional estrogen receptor. Science 1994;266:1524–1528.
43. Hou Q, Gorski J. Estrogen receptor and progesterone receptor genes are expressed differentially in mouse embryos during preimplantation development. Proc Natl Acad Sci USA 1993;90:9460–9464.
44. Bachrach LK. Bone mineralization in childhood and adolescence. Current Opinion Pediat 1993;5:467–473.

12

Molecular Genetics of Thyroid Cancer

Evidence That Inactivation of Tumor Suppressor Genes Occurs at Late Stages of Tumor Progression

Laura S. Ward, MD and James A. Fagin, MD

CONTENTS

INTRODUCTION

Cancer occurs because of inherited and/or acquired genetic damage altering either the expression or biochemical properties of genes involved in the regulation of cell growth or differentiation *(1–4)*. In addition, disruption of the genetic program controlling cell death may result in prolongation of cellular life span and greater predisposition to accumulate further gene mutations. The cell needs to breach a series of physiological barriers in order to escape normal growth control and progress toward the end point of malignancy. These sequential hurdles conspire to assure that successful completion of the tumorigenic process is a rarely achieved event. Mutations of either oncogenes or tumor suppressor genes are thought to confer cells with a growth advantage that allows clonal expansion, and this expansion in turn increases the probability of additional mutations. In humans, indirect measurements based on age-dependent tumor incidence predicts that, on average, the accumulation of five to six different successive mutational steps is necessary to drive a normal cell to a highly malignant phenotype *(2)*.

GENES INVOLVED IN TUMORIGENESIS

The nature of many of these genetic aberrations and of the controls regulating growth is now becoming unraveled. According to their mechanism of action, genes subject to

From: *Molecular and Cellular Pediatric Endocrinology*
Edited by: S. Handwerger © Humana Press Inc., Totowa, NJ

mutations in human cancer can be classified as oncogenes, tumor suppressor genes, and genes controlling cell death *(5)*. Activating mutations of proto-oncogenes, through either chromosomal translocation, gene amplification, retroviral insertion, or point mutations, may induce cell growth or transformation in a variety of human tissues *(1–5)*. These mutations usually act in a dominant fashion, that is, a disruption of one allele is sufficient to evoke the neoplastic phenotype. Tumor suppressor genes (TSG) act by inhibiting or preventing the expression of the tumorigenic phenotype *(1–5)*. In contrast to oncogene mutations, TSG tend to act in a recessive manner, that is, both alleles must be mutated for the loss-of-function phenotype to be fully expressed. Even if one abnormal allele is inherited, as occurs in familial retinoblastoma, the normal remaining allele is sufficient to protect against tumor development *(6)*. For the transformed phenotype to emerge, the normal allele must be either lost by deletion or inactivated by more discrete mutations *(6)*. For most human cancers, the more frequently mutated genes are the TSG, with the notable exception of the leukemias and lymphomas.

A third class of genes acts by interfering with the control of programmed cell death (for example bcl2). The process of cell death is, under physiological conditions, a well-controlled event, responding to specific signals and requiring the expression of certain genes. The bcl2 gene family is a complex group of genes that determines the apoptotic susceptibility of different cell types, and act as potent determinants of programmed cell death. Overexpression of bcl2 through translocations in follicular lymphomas is associated with marked inhibition of apoptosis, and presumably with a predisposition to transformation through accumulation of genetic damage in cells that are not cleared from the cell population *(7)*. In this chapter, we will discuss the current knowledge of the role that tumor suppressor genes may play in the development and progression of human thyroid tumors.

MOLECULAR GENETICS OF HUMAN THYROID TUMORS

Tumors of the thyroid gland are common among the general population. Approximately 10% of individuals will develop a clinically palpable thyroid nodule during their lifetime, but only a minority of these are malignant *(8)*. The thyroid follicular cell can give rise to both benign and malignant neoplasms. There is evidence that at least some benign follicular adenomas have the potential for malignant transformation *(9,10)*. A sequence of genetic events associated with the gradual progression toward thyroid cancer has been proposed *(5,9)*. Activating mutations of ras proto-oncogenes are thought to occur early in the evolution of thyroid neoplasms, and appear to be more prevalent in follicular adenomas and carcinomas than in papillary carcinomas. By contrast, rearrangements leading to the illegitimate expression of the C-terminal fragment of the ret proto-oncogene containing the intracytoplasmatic portion of this membrane receptor, are found only in thyroid cancers of the papillary subtype. They are particularly prevalent in pediatric thyroid cancers, and in those arising in children exposed to radiation after the Chernobyl nuclear accident *(11)*.

There have been a number of studies focusing on the role of tumor suppressor genes in thyroid neoplasms. We will first review the current knowledge on the prevalence of allelic losses in these tumors, as deletion of genetic material provides an important clue to the chromosomal localization of potential TSG. Subsequently, we will discuss present information on the role of known tumor suppressor genes, such as p53, RB, p16, and APC, in thyroid tumor evolution.

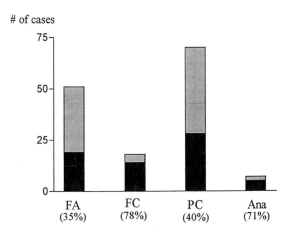

Fig. 1. Chromosomal abnormalities observed in cytogenetic studies of follicular adenomas (FA), follicular carcinomas (FC), papillary carcinomas (PC), and anaplastic carcinomas (Ana) of the thyroid. Dark portion of bar represents number of samples with a detectable cytogenetic lesion. Data summarized from refs. *12–18*.

Loss of function of TSG requires structural inactivation of both alleles. One of these is frequently lost as part of a large deletion of chromosomal material. Hence, efforts to identify consistent regions of chromosome loss in a given tumor type are a standard way to localize and eventually identify TSG. We will outline the major findings using the various strategies to identify regions of genetic loss in thyroid tumors; that is, cytogenetics, comparative genomic hybridization, and molecular approaches to identify loss of heterozygosity.

Cytogenetics

Cancer cytogenetics is the investigation of chromosome changes in tumors, and has been one of the tools used to localize TSG. In general, this approach has been more valuable for the analysis of hematological malignancies and less so for solid tumors. Since the Philadelphia chromosome was found associated with chronic myeloid leukemia, many chromosome changes observed in different tumors have provided valuable clues as to the location of genes involved in oncogenesis. In human thyroid neoplasms, cytogenetic studies have yielded abnormal karyotypes in 37–78% of the tumors analyzed *(12–18)*. In Fig. 1, we summarize the prevalence of cytogenetic abnormalities in benign and malignant human thyroid tumors. Structural aberrations were found more commonly in cancers with more aggressive behavior, such as follicular and anaplastic carcinomas. Abnormalities involving the short arm of chromosome 3 were more prevalent in follicular carcinomas, while chromosome 10q abnormalities were more commonly associated with papillary carcinomas *(13,15)*. Among the genes that could be important for the development of thyroid neoplasia on chromosome 10q is the RET proto-oncogene, that is subject to rearrangements in human papillary carcinomas. Mutations of RET also confer predisposition to multiple endocrine neoplasia Type-II (MEN IIA). We performed cytogenetic analysis on six follicular adenomas and three papillary carcinomas. Three follicular adenomas showed abnormalities: a 3;7 translocation, a 8;11 translocation and a chromosome 8 trisomy in the third case. One of the papillary carcinomas presented a deletion on chromosome 10q23–q26. This region is far from the RET/PTC rearrangement (RET is located at 10q11–q12), but is close to the Cowden's disease gene locus, recently located on chromosome 10q22–23 *(19,20)*. Cowden's disease is a familial syndrome characterized by tumors of the skin, oral mucosa, breast, and intestinal epithelium. Thyroid abnormalities, benign and malignant, occur in more than 60% of the cases *(21)*. In all the other cases the karyotype was considered normal.

Comparative Genomic Hybridization

There is considerable difficulty in obtaining reliable information on chromosome structure in solid neoplasms by standard cytogenetic techniques. When high-quality metaphase spreads are unavailable, and/or where karyotyping is hindered by the complex nature of the chromosomal abnormalities, changes in allelic dosage (i.e., deletions, amplification) can be detected by comparative genomic hybridization (CGH), a novel approach that permits the identification and mapping of regions of gain or loss of DNA by comparing DNA extracted from malignant and normal cells *(22)*. This is an unbiased technique that identifies regions of amplification or deletion in tumors by hybridizing differentially labeled tumor DNA and normal DNA to a normal metaphase spread. Amplified regions are identified by preferential hybridization of the differentially tagged tumor DNA to specific chromosome regions, that are then mapped by simultaneous comparison to conventionally banded chromosomes. In our studies, four regions (1p36, 1q42, 2p21, and 19q13.1) were demonstrated to be amplified in 40% or more of the thyroid neoplasms studied, and one region (16q12–13) was found to be consistently deleted *(23)*. LOH in this region was confirmed by PCR of markers bracketing microsatellite polymorphisms. This region of chromosome 16 has been postulated to harbor a TSG important in the evolution of breast and prostate cancer. In general, however, CGH may not provide adequate resolution for detection of relatively discrete regions of deletion to make it a powerful tool to identify the location of TSG.

Identification of Loss of Heterozygocity Based on Allelic Polymorphism

The first approach to detect loss of specific alleles in tumor DNA was based on distinction of the maternal and paternal copy through restriction fragment length polymorphisms *(24)*. The frequency of heterozygocity with this strategy, however, was always <50%, making these analyses more cumbersome. Recent technologies based on examination of hypervariable DNA regions have increased the power of these studies. Microsatellites and minisatellites are highly polymorphic regions containing variable numbers of tandem repeats, which are widely distributed throughout the genome, and have a frequency of heterozygosity of 75% or more. Polymorphism at these sites can be revealed by PCR using primers flanking the tandem repeats *(25)*. We summarize all the published literature on LOH data obtained with any of these approaches in Figs. 2 and 3 *(15,26–31)*. The overall prevalence of genetic loss in thyroid tumors is relatively low, particularly when compared to other forms of human malignancies, such as colorectal cancers *(32)*. However, follicular carcinomas and anaplastic carcinomas have much higher prevalence of LOH as compared to follicular adenomas, suggesting that these tumors have greater degree of genomic instability. It is also quite striking that papillary carcinomas have a very low prevalence of LOH. This suggests that large-scale chromosomal instability is not a major feature of these tumors, which correlates well with their favorable prognosis. Alternatively, the prevalence of LOH may be underestimated in

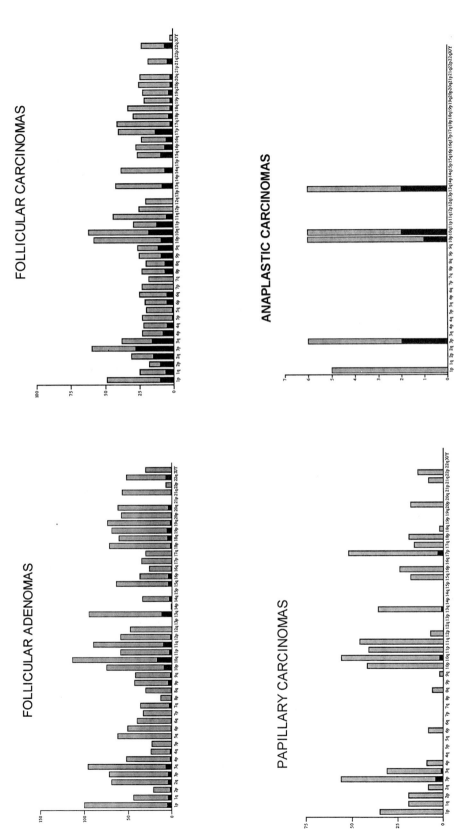

Fig. 2. Cases of LOH in each chromosome arm (black portion of bar) versus the total number of cases reported in (gray bar) in refs. *15,26–31.* Reprinted with permission from Ward et al. J Endocrinol Metab 1998;83:525–530.

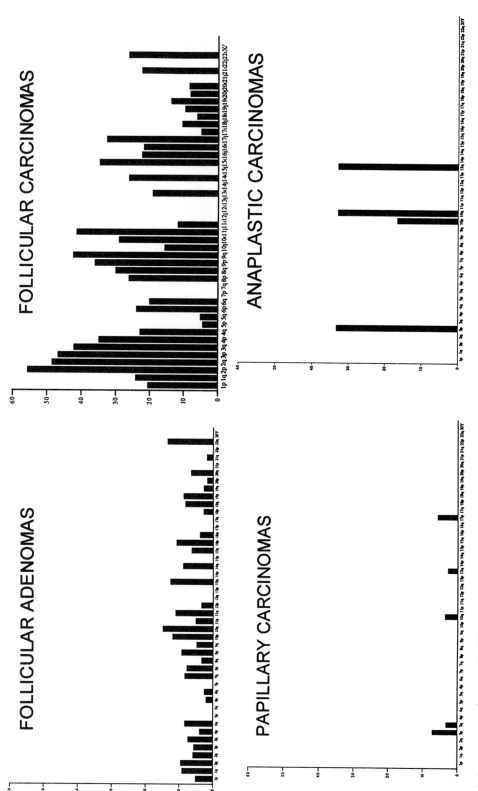

Fig. 3. Percentage of cases of LOH reported in each chromosome arm based on refs. *15,26–31*. Reprinted with permission from Ward et al. J Clin Endocrinol Metab 1998;83:525–530.

these tumors because of stromal contamination of the samples. It is also possible that loss-of-function of TSG alleles in papillary carcinomas may occur as a result of deletion of more discrete chromosome regions, or even through a point mutation, and the probes used in most of the previous reports were not sufficiently close to detect them. Two studies have described LOH at chromosome 3 in follicular carcinomas, consistent with cytogenetic findings *(15,29)*. Many other types of tumors also show deletions on chromosome 3. The 3p21–p25 region harbors the Von Hippel Lindau gene (VHL), and possibly other tumor suppressor genes. However, a recent report could not confirm mutations in exons 1–3 of the VHL gene in thyroid tumors *(30)*. Moreover, in an analysis of 28 follicular carcinomas Tung et al. found only a 30.4% rate of LOH in 23 follicular carcinomas informative for 3p, lower than the LOH rate they found in many other chromosomes *(31)*. Loss of genetic material has also been observed on chromosome 11q13 in follicular, but not papillary neoplasms, within the region containing the gene that confers predisposition to multiple endocrine neoplasia type I (MEN I) *(26)*. Taken together, the data presented in Figs. 1–3 make a compelling case for allelic losses arising as late events in thyroid tumor progression. Besides the studies attempting to define regions of allelic loss that may harbor TSG important in thyroid tumor evolution, several groups have examined thyroid tumors for structural or functional abnormalities of known tumor suppressors.

p53

p53 is a nuclear protein that exerts an important role in the negative control of cellular proliferation, and in masterminding signaling cascades important in DNA repair and/or apoptosis *(33–35)*. For example, when severe damage to DNA has occurred, p53 arrests the cell cycle, presumably allowing DNA repair to take place or, alternatively, initiating the pathway toward programmed cell death *(34)*. Cell cycle progression is controlled, in part, by cyclin-dependent kinases (CDKs) at the transition of both G1 to S and G2 to M phases *(35)*. Deregulation of the factors that positively or negatively influence CDK activity can allow aberrant progression of the cell cycle and favor development of a tumor cell. p53 binds to the promoter of the p21 gene and activates its transcription. Since p21 is a CDK inhibitor, activation of its expression and function results in cell cycle blockage at the G1 phase. Mutations of p53 alone can immortalize some cell lines. Mice with homozygous disruption of the p53 gene have increased incidence of multiple tumor types *(36)*. Mutations of p53 have been reported with high frequency in many cancer types and are believed to be a major determinant of the phenotype of many forms of cancer *(37,38)*. Conversely, expression of the wild-type protein suppresses growth and/or induces apoptosis of many transformed cells bearing deleted or mutant p53 genes *(34,39)*. Many studies, both with immunocytochemistry and genetic analysis, have shown that p53 mutations are highly prevalent in poorly differentiated and undifferentiated thyroid carcinomas, as well as thyroid cancer cell lines *(41–46)*. However, they are not found in benign tumors and are infrequent in well-differentiated cancer, suggesting that mutational inactivation of p53 occurs at a late stage of thyroid tumor progression. Interestingly, there is a low rate of LOH in chromosome 17p (Fig. 2). There is also evidence that p53 may interfere with thyroid cell differentiation. Introduction of a mutated p53 markedly impairs the differentiated gene expression of PCC13 thyroid cells *(46)*. By contrast, wild-type p53 reintroduction into an undifferentiated thyroid carcinoma cell line leads to reexpression of thyroid peroxidase, a characteristic differentiated marker of the thyroid cell *(47)*.

RB

Since RB plays a key role in the control of the G1/S interphase of the cell cycle, it is tempting to speculate that RB and related proteins might constitute primary targets for mutations in human thyrocytes. RB is a substrate for phosphorylation by CDK. After phosphorylation, RB releases E2F transcription factors, which promote the expression of genes that control cell cycle progression *(35)*. Inactivation of one of the RB alleles in transgenic mice leads to a high incidence of pituitary tumors *(48)*. Transgenic mice that overexpress SV40 T antigen ubiquitously (a viral oncogene product that binds and inactivates the RB and p53 gene products) develop a syndrome similar to multiple endocrine neoplasia *(49)*. These mice develop thyroid follicular, pancreatic, pituitary, adrenal, and testicular tumors. By contrast, transgenic mice exhibiting thyroid-specific expression of T antigen develop undifferentiated thyroid cancer *(50)*. Transgenic mice expressing the E7 protein (an oncogene whose action is attributed in part to its interaction with RB) in thyroid follicular cells develop well-differentiated goiters. These glands show foci of more actively proliferating cells that become invasive and ultimately tend to lose their differentiated properties. Old mice display secondary tumors similar to human differentiated follicular and papillary carcinomas *(50)*. RB is expressed uniformly in the normal thyroid epithelium *(51)*. Zou et al. found deletions of RB gene exon 21 in 27 of 46 (59%) thyroid neoplasms *(52)*. However, Holm and Nesland found that RB immunoreactivity was not lost in any case of 131 thyroid tumors they examined *(45)*. Furthermore, different molecular studies of chromosome 13 also do not signal this region as an important site of LOH (Figs. 2 and 3). The role of other cell cycle proteins that interact with RB in thyroid tumors has not been fully explored.

APC

Mutations of the APC gene confer predisposition to familial adenomatous polyposis coli. This gene is also involved in sporadic colorectal tumorigenesis. As papillary thyroid carcinomas occur more frequently in patients with familial adenomatous polyposis, there has been considerable interest in exploring whether APC may play a role in thyroid tumor formation *(53)*. We examined 80 human thyroid neoplasms for LOH of the APC locus, located on chromosome 5q21 *(54)*. Only two cases, a follicular adenoma and a multinodular goiter, showed LOH. We also examined the DNA from 83 benign and malignant tumors and four thyroid carcinoma cell lines using SSCP and five different sets of overlapping primers. Only one mutation was detected in an anaplastic carcinoma and in the ARO cell line, a cell line derived from an anaplastic carcinoma *(54)*. Lack of significant involvement of APC in thyroid tumors was also reported by Curtis et al. who studied 16 papillary carcinomas, and Colletta et al. who investigated 26 thyroid tumors of different histological types *(55,56)*.

P16

The p16 gene is located on chromosome 9p21. It acts as an inhibitor of cyclin-dependent kinase 4 (CDK4), and thus blocks progression through the G1-S boundary of the cell cycle *(57,58)*. Homozygous deletions and mutations of p16 have been demonstrated in many malignancies of the head and neck, esophagus, pancreas, brain and lung carcinomas, T-cell acute lymphoblastic leukemias and a large variety of cell lines *(58–60)*. Tung et al. reported loss of 9p sequences in a significant proportion of follicular (27%) and anaplastic carcinomas of the thyroid (two out of four cases), but not in papillary carcinomas *(61)*. Calabro et al. found abnormalities of p16 in five out of the seven thyroid cell lines they examined *(62)*. However, they found neither deletions nor point mutations in 31 thyroid tumors. We examined 20 thyroid tumors and four human thyroid carcinoma cell lines (ARO, FRO, WRO, and NPA) for gene deletions and point mutations of p16 *(63)*. Although, three of our four cell lines showed mutational alterations, deletions, and/or point mutations, only 1 out of 12 papillary carcinomas presented a point mutation. No mutations were found in eight follicular adenomas. These findings suggest that although loss of p16 function gives cells in culture a selective growth advantage, it does not appear to be directly involved in thyroid tumor development. However, it is conceivable that these genes may be involved in the late stages of thyroid carcinogenesis.

The role of many other TSG genes, such as BRCA1, DCC, VHL, NF1 and NF2, FHIT, WT1, RCC, NB1, MLM, BCNS, and LC1, have not been studied in thyroid cancer. Likewise, we still lack a better understanding of the role of genes involved in tumor progression and metastasis. As more of these genetic defects are identified, it is likely that this will result in better diagnostic and prognosis markers, and ultimately, on more specific biological therapies aimed at precise biochemical targets in the damaged tumor cells.

ACKNOWLEDGMENT

This work was supported in part by NIH grants CA50706 and CA72597. J. A. F. is a recipient of an Established Investigator Award from the American Heart Association and Bristol Myers Squibb.

REFERENCES

1. Bishop JM. The molecular genetics of cancer. Science 1987;235:305–311.
2. Weinberg R. Oncogenes, antioncogenes, and the molecular bases of multistep carcinogenesis. Cancer Res 1989;49:3713–3721.
3. Smith JR, Pereira-Smith OM. Replicative senescence: implications for in vivo aging and tumor suppression. Science 1996;273:63–67.
4. Knudson AG. Antioncogenes and human cancer. Proc Natl Acad Sci USA 1993;90:10,914–10,921.
5. Fagin JA. Molecular pathogenesis of human thyroid neoplasms. Thyroid Today 1994;17:1–7.
6. Knudson AG. Mutation and cancer: statistical study of retinoblastoma. Proc Natl Acad Sci USA 1971;68:820.
7. Chittenden T, Harrington EA, O'Connor R, Flemington C, Lutz RJ, Evan GI, Guild BC. Induction of apoptosis by the Bcl-2 homologue Bak. Nature 1995;374:733–739.
8. Williams ED. The etiology of thyroid tumors. Clin Endocrin Metab 1979;8:193–207.
9. Nadir RF, Yufei S, Minjing Z. Molecular basis of thyroid cancer. Endocrine Rev 1994;15:202–232.
10. Mazzaferri EL. Management of a solitary thyroid nodule. N Engl J Med 1993;328:553–559.
11. Nikiforov YE, Rowland JM, Bove KE, Monforte-Munoz H, Fagin JA. Distinct pattern of RET oncogene rearrangements in morphological variants of radiation-induced and sporadic thyroid papillary carcinomas in children. Cancer Res 1997;57:1690–1694.
12. Teyssier JR, Liautaud-Roger D, Ferre D, Patey M, Dufer J. Chromosomal changes in thyroid tumors. Relation with DNA content, karyotypic features and clinical data. Cancer Genet Cytogenet 1990;50: 249–263.
13. Jenkins RB, Hay ID, Herath JF, Schultz CG, Spurbeck JL, Grant CS, et al. Frequent occurrence of cytogenetic abnormalities in sporadic nonmedullary thyroid carcinoma. Cancer (Phila) 1990;66: 1213–1220.
14. Roque L, Castedo S, Clode A, Soares J. Deletion of 3p25 → pter in a primary follicular thyroid carcinoma and its metastasis. Genes, Chromosomes Cancer 1993;8:199–203.
15. Herrmann MA, Hay ID, Bartelt DH, Ritland SR, Dahl RJ, Grant CS, Jenkins RB. Cytogenetic and molecular genetic studies of follicular and papillary thyroid tumors. J Clin Invest 1991; 88:1596–1604.

16. Bondeson L, Bengtsson A, Bondeson AG, Dahlenfors R, Grimelius L, Wedell B, Mark J. Chromosome studies in thyroid neoplasia. Cancer 1989;64:680–685.

17. van den Berg E, van Doormaal JJ, Oosterhuis JV, de Jong B, Wiersema J, Vos AM, et al. Chromosomal aberrations in follicular thyroid carcinoma. Cancer Genet Cytogenet 1991;54:215–222.

18. Roque L, Clode AL, Gomes P, Rosa-Santos J, Soares J, Castedo S. Cytogenetic findings in 31 papillary thyroid carcinomas. Genes Chromosomes Cancer 1995;13:157–162.

19. Donghi R, Sozzi G, Pierotti MA, Biunno I, Miozzo M, Fusco A, et al. The oncogene associated with human papillary thyroid carcinoma (PTC) is assigned to chromosome 10q11-q12 in the same region as multiple endocrine neoplasia 2A (MEN2). Oncogene 1989;4:521–523.

20. Nelen MR, Padberg GW, Peeters EA, Lin AY, van den Helm B, Frants RR, et al. Localization of the gene for Cowden's disease to chromosome 10q22-23. Nature Genet 1996;13:114–116.

21. Starink TM, van der Veen JP, Arwert F, de Waal LP, de Lange GG, Gille JJ, Eriksson AW. The Cowden syndrome: A clinical and genetic study in 21 patients. Clin Genet 1986;29:222–233.

22. Kallioniemi A, Kallioniemi O-P, Sudar D, Rutovitz D, Gray JW, Waldman F, Pinkel D. Comparative genomic hybridization for molecular cytogenetic analysis of solid tumors. Science 1992;258:818–820.

23. Chen XN, Knauf JA, Gonsky R, Wang M, Lai EH, Chissoe S, Fagind A, Korenberg JR. From amplification to gene in thyroid cancer: a high resolution mapped BAC resource for cancer chromosome aberrations guides gene discovery after comparative genomic hybridization. Am J Hum Genet 1998; in press.

24. Hansen MF, Cavenee WK. Genetics of cancer predisposition. Cancer Res 1987;47:5518–5527.

25. Orita M, Suzuki Y, Sekiya T, Hayashi K. Rapid and sensitive detection of point mutations and DNA polymorphisms using the polymerase chain reaction. Genomics 1989;5:874–879.

26. Matsuo KS, Tang H, Fagin JA. Allelotype of human thyroid tumors: loss of chromosome 11q13 sequences in follicular neoplasms. Mol Endocrinol 1991;5:1873–1879.

27. Kubo K, Yoshimoto K, Yokogoshi Y, Tsuyuguchi M, Saito S. Loss of heterozygosity on chromosome 1p in thyroid adenoma and medullary carcinoma, but not in papillary carcinoma. Jpn J Cancer Res 1991;82:1097–1103.

28. Zedenius J, Wallin G, Svensson A, Grimelius L, Hoog A, Lundell G, et al. Allelotyping of follicular thyroid tumors. Hum Genet 1995;96:27–32.

29. Zedenius J, Wallin G, Svensson A, Bovee J, Hoog A, Backdahl M, Larsson C. Deletions of the long arm of chromosome 10 in progression of follicular thyroid tumors. Hum Genet 1996;97:299–303.

30. Grebe SKG, Hay ID, Jenkins RB, Wu S-C, Maciel L, Eberhardt NL. Frequent loss of heterozygosity on the distal portions of chromosomes 3p and 17p in follicular thyroid carcinoma is rarely associated with mutations in the known tumor suppressor genes VHL and p53. Thyroid 1996;137:S70–79 (abstract).

31. Tung WS, Shevlin DW, Kaleem Z, Tribune DJ, Wells SA, Goodfellow PJ. Allelotype of follicular carcinomas reveals genetic instability consistent with frequent nondisjunctional chromosomal loss. Genes, Chromosomes Cancer, 1997, in press.

32. Ward LS, Brenta G, Medvedovic M, Fagin JA. Studies of allelic loss in thyroid tumors reveal major differences in chromosome instability between papillary and follicular carcinomas. J Clin Endocrinol Metab 1998;83:525–530.

33. Levine AJ. p53, the cellular gatekeeper for growth and division. Cell 1997;88:323–331.

34. Yonish-Rouach E, Resnitzky D, Lotem J, Sachs L, Kimchi A, Oren M. Wild-type p53 induces apoptosis of myeloid leukemic cells that is inhibited by interleukin-6. Nature, 1991;352:345–347.

35. Paulovich AG, Toczyski DP, Hartwell LH. When checkpoints fail. Cell 1997;83:315–321.

36. Donehower LA, Harvey M, Slagle BL, McArthur MJ, Montgomery CA, Butel JS, Bradley A. Mice deficient for p53 are developmentally normal but susceptible to spontaneous tumours. Nature 1992;356:215–221.

37. Nigro JM, Baker SJ, Presinger AC, et al. Mutations in the p53 gene occur in diverse human tumor types. Nature 1989;342:705–708.

38. Harris CC, Hollstein M. Clinical implications of the p53 tumor-suppressor gene. N Engl J Med 1993;329:1318–1327.

39. Baker SJ, Markowitz S, Fearon ER, Wilson JK, Vogelstein B. Suppression of human colorectal carcinoma cell growth by wild-type p53. Science (Washington DC) 1990;249:912–915.

40. Ito T, Seyama S, Mizuno T, Tsuyama T, Hayashi T, Hayashi Y, et al. Unique association of p53 mutations with undifferentiated but not with differentiated carcinomas of the thyroid gland. Cancer Res 1992;52:1369–1372.

41. Fagin JA, Matsuo K, Karmakar A, Chen DL, Tang SH, Koeffler HP. High prevalence of mutations of the p53 gene in poorly differentiated human thyroid carcinomas. J Clin Invest 1993;91:179–184.

42. Donghi R, Longoni A, Pilotti S, Michieli P, Della Porta G, Pierotti MA. p53 mutations are restricted to poorly differentiated and undifferentiated carcinomas of the thyroid gland. J Clin Invest 1993; 91:1753–1760.

43. Dobashi Y, Sakamoto A, Sugimura H, Merney M, Mori M, Oyama T, Machinami R. Overexpression of p53 as a possible factor in human thyroid carcinoma. Am J Surg Pathol 1993;17:375–381.

44. Jossart GH, Epstein HD, Shaver JK, Weier HU, Greulich KM, Tezelman S, et al. Immunocytochemical detection of p53 in human thyroid carcinomas is associated with mutation and immortalization of cell lines. J Clin Endocrinol Metab 1996;81:3498–3504.

45. Holm R, Nestland JM. Retinoblastoma and p53 tumor suppressor gene protein expression in carcinomas of the thyroid gland. J Pathol 1994;172:267–272.

46. Battista S, Martelli ML, Fedele M, Chiappetta G, Trapasso F, De Vita G, et al. A mutated p53 alters differentiation of thyroid cells. Oncogene 1995;72:2029–2037.

47. Fagin JA, Tang S-H, Zeki K, Di Lauro R, Fusco A, Gonsky R. Reexpression of thyroid peroxidase in a derivative of an undifferentiated thyroid carcinoma cell line by introduction of wild-type p53. Cancer Res 1996;56:765–771.

48. Jacks T, Fazeli A, Schmitt EM, et al. Effects of an RB mutation in the mouse. Nature 1992;359:259–300.

49. Reynolds RK, Hoekzema GS, Vogel J, et al. Multiple endocrine neoplasia induced by the promiscuous expression of a viral oncogene. Proc Natl Acad Sci USA 1988;85:3135–3139.

50. Ledent C, Marcotte A, Dumont JE, Vassart G, Parmentier M. Differentiated carcinomas develop as a consequence of the thyroid specific expression of a thyroglobulin-human papillomavirus type 16 E7 transgene. Oncogene 1995;10:1789–1797.

51. Cordon-Cardo C, Richon VM. Expression of the retinoblastoma protein is regulated in normal human tissues. Am J Pathol 1994;144:500–510.

52. Zou MU, Shi YF, Farid NR. Retinoblastoma gene defects are central to thyroid carcinogenesis. Endocrine Soc Meet 1993, abstr 162.

53. Bell B, Mazzaferri EL. Familial adenomatous polyposis (Gardner's syndrome) and thyroid carcinoma. A case report and review of the literature. Dig Dis Sci 1993;38:185–189.

54. Zeki K, Spambalg D, Sharifi N, Gonsky R, Fagin JA. Mutations of the adenomatous polyposis coli gene in sporadic thyroid neoplasms. J Clin Endorinol Metab 1994;79:1317–1321.

55. Curtis L, Wyllie AH, Shaw JJ, Williams GT, Radulescu A, DeMicco C, et al. Evidence against involvement of APC mutation in papillary carcinoma. Eur J Cancer 1994;30:984–987.

56. Colletta G, Sciacchitano S, Palmirotta R, Ranieri A, Zanella E, Cama A, et al. Analysis of adenomatous polyposis coli gene in thyroid tumours. Br J Cancer 1994;70:1085–1088.

57. Serrano M, Hannon GJ, Beach D. A new regulatory motif in cell-cycle control causing specific inhibition of cyclin D/CDK4. Nature 1993;366:704–707.

58. Kamb A, Gruis N, Weaver-Feldhaus J, et al. A cell cycle regulator potentially involved in genesis of many tumor types. Science 1994;264:436–440.

59. Liggett WH, Sewell DA, Rocco J, Ahrendt SA, Koch W, Sidransky D. p16 and p16 beta are potent growth suppressors of head and neck squamous carcinoma cells in vitro. Cancer Res 1996;56: 4119–4123.

60. Nobori T, Miura K, Wu D, Lois A, Takabayashi K, Carson D. Deletions of the cyclin-dependent kinase-4 inhibitor gene in multiple human cancers. Nature 1994;368:753–756.

61. Tung WS, Shevlin DW, Bartsch D, Norton JA, Wells SA, Goodfellow PJ. Infrequent CDKN2 mutation in human differentiated thyroid cancers. Mol Carcinog 1996;15:5–10.

62. Calabro V, Strazzullo M, La Mantia G, Fedele M, Paulin C, Fusco A. Status and expression of the p16 gene in human thyroid tumors and thyroid-tumor cell lines. Int J Cancer 1996;67:29–34.

63. Elisei R, Shiohara M, Koeffler HP, Fagin JA. Genetic and epigenetic alterations of the cyclin dependent kinase inhibitors p15[INK4b] and p16[INK4a] in human thyroid carcinoma cell lines, and in primary human cancers. Cancer 1998; in press.

13 The Molecular Basis of Mineralocorticoid Action

Perrin C. White, MD

CONTENTS

PHYSIOLOGY OF MINERALOCORTICOID ACTION

Mineralocorticoids, or salt retaining steroids, help control intravascular volume by regulating sodium resorption in target tissues such as the kidney, colon, and salivary glands.

Although the bulk of sodium resorption from the renal glomerular filtrate occurs in the proximal tubule and the thin ascending limb of the loop of Henle, regulated sodium resorption takes place in the distal convoluted tubule and cortical collecting duct *(1)*. The first step in sodium resorption is by passive diffusion through sodium-permeable channels in the apical membranes of epithelial cells lining the tubules. This is driven by an electrochemical gradient generated by a sodium/potassium ATPase located in the basolateral cell membrane.

The most important regulator of sodium resorption is the renin-angiotensin-aldosterone system (Fig. 1). The classic regulatory pathway of this system begins in the renal juxtaglomerular apparatus, where stretch receptors in the afferent arteriole respond to a fall in intravascular volume by stimulating secretion of renin, a proteolytic enzyme that cleaves angiotensinogen to produce a decapeptide, angiotensin I. This is converted by a widely distributed angiotensin converting enzyme to the octapeptide, angiotensin II. Angiotensin II activates aldosterone biosynthesis in the zona glomerulosa of the adrenal cortex through effects on steroidogenic enzymes that are mediated by a specific receptor.

Aldosterone, in turn, increases the apparent number of sodium channels in the epithelium of the distal tubule. This may reflect an increase in the percentage of time that each

From: *Molecular and Cellular Pediatric Endocrinology*
Edited by: S. Handwerger © Humana Press Inc., Totowa, NJ

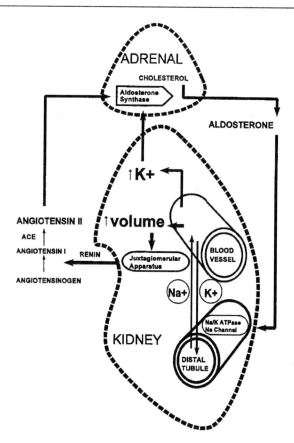

Fig. 1. Regulation of intravascular volume and plasma potassium concentrations by the renin-angiotensin-aldosterone system *(103)*. Decreased intravascular volume increases renin secretion by the juxtaglomerular apparatus leading to increased conversion of angiotensinogen to angiotensin II. Angiotensin II acts on the adrenal zona glomerulosa to increase the activity of aldosterone synthase and therefore aldosterone secretion. Hyperkalemia also increases activity of aldosterone synthase. Aldosterone acts on the renal distal tubule to increase sodium (Na^+) resorption and potassium (K^+) excretion. ACE, angiotensin converting enzyme; Na/K ATPase, sodium-potassium dependent adenosine triphosphatase.

channel stays open *(2)*, and/or an increase in the actual number of channels *(3)*, although the signaling pathways by which aldosterone acts are not well-understood. Aldosterone also increases synthesis of the sodium/potassium ATPase *(4)*.

MINERALOCORTICOID BIOSYNTHESIS

Pathways

Aldosterone is synthesized from cholesterol in the zona glomerulosa (the outermost zone) of the adrenal cortex (Fig. 2). This process requires five enzymatic conversions. The side-chain of cholesterol is cleaved in mitochondria by cholesterol desmolase (CYP11A) to yield pregnenolone. This is converted to progesterone by 3β-hydroxy-steroid dehydrogenase (3β-HSD) in the endoplasmic reticulum and then to deoxycorticosterone by 21-hydroxylase (CYP21). In mitochondria, deoxycorticosterone is

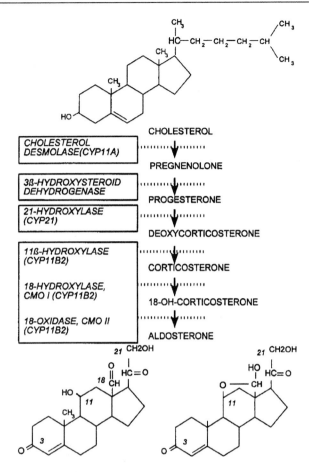

Fig. 2. Pathway of aldosterone biosynthesis. The planar structures of cholesterol **(Bottom)** and aldosterone **(Top)** are shown. Aldosterone exists in two conformations (18-aldehyde and hemiacetal) that are freely interconvertible; the hemiacetal predominates under physiological conditions. The enzymes responsible for each biosynthetic step are listed in boxes on the left; the last three steps of aldosterone biosynthesis are mediated by a single enzyme, aldosterone synthase (CYP11B2).

successively hydroxylated at the 11β and 18 positions to corticosterone and 18-hydroxycorticosterone, respectively, and further oxidized at the 18-position to aldosterone. These last three steps are all catalyzed by the same enzyme, a cytochrome P450 termed aldosterone synthase (CYP11B2) *(5,6)*. Probably all three steps take place in succession without release of the steroid molecule from the enzyme. This enzyme is normally expressed only in the zona glomerulosa; the zona fasciculata expresses a distinct isozyme of 11β-hydroxylase, CYP11B1, that is required for cortisol biosynthesis.

Regulation

The rate of aldosterone synthesis, which is normally 100–1000-fold less than that of cortisol synthesis, is regulated mainly by angiotensin II and potassium levels with ACTH having only a short-term effect *(7)*.

CYP11B2 is expressed at very low levels in the normal adrenal gland compared to CYP11B1 *(5,8)* but is present at increased levels in aldosterone secreting tumors *(5,6)*. CYP11B1 and CYP11B2 are expressed, respectively, in the zonae fasciculata and glomerulosa in a mutually exclusive manner when examined by *in situ* hybridization of normal human adrenal cortex *(9)*.

Angiotensin II markedly increases CYP11B2 expression in primary cultures of human zona glomerulosa cells *(5)* and in NCI-H295 human adrenocortical carcinoma cells *(10)*; potassium also increases CYP11B2 levels in the latter cells. Angiotensin II acts by occupying a specific G protein-coupled receptor *(11,12)*, activating phospholipase C. The latter protein hydrolyses phosphatidylinositol bisphosphate to produce inositol triphosphate and diacylglycerol, which raise intracellular calcium levels. In contrast, potassium increases calcium influx through specific membrane channels. In either case, calcium activates kinases that presumably phosphorylate transcription factors to regulate gene expression. Although it has been presumed that protein kinase C is one such kinase, experiments with inhibitors and agonists suggest that this kinase does not play a major role in regulation of CYP11B2 transcription *(13)*.

The 5' flanking region of the CYP11B2 gene *(8)* contains a cAMP response element and at least two recognition sites for steroidogenic factor-1 (SF-1) *(14,15)*. Factors binding cAMP response elements (CREB) *(16)* have been identified. SF-1 (also called Ad4BP) is an orphan nuclear receptor; i.e., it is a member of the steroid and thyroid hormone receptor superfamily but its ligand is not known. Both the cAMP response elements and the most proximal SF-1 site are critical for both basal and calcium-stimulated transcription of human CYP11B2, suggesting that phosphorylation of CREB and/or SF-1 may be a mechanism by which CYP11B2 is regulated *(13)*. In addition, this SF-1 site is known to bind additional protein factors, such as the orphan nuclear receptor, COUP-TF. As yet, the genetic elements responsible for the differential regulation of CYP11B1 and CYP11B2 in the zonae fasciculata and glomerulosa have not been identified.

Pathophysiology

CONGENITAL ADRENAL HYPERPLASIA

Congenital adrenal hyperplasia, the inherited inability to synthesize cortisol, may be associated with either decreased or increased mineralocorticoid activity depending on the metabolic defect involved.

Two-thirds of patients with classic 21-hydroxylase deficiency are unable to synthesize adequate amounts of aldosterone and are said to have the "salt-wasting" form of the disorder. This represents by far the most frequent defect in aldosterone biosynthesis *(17,18)*. In contrast, two thirds of cases of 11β-hydroxylase deficiency, the second most common cause of congenital adrenal hyperplasia, are associated with hypertension *(19,20)*. The reason for this is not well understood; serum levels of deoxycorticosterone, a weak mineralocorticoid, are elevated in this disorder, but blood pressure and deoxycorticosterone levels are poorly correlated in patients *(19,21)*.

ALDOSTERONE SYNTHASE DEFICIENCY

Clinical Features. Rare patients have aldosterone deficiency with entirely normal cortisol and sex steroid synthesis *(22,23)*, as a result of disruption of the final steps of aldosterone biosynthesis (conversion of corticosterone to aldosterone) *(24)*. This leads to excessive sodium excretion and potassium retention in the renal distal tubule and cortical collecting duct, causing hyponatremia and hyperkalemia. Plasma renin activity is markedly elevated in affected infants and young children, but it may be normal in adults.

Two forms of aldosterone synthase (also termed corticosterone methyloxidase) deficiency are recognized *(25)*. These syndromes have identical clinical features but differ in profiles of secreted steroids. In particular, whereas excretion of 18-hydroxycorticosterone is mildly decreased in Type-I deficiency, urinary and serum levels of this steroid are dramatically increased in patients with Type-II deficiency *(26)*.

Genetics. All patients with aldosterone synthase deficiency carry mutations in CYP11B2. Two kindreds with Type-I deficiency have mutations that destroy enzymatic activity *(27)*. Most kindreds with Type-II deficiency are Jews of Iranian origin who are all homozygous for the same two missense mutations, R181W and V386A. These mutations together yield an enzyme with normal 11β-hydroxylase activity, markedly decreased 18-hydroxylase activity and almost undetectable 18-oxidase activity. Although this would suggest that Type-I and Type-II deficiencies represent allelic variants, one kindred with Type-II deficiency has been described that has mutations on both chromosomes that completely inactive the enzyme *(28)*. In this kindred, at least, the enzymatic source of 18-hydroxycorticosterone is not obvious; perhaps the amount of 18-hydroxylase activity present in CYP11B1 (which normally expresses very low levels of this activity) is itself subject to allelic variation *(29)*.

GLUCOCORTICOID SUPPRESSIBLE HYPERALDOSTERONISM

Clinical Features. Glucocorticoid suppressible hyperaldosteronism (also called dexamethasone-suppressible hyperaldosteronism or glucocorticoid remediable aldosteronism) is a rare form of hypertension inherited in an autosomal dominant manner with high penetrance *(30,31)*. It is characterized by moderate hypersecretion of aldosterone, suppressed plasma renin activity, and rapid reversal of these abnormalities after administration of glucocorticoids. Hypokalemia is usually mild and may be absent. Elevation of 18-oxocortisol is the most consistent and reliable biochemical marker of the disease, although it may also be elevated in cases of primary aldosteronism *(32,33)*. This steroid may be of pathophysiologic significance; it is an agonist for the mineralocorticoid receptor and has been shown to raise blood pressure in animal studies *(34)*.

Once an affected individual has been identified in a kindred, additional cases may be ascertained within that kindred using biochemical (18-oxocortisol levels) or genetic *(see below)* markers *(35)*. Affected individuals have blood pressures that are markedly elevated as compared to unaffected individuals in the same kindred, although some patients may in fact have normal blood pressures. Some affected kindreds have remarkable histories of early (before age 45) death from strokes in many family members *(35,36)*. Steroid biosynthesis is otherwise normal so that affected individuals have normal growth and sexual development.

Whereas most laboratory and clinical abnormalities are suppressed by treatment with glucocorticoids, infusion of ACTH exacerbates these problems *(37,38)*. This suggests that aldosterone is being inappropriately synthesized in the zona fasciculata and is being regulated by ACTH. Moreover, 18-hydroxycortisol and 18-oxocortisol, steroids that are characteristically elevated in this disorder, are 17α-hydroxylated analogs of 18-hydroxycorticosterone and aldosterone, respectively. Because 17α-hydroxylase is not expressed in the zona glomerulosa, the presence of large amounts of a 17α-hydroxy, 18-oxosteroid suggests that an enzyme with 18-oxidase activity (i.e., aldosterone synthase, CYP11B2) is abnormally expressed in the zona fasciculata *(39)*.

Genetics. CYP11B2 and CYP11B1 are normally about 40 kb apart on chromosome 8q22, but all patients with glucocorticoid suppressible hyperaldosteronism have a chromosome that carries three CYP11B genes instead of the normal two *(40–42)*. The middle gene on this chromosome is a chimera with 5' and 3' ends corresponding to CYP11B1 and CYP11B2, respectively. The chimeric gene is flanked by presumably normal CYP11B2 and CYP11B1 genes. In all kindreds analyzed thus far, the breakpoints (the points of transition between CYP11B1 and CYP11B2 sequences) are located between intron 2 and exon 4. As the breakpoints are not identical in different kindreds, these must represent independent mutations.

The chromosomes carrying chimeric genes are presumably generated by unequal crossing over. The high homology (93% identity) and proximity of the CYP11B1 and CYP11B2 genes makes it possible for them to become misaligned during meiosis. If this occurs, crossing over between the misaligned genes creates two chromosomes, one of which carries one CYP11B gene (i.e., a deletion) whereas the other carries three CYP11B genes.

The invariable presence of a chimeric gene in patients with this disorder suggests that this gene is regulated like CYP11B1 (expressed at high levels in the zona fasciculata and regulated primarily by ACTH) because it has transcriptional regulatory sequences identical to those of CYP11B1. Recently, abnormal expression of the chimeric gene in the zona fasciculata was directly demonstrated by *in situ* hybridization studies of an adrenal gland from a patient with this disorder *(9)*.

If the chimeric gene has enzymatic activity similar to that of CYP11B2, a single copy of such an abnormally regulated gene should be sufficient to cause the disorder, consistent with the known autosomal dominant mode of inheritance of this syndrome. In fact, chimeric enzymes with amino termini from CYP11B1 and carboxyl termini from CYP11B2 have 18-oxidase activity only if at least the region encoded by exons 5–9 corresponds to CYP11B2 *(41)*. This is entirely consistent with the observation that no breakpoints in glucocorticoid suppressible hyperaldosteronism alleles occur after exon 4. The chimeric enzymes either have strong 18-oxidase activity or none detectable and there does not appear to be any location of crossover that yields an enzyme with an intermediate level of 18-oxidase activity. Thus, there is no evidence for allelic variation in this disorder (i.e., variations in clinical severity are unlikely to be the result of different crossover locations).

Although it originally seemed possible that a "mild" form of glucocorticoid suppressible hyperaldosteronism might be a common etiology of essential hypertension, the lack of allelic variation in this disorder makes this unlikely. However, other polymorphisms in the 5' flanking region of CYP11B2 have been documented *(40,43)*, although none has been shown to affect expression of the gene. If any does influence regulation of CYP11B2, it might be a risk factor for the development of hypertension.

Other factors such as kallikrein levels may affect the development of hypertension in this disorder *(44)*. One study found that blood pressure in persons with glucocorticoid suppressible hyperaldosteronism is higher when the disease is inherited from the mother than when it is paternally inherited *(45)*. It is theoretically possible that the gene is imprinted (i.e., the maternal and paternal copies are expressed differently), but it seems more likely that exposure of the fetus to elevated levels of maternal aldosterone subsequently exacerbates the hypertension.

It is notable that many kindreds with glucocorticoid suppressible hyperaldosteronism are of Anglo-Irish extraction *(41,42)*. Moreover, the chromosomes carrying chimeric genes tend to occur in association with specific polymorphisms in the CYP11B genes *(42,45)*, even though the duplications generating the chimeric genes are apparently independent events. This suggests that one of these polymorphisms is, or is in linkage disequilibrium with, a structural polymorphism that predisposes to unequal crossing over during meiosis. Such features might include sequences similar to *chi* sites in bacteriophage lambda; this type of sequence has been postulated to increase the frequency of recombination in the CYP21 genes *(46)*.

MINERALOCORTICOID RECEPTOR

Structure and Genetics

Although membrane receptors for aldosterone may exist *(47)*, most effects of aldosterone are mediated by a specific nuclear receptor referred to as the mineralocorticoid or "Type 1 steroid" receptor. This receptor is expressed at high levels in renal distal tubules and cortical collecting ducts but also in other mineralocorticoid target tissues, including salivary glands and the colon. It is also found at multiple sites in the brain and at low levels in the myocardium and in the peripheral vasculature.

As is the case with the glucocorticoid receptor, the unliganded mineralocorticoid receptor is located mainly in the cytoplasm *(48)*. Once liganded, the receptor is translocated to the nucleus.

The mineralocorticoid receptor has a high degree of sequence identity with the glucocorticoid or "type 2" receptor *(49)*. The carboxyl terminus is a ligand binding domain that is 57–60% identical in amino acid sequence in the two receptors. In fact, the mineralocorticoid receptor has high affinity for both mineralocorticoids and glucocorticoids. One mechanism by which these ligands are distinguished is discussed in the next section.

The center of the molecule contains a DNA binding domain consisting of two "zinc fingers;" this region is also involved in dimerization of liganded receptors. The amino acid sequences of the mineralocorticoid and glucocorticoid receptors are 94% identical in this region.

Given the high degree of sequence identity in the DNA binding domains of the glucocorticoid and mineralocorticoid receptors, it would be expected that these receptors would bind similar or identical DNA sequences, and indeed both bind "glucocorticoid response elements" in vitro consisting of imperfect inverted repeats of 6 bp separated by 3 bp. This raises the obvious question of how glucocorticoids and mineralocorticoids can have distinct biological effects. Moreover, functional glucocorticoid response elements have not been documented in known mineralocorticoid genes. Possibly the mineralocorticoid receptor also binds to nonclassic response elements or perhaps transactivates certain genes without directly binding to DNA.

These receptors are least similar (<15% identical) in their amino terminal domains. In the glucocorticoid receptor, this region is known to interact with other nuclear transcription factors such as AP-1[50] (Fig. 3). Thus, most glucocorticoid responsive promoters probably contain complex or composite response elements that interact with both the glucocorticoid receptor and with additional transactivating factors that themselves interact with the receptor. In addition, the glucocorticoid receptor demonstrates cooperativity, so that several glucocorticoid response elements can act synergistically to increase tran-

LUMEN   INTERSTITIUM

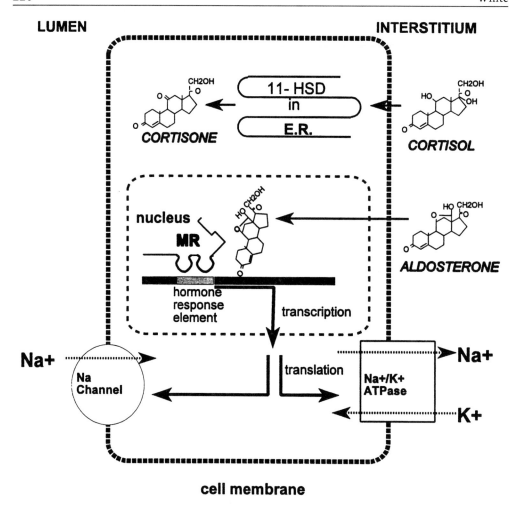

cell membrane

Fig. 3. Schematic of mineralocorticoid action. Aldosterone occupies nuclear receptors (MR) that bind to hormone response elements (probably as dimers, not shown). This increases transcription of genes and directly or indirectly increases activities of apical sodium (Na) channels and the basolateral sodium-potassium (Na/K) ATPase. This increases resorption of sodium from and excretion of potassium into the tubular lumen. Cortisol, which circulates at higher levels than aldosterone, cannot occupy the receptor because it is oxidized to cortisone by 11β-hydroxysteroid dehydrogenase(11-HSD).

scription. In contrast, interactions of the large amino terminal region of the mineralocorticoid receptor with other transacting factors have not been demonstrated and indeed this region seems to be inhibitory to transactivation *(51)*. However, it is possible that the receptor has not been tested in a system where appropriate transactivating factors are available. Similarly, cooperativity has not been observed *(51)*.

Many nuclear receptors form both homodimers and heterodimers on DNA, often with different transactivation properties. The mineralocorticoid and glucocorticoid receptors form heterodimers that have synergistic and antisynergistic properties in different systems *(52)*. The A isoform of the progesterone receptor acts as a ligand-dependent inhibitor of the mineralocorticoid receptor, but this does not require direct interactions between the receptors and instead may involve competition between these receptors for a common transactivating factor *(53)*.

The gene encoding the mineralocorticoid receptor is located on chromosome 4q31.1–31.2. There are two alternative untranslated first exons that are driven by different promoters. The more proximal promoter is constitutive and is by far the stronger; the more distal promoter is positively regulated by mineralocorticoids, suggesting that there may be a positive feedback mechanism increasing the transcriptional effects of mineralocorticoids *(54,55)*.

Mechanisms Conferring Ligand Specificity

When cDNA encoding the mineralocorticoid receptor was cloned and expressed *(49)*, it became apparent that this receptor had very similar binding affinities for aldosterone and for glucocorticoids such as corticosterone and cortisol. This was consistent with observations that this receptor in the rat hippocampus had identical affinities for aldosterone and corticosterone *(56)*, but it was difficult to reconcile with the fact that corticosterone and cortisol are relatively weak mineralocorticoids in vivo.

It is now apparent that an important mechanism conferring ligand specificity on the mineralocorticoid receptor in vivo is the activity of 11β-hydroxysteroid dehydrogenase (11-HSD). This enzyme is expressed in mineralocorticoid target tissues and oxidizes active glucocorticoids such as cortisol to inactive steroids such as cortisone. Aldosterone is not a substrate for this enzyme and thus has unimpeded access to mineralocorticoid receptors *(57–59)* (Fig. 3).

There are two distinct isozymes of 11-HSD. Both are members of the "short chain dehydrogenase" family. These enzymes all have a highly conserved nucleotide cofactor binding domain near the amino terminus; the cofactor functions as an electron acceptor for dehydrogenation (NAD^+ or $NADP^+$) and as an electron donor for reduction (NADH or NADPH). Completely conserved tyrosine and lysine residues toward the carboxyl terminus function in catalysis to facilitate a hydride (a proton plus two electrons) transfer from the 11α position to $NADP^+$ or NAD^+ 60.

The liver (L) or Type-1 isozyme requires $NADP^+$ as a cofactor, has an affinity for steroids in the micromolar range *(61)*, and is expressed at highest levels in the human liver *(62)*. It catalyzes both dehydrogenation and reduction (conversion of cortisone to cortisol) *(63)* and probably functions mainly as a reductase in vivo.

The kidney (K) or Type-2 isozyme is expressed in mineralocorticoid target tissues, particularly the distal nephron, and in the placenta. This isozyme is NAD^+ dependent, has a very high (10–100 nM) affinity for steroids, and only catalyzes dehydrogenation *(64,65)*. The two isozymes are only 21% identical in amino acid sequence *(66,67)*. The corresponding genes map to different chromosomes (HSD11L on chromosome 1 and HSD11K on chromosome 16q22) and have different intron–exon organizations, suggesting that the two isozymes are only distantly related *(62,68)*.

Pathophysiology

SYNDROME OF APPARENT MINERALOCORTICOID EXCESS (AME)

Clinical Features. AME is a syndrome inherited in an autosomal recessive manner in which children develop hypertension, hypokalemia, and low-plasma renin activity. A low salt diet or blockade of mineralocorticoid receptors with spironolactone ameliorate the hypertension whereas ACTH and hydrocortisone exacerbate it. Levels of all known mineralocorticoids are low *(69,70)*. These findings suggest that cortisol (i.e., hydrocortisone) acts as a stronger mineralocorticoid than is normally the case. Indeed, plasma cortisol half-life is prolonged in patients with AME *(69)*. Very low levels of cortisone metabolites are excreted in the urine as compared to cortisol metabolites, indicating a marked deficiency in 11-HSD, the enzyme catalyzing the conversion of cortisol to cortisone. However, 11-reduction is unimpaired *(71)*.

Similar but milder abnormalities occur with licorice intoxication, including abuse of licorice-flavored chewing tobacco *(57)*. The active component of licorice, glycyrrhetinic acid, inhibits 11-HSD in isolated rat kidney microsomes *(72)*. Thus, it appears that licorice intoxication is a reversible pharmacological counterpart to the inherited syndrome of apparent mineralocorticoid excess.

Genetics. All patients with AME are homozygotes or compound heterozygotes for mutations in the HSD11K (HSD11B2) gene encoding the kidney isozyme of 11-HSD. These mutations all affect enzymatic activity or pre-mRNA splicing, thus confirming in its entirety the hypothesis that 11-HSD protects the mineralocorticoid receptor from high concentrations of cortisol *(73,74)*.

Although the number of patients with AME is small, sufficient data now exist to demonstrate a statistically significant correlation between degree of enzymatic impairment and biochemical severity as measured by urinary cortisol:cortisone metabolite ratios *(75)*. This correlation is most obvious for partially active mutants. Because of the small numbers of patients, and the possible confounding effects of prior antihypertensive therapy, it is difficult to correlate biochemical severity with measures of clinical severity, although anecdotal reports suggest that mutations that do not destroy activity may be associated with milder disease *(73,74)*. With the elucidation of the molecular genetic basis of this disorder, ascertainment of additional cases may permit these questions to be answered.

MINERALOCORTICOID ACTIONS

Sodium-Potassium (Na,K)-ATPase

STRUCTURE AND FUNCTION

The Na,K-ATPase maintains the electrochemical transmembrane gradient that is an essential feature of all living cells. It consists of a large (110 kDa) catalytic α subunit and a smaller β subunit (35 kDa polypeptide, 55 kDa including glycosylation). The α subunit contains 10 transmembrane domains; most of the remainder of the molecule is cytoplasmic with very few residues on the extracellular surface of the membrane. In contrast, the β subunit contains a single transmembrane domain and most of the polypeptide is extracellular (reviewed in *[76,77]*).

There are three isoforms of the α subunit encoded by distinct genes. The $\alpha 1$ isoform is ubiquitously expressed and is the predominant isoform in the kidney. The $\alpha 2$ isoform is expressed mainly in skeletal muscle and the $\alpha 3$ isoform in the nervous system and heart. There are two β subunit isoforms, with the $\beta 1$ isoform being ubiquitous and the $\beta 2$ isoform expressed mostly in the nervous system.

In the first step in ion transport by the Na,K-ATPase, three Na^+ ions bind to the cytoplasmic surface of the α subunit, probably to negatively charged residues within the several of the transmembrane helices. This is followed by hydrolysis of ATP and phosphorylation of the enzyme in the very large third cytoplasmic loop. Phosphorylation triggers a shift from the "E1" to the "E2" conformation, resulting in translocation and release of the Na^+ ions at the extracellular surface. In their stead, two K^+ ions are then bound, leading to dephosphorylation of the enzyme and a shift from the E2 back to the E1 conformation. The K^+ ions are finally released to the cytoplasm, and the enzyme is ready for another cycle.

The β subunit does not seem to be involved in this process, but it is required to produce an active enzyme. Possibly it is required for proper posttranslational modifications, targeting and/or stability of the α subunit. It may also stabilize the E2 conformation. The genes encoding both the α1 (ATP1A1) and β1 (ATP1B1) subunits are located on chromosome 1, but are not known to be closely linked.

REGULATION

Transcriptional. Both the α1 and β1 subunit genes are regulated by intracellular sodium concentration. They are also upregulated by both glucocorticoids and mineralocorticoids via both the glucocorticoid and mineralocorticoid receptors. In mammalian cells, this upregulation is on the transcriptional level, and no synthesis of additional protein factors is required (78). In addition, vasopressin increases Na,K-ATPase expression via increased levels of cAMP generated by the G protein coupled vasopressin receptor (79).

The DNA-protein interactions mediating regulation by mineralocorticoids have not been identified. Constitutive expression of the subunit gene is controlled by the proximal 120 bp of the 5' flanking region. This region includes two "GC boxes" that bind the Sp1 transcription factor, and a cAMP response element that binds at least two transcription factors of the "leucine zipper" type, CREB and ATF-1 (80).

The subunits of the enzyme have a half-life of approx 1 d and these transcriptional effects take several hours to significantly increase expression of the subunits. More rapid regulation of the NA,K-ATPase seems to be mediated by activation of already synthesized, inactive receptors. The mechanisms by which this occurs are not understood.

Endogenous Cardiac Glycosides. Cardiac glycosides, such as digoxin and ouabain, inhibit the Na,K-ATPase by binding to specific residues in the first extracellular loop. Related compounds, the bufenolides, exists in toad poisons. There is substantial evidence that related biologically active compounds exist in mammals. Cross reactivity with antisera to ouabain and digoxin has also been observed. These compounds have been noted in urine from hypertensive humans and animals, in human cord blood and placentas, and in the mammalian heart and adrenal glands (81). Mass spectroscopic analysis suggests that the compound in human placenta is a dihydropyrone-substituted steroid, which suggests that it is closely related to the bufenolides (82). The biosynthetic pathway to such a compound in mammals is not obvious.

Such a compound could have significant effects on intracellular calcium stores and thus on myocardial contractility (83). By inhibiting the Na,K-ATPase, it could lead to compensatory increases in activity of the renin-angiotensin system and in aldosterone secretion, and could thus be an important mechanism in the development of essential hypertension. Exploration of these possibilities awaits elucidation of the precise structure(s) of the active compound(s) and synthesis of adequate quantities for physiological studies.

Sodium Channel

STRUCTURE AND FUNCTION

The epithelial sodium channel consists of three subunits (α, β, and γ) that share 35% sequence identity *(84,85)*. Each consists of two transmembrane segments joined by a large extracellular domain. The C-terminal cytoplasmic region of each subunit is rich in proline residues. In the α subunit, this region binds to the *src*-homology 3 (SH3) domain of α-spectrin and mediates localization to the apical side of epithelial cells *(86)*.

When the cRNA encoding each subunit is injected into *Xenopus* oocytes, the α subunit alone generates a small sodium current. The β and γ subunits do not generate a sodium current either alone or together, but each increases the sodium current by three- to fivefold over that observed with injection of only the cRNA encoding the α subunit *(85)*. When cRNAs for all three subunits were injected together, the observed current is more than 100 times greater than that seen with the α subunit alone. Thus, β and γ are regulatory subunits. Although the optimum stoichiometry has not been determined, it seems likely that the functional sodium channel contains the α, β, and γ subunits in equimolar ratios. The channel could consist of one of each subunit and thus contain six transmembrane domains, but other regulated channels, such as the cystic fibrosis transmembrane conductance regulator (CFTR) and the sodium–calcium exchanger, contain 12 transmembrane domains. If the sodium channel has a similar organization, this would require two of each subunit.

Recently cDNA encoding a novel δ subunit was isolated. This subunit is expressed in gonads, pancreas and brain but not in the kidney. The δ subunit forms an active complex with the β and γ subunits and thus can substitute for the α subunit, although its behavior is different with regard to conductance, ionic specificity, and sensitivity to amiloride *(87)*.

REGULATION

The sodium channel is regulated by several parallel pathways *(88)*. Protein kinase A phosphorylates the channel and increases single channel open probability. Cholera toxin can thus increase channel activity through cAMP signalling pathways. In addition, G proteins (e.g., $G\alpha_{i3}$) interact directly with the channel to inhibit it. Pertussin toxin increases channel activity by ADP-ribosylating $G\alpha_i$, causing it to associate with $G\beta\gamma$ subunits and thus inhibiting its association with the channel. The protein kinase A and G protein-mediated pathways interact in a complex, but usually mutually inhibitory manner. All of these mechanisms can rapidly regulate channel activity. In addition, aldosterone leads to sustained increases in synthesis of channel subunits.

Pathophysiology

LIDDLE'S SYNDROME

Clinical Features. Patients with Liddle's syndrome, an inherited autosomal-dominant disorder with high penetrance, have signs of mineralocorticoid excess including hypertension and usually, but not always, hypokalemic alkalosis. However, levels of aldosterone and other known mineralocorticoids are subnormal. Blockade of the mineralocorticoid receptor with spironolactone does not ameliorate these problems, but sodium restriction combined with the potassium sparing diuretic triamterine is effective in reducing blood pressure and increasing serum potassium levels *(89,90)*.

A number of affected subjects have died in their 30s of hypertensive vascular disease. The index case developed chronic renal failure necessitating a renal transplant. After transplantation, her hypokalemia resolved and her blood pressure decreased to near normal levels *(90)*.

These features suggest that there is a structural abnormality in the kidney in this disorder rather than abnormal levels of any circulating humoral factor. The improvement in signs of mineralocorticoid excess with triamterine, an agent that inhibits the sodium channel in the renal distal tubule and collecting duct, suggests that the abnormality is one of regulation of the sodium channel. This has been demonstrated by genetic studies.

Genetics. In most kindreds, the disease is linked genetically to the *SCNN1B* gene encoding the β subunit of the epithelial sodium channel on chromosome 16p12–13 *(89,91)*. Several kindreds carry nonsense or frameshift mutations that leave both trans-membrane domains intact but delete almost the entire C-terminal cytoplasmic domain. Expression of the truncated β subunit in *Xenopus* oocytes together with wild-type α and γ subunits increases channel activity threefold over that seen when the wild-type β sub-unit was used *(92)*. Missense mutations have also been identified *(93,94)* in the cytoplas-mic C terminal domain including P616–Y618, which thus seems to be an important regulatory site that when mutated or deleted leads to constitutive activation of the recep-tor. Analogous mutations in the *SCNN1G* gene on chromosome 12p13.1–pter that encodes the γ subunit have been detected in a kindred with Liddle's syndrome and lead to the identical clinical phenotype *(95)*. Thus, the β and γ subunits apparently act equivalently and synergistically to regulate the epithelial sodium channel.

Because activating mutations in the genes encoding the β and γ subunits cause severe hypertension, it is plausible that milder activating mutations might underlying some cases of essential hypertension. At this time, however, no studies have demonstrated any linkage of the *SCNN1B* or *SCNN1G* genes to milder forms of hypertension.

PSEUDOHYPOALDOSTERONISM

Clinical Features. If activating mutations in the regulatory subunits of the epithelial sodium channel lead to signs and symptoms of aldosterone excess with suppressed renin and aldosterone levels, one might expect that mutations that cause loss of function of one of the three subunits of the receptor would lead, conversely, to signs of mineralocorticoid deficiency, such as hyponatremia, hypovolemia, hyperreninemia, and hyperkalemia. Pseudohypoaldosteronism is such a condition.

Patients with pseudohypoaldosteronism present shortly after birth with signs of min-eralocorticoid deficiency, but with markedly elevated plasma concentrations of aldoster-one and renin. Because these patients are resistant to mineralocorticoids, they must be treated with supplemental sodium chloride. Signs and symptoms of aldosterone resis-tance decrease with age in many patients so that concentrations of aldosterone fall and salt supplements may be discontinued when a patient is a few years old. Other patients, however, are resistant to therapy and they may die in infancy from hyperkalemia.

Sporadic, autosomal dominant and recessive forms of pseudohypoaldosteronism are recognized. In patients with the autosomal dominant form, aldosterone resistance is confined to the renal tubule and is less severe than in patients with the autosomal-reces-sive form. In patients with the recessive form, the resistance is expressed in both the renal tubules and other aldosterone target tissues including salivary and sweat glands and the colon *(96)*.

Genetics. Because patients were resistant to mineralocorticoids, it was initially assumed that the defect lay in the mineralocorticoid receptor itself. This hypothesis was supported by studies demonstrating reduced numbers of mineralocorticoid receptors in peripheral blood mononuclear leukocytes *(97).* However, no mutation affecting function was detected in any of seven unrelated patients with pseudohypoaldosteronism *(98–100).* Presumably, patients with this disorder have decreased numbers of mineralocorticoid receptors because elevated blood levels of aldosterone downregulate the receptor.

Instead, at least the autosomal recessive form of the disorder segregates with the genes encoding the various subunits of the epithelial sodium channel *(101),* and nonsense, frameshift, and missense mutations in the α or β subunits have been identified in five kindreds with this disorder *(102).* Thus, Liddle's syndrome and pseudohypoaldosteronism represent allelic variants.

ACKNOWLEDGMENT

This work was supported by the National Institutes of Health under Grants DK37867 and DK42169.

REFERENCES

1. Berry CA, Ives HF, Rector FC. Renal transport of glucose, amino acids, sodium, chloride and water. In Brenner BM, ed. The kidney. 5th edition. Saunders, Philadelphia, PA, 1996, pp. 334–370.
2. Duchatelle P, Ohara A, Ling BN, Kemendy AE, Kokko KE, Matsumoto PS, Eaton DC. Regulation of renal epithelial sodium channels. Mol Cell Biochem 1992;114:27–34.
3. Palmer LG, Frindt G. Regulation of apical membrane Na and K channels in rat renal collecting tubules by aldosterone. Semin Nephrol 1992;12:37–43.
4. Horisberger JD, Rossier BC. Aldosterone regulation of gene transcription leading to control of ion transport. Hypertension 1992;19:221–227.
5. Curnow KM, Tusie-Luna MT, Pascoe L, Natarajan R, Gu JL, Nadler JL, White PC. The product of the CYP11B2 gene is required for aldosterone biosynthesis in the human adrenal cortex. Mol Endocrinol 1991;5:1513–1522.
6. Kawamoto T, Mitsuuchi Y, Ohnishi T, Ichikawa Y, Yokoyama Y, Sumitomo H, et al. Cloning and expression of a cDNA for human cytochrome P-450aldo as related to primary aldosteronism. Biochem Biophys Res Commun 1990;173:309–316.
7. Quinn SJ, Williams GH. Regulation of aldosterone secretion. Annu Rev Physiol 1988;50:409–426.
8. Mornet E, Dupont J, Vitek A, White PC. Characterization of two genes encoding human steroid 11 beta-hydroxylase (P-450(11) beta). J Biol Chem 1989;264:20,961–20,967.
9. Pascoe L, Jeunemaitre X, Lebrethon MC, Curnow KM, Gomez-Sanchez CE, Gasc JM, et al. Glucocorticoid-suppressible hyperaldosteronism and adrenal tumors occurring in a single French pedigree. J Clin Invest 1995;96:2236–2246.
10. Bird IM, Hanley NA, Word RA, Mathis JM, McCarthy JL, Mason JI, Rainey WE. Human NCI-H295 adrenocortical carcinoma cells: a model for angiotensin-II-responsive aldosterone secretion. Endocrinology 1993;133:1555–1561.
11. Sasaki K, Yamamo Y, Bardhan S, Iwai N, Murray JJ, Hasegawa M, et al. Cloning and expression of a complementary cDNA encoding a bovine adrenal angiotensin II type-1 receptor. Nature 1991;351:230–233.
12. Curnow KM, Pascoe L, White PC. Genetic analysis of the human type-1 angiotensin II receptor. Mol Endocrinol 1992;6:1113–1118.
13. Clyne CD, Zhang Y, Slutsker L, Mathis JM, White PC, Rainey WE. Angiotensin II and potassium regulate human CYP11B2 transcription through common cis elements. Mol Endocrinol 1997, in press.
14. Lala DS, Rice DA, Parker KL. Steroidogenic factor I, a key regulator of steroidogenic enzyme expression, is the mouse homolog of fushi tarazu-factor I. Mol Endocrinol 1992;6:1249–1258.
15. Honda S, Morohashi K, Nomura M, Takeya H, Kitajima M, Omura T. Ad4BP regulating steroidogenic P-450 gene is a member of steroid hormone receptor superfamily. J Biol Chem 1993;268:7494–7502.

16. Meyer TE, Habener JF. Cyclic adenosine 3',5'-monophosphate response element binding protein (CREB) and related transcription-activating deoxyribonucleic acid-binding proteins. Endocr Rev 1993;14:269–290.

17. White PC, New MI. Genetic basis of endocrine disease 2: congenital adrenal hyperplasia due to 21-hydroxylase deficiency. J Clin Endocrinol Metab 1992;74:6–11.

18. Speiser PW, Dupont J, Zhu D, Serrat J, Buegeleisen M, Tusie-Luna MT, et al. Disease expression and molecular genotype in congenital adrenal hyperplasia due to 21-hydroxylase deficiency. J Clin Invest 1992;90:584–595.

19. Rosler A, Leiberman E, Sack J, Landau H, Benderly A, Moses SW, Cohen T. Clinical variability of congenital adrenal hyperplasia due to 11 beta-hydroxylase deficiency. Hormone Res 1982;16:133–141.

20. Rosler A, Leiberman E, Cohen T. High frequency of congenital adrenal hyperplasia (classic 11 beta-hydroxylase deficiency) among Jews from Morocco. Am J Med Genet 1992;42:827–834.

21. Zachmann M, Tassinari D, Prader A. Clinical and biochemical variability of congenital adrenal hyperplasia due to 11 beta-hydroxylase deficiency. A study of 25 patients. J Clin Endocrinol Metab 1983;56:222–229.

22. Visser HKA, Cost WS. A new hereditary defect in the biosynthesis of aldosterone: Urinary C21-corticosteroid pattern in three related patients with a salt-losing syndrome, suggesting an 18-oxidation defect. Acta Endocrinol (Copenh) 1964;47:589–612.

23. Ulick S, Gautier E, Vetter KK, Markello JR, Yaffe S, Lowe CU. An aldosterone biosynthetic defect in a salt-losing disorder. J Clin Endocrinol Metab 1964;24:669–672.

24. Veldhuis JD, Melby JC. Isolated aldosterone deficiency in man: acquired and inborn errors in the biosynthesis or action of aldosterone. Endocr Rev 1981;2:495–517.

25. Ulick S. Diagnosis and nomenclature of the disorders of the terminal portion of the aldosterone biosynthetic pathway. J Clin Endocrinol Metab 1976;43:92–96.

26. Ulick S, Wang JZ, Morton DH. The biochemical phenotypes of two inborn errors in the biosynthesis of aldosterone. J Clin Endocrinol Metab 1992;74:1415–1420.

27. Mitsuuchi Y, Kawamoto T, Miyahara K, Ulick S, Morton DH, Naiki Y, et al. Congenitally defective aldosterone biosynthesis in humans: inactivation of the P450C18 gene (CYP11B2) due to nucleotide deletion in CMO I deficient patients. Biochem Biophys Res Commun 1993;190:864–869.

28. Zhang G, Rodriguez H, Fardella CE, Harris DA, Miller WL. Mutation T318M in the CYP11B2 gene encoding P450c11AS (aldosterone synthase) causes corticosterone methyl oxidase II deficiency. Am J Hum Genet 1995;57:1037–1043.

29. Russell DW, White PC. Four is not more than two. Am J Hum Genet 1995;57:1002–1005.

30. Sutherland DJ, Ruse JL, Laidlaw JC. Hypertension, increased aldosterone secretion and low plasma renin activity relieved by dexamethasone. Can Med Assoc J 1966;95:1109–1119.

31. New MI, Peterson RE. A new form of congenital adrenal hyperplasia. J Clin Endocrinol Metab 1967;27:300–305.

32. Gomez-Sanchez CE, Gill JR, Jr., Ganguly A, Gordon RD. Glucocorticoid-suppressible aldosteronism: a disorder of the adrenal transitional zone. J Clin Endocrinol Metab 1988;67:444–448.

33. Hamlet SM, Gordon RD, Gomez-Sanchez CE, Tunny TJ, Klemm SA. Adrenal transitional zone steroids, 18-oxo and 18-hydroxycortisol, useful in the diagnosis of primary aldosteronism, are ACTH-dependent. Clin Exp Pharmacol Physiol 1988;15:317–322.

34. Hall CE, Gomez-Sanchez CE. Hypertensive potency of 18-oxocortisol in the rat. Hypertension 1986;8:317–322.

35. Rich GM, Ulick S, Cook S, Wang JZ, Lifton RP, Dluhy RG. Glucocorticoid-remediable aldosteronism in a large kindred: clinical spectrum and diagnosis using a characteristic biochemical phenotype. Ann Intern Med 1992;116:813–820.

36. O'Mahony S, Burns A, Murnaghan DJ. Dexamethasone-suppressible hyperaldosteronism: a large new kindred. J Hum Hypertens 1989;3:255–258.

37. Oberfield SE, Levine LS, Stoner E, Chow D, Rauh W, Greig F, et al. Adrenal glomerulosa function in patients with dexamethasone-suppressible hyperaldosteronism. J Clin Endocrinol Metab 1981;53:158–164.

38. Ganguly A, Weinberger MH, Guthrie GP, Fineberg NS. Adrenal steroid responses to ACTH in glucocorticoid-suppressible aldosteronism. Hypertension 1984;6:563–567.

39. White PC. Defects in cortisol metabolism causing low-renin hypertension. Endocr Res 1991;17:85–107.

40. Lifton RP, Dluhy RG, Powers M, Rich GM, Cook S, Ulick S, Lalouel JM. A chimaeric 11 beta-hydroxylase/aldosterone synthase gene causes glucocorticoid-remediable aldosteronism and human hypertension. Nature 1992;355:262–265.

41. Pascoe L, Curnow KM, Slutsker L, Connell JM, Speiser PW, New MI, White PC. Glucocorticoid-suppressible hyperaldosteronism results from hybrid genes created by unequal crossovers between CYP11B1 and CYP11B2. Proc Natl Acad Sci USA 1992;89:8327–8331.

42. Lifton RP, Dluhy RG, Powers M, Rich GM, Gutkin M, Fallo F, Gill JR, Jr., et al. Hereditary hypertension caused by chimaeric gene duplications and ectopic expression of aldosterone synthase. Nat Genet 1992;2:66–74.

43. White PC, Slutsker L. Haplotype analysis of CYP11B2. Endocr Res 1995;21:437–442.

44. Dluhy RG, Lifton RP. Glucocorticoid-remediable aldosteronism (GRA): diagnosis, variability of phenotype and regulation of potassium homeostasis. Steroids 1995;60:48–51.

45. Jamieson A, Slutsker L, Inglis GC, Fraser R, White PC, Connell JM. Glucocorticoid-suppressible hyperaldosteronism: effects of crossover site and parental origin of chimaeric gene on phenotypic expression. Clin Sci 1995;88:563–570.

46. Amor M, Parker KL, Globerman H, New MI, White PC. Mutation in the CYP21B gene (Ile-172—Asn) causes steroid 21-hydroxylase deficiency. Proc Natl Acad Sci USA 1988;85:1600–1604.

47. Wehling M. Nongenomic aldosterone effects: the cell membrane as a specific target of mineralocorticoid action. Steroids 1995;60:153–156.

48. Robertson NM, Schulman G, Karnik S, Alnemri E, Litwack G. Demonstration of nuclear translocation of the mineralocorticoid receptor (MR) using an anti-MR antibody and confocal laser scanning microscopy. Mol Endocrinol 1993;7:1226–1239.

49. Arriza JL, Weinberger C, Cerelli G, Glaser TM, Handelin BL, Housman DE, Evans RM. Cloning of human mineralocorticoid receptor complementary DNA: structural and functional kinship with the glucocorticoid receptor. Science 1987;237:268–275.

50. Pearce D, Yamamoto KR. Mineralocorticoid and glucocorticoid receptor activities distinguished by nonreceptor factors at a composite response element. . Science 1993;259:1161–1165.

51. Rupprecht R, Arriza JL, Spengler D, Reul JM, Evans RM, Holsboer F, Damm K. Transactivation and synergistic properties of the mineralocorticoid receptor: relationship to the glucocorticoid receptor. Mol Endocrinol 1993;7:597–603.

52. Liu W, Wang J, Sauter NK, Pearce D. Steroid receptor heterodimerization demonstrated in vitro and in vivo. Proc Natl Acad Sci USA 1995;92:12,480–12,484.

53. McDonnell DP, Shahbaz MM, Vegeto E, Goldman ME. The human progesterone receptor A-form functions as a transcriptional modulator of mineralocorticoid receptor transcriptional activity. J Steroid Biochem Mol Biol 1994;48:425–432.

54. Zennaro MC, Keightley MC, Kotelevtsev Y, Conway GS, Soubrier F, Fuller PJ. Human mineralocorticoid receptor genomic structure and identification of expressed isoforms. J Biol Chem 1995; 270:21,016–21,020.

55. Zennaro MC, le Menuet D, Lombes M. Characterization of the human mineralocorticoid receptor gene 5'-regulatory region: evidence for differential hormonal regulation of two alternative promoters via nonclassical mechanisms. Mol Endocrinol 1996;10:1549–1560.

56. Krozowski ZS, Funder JW. Renal mineralocorticoid receptors and hippocampal corticosterone binding species have identical intrinsic steroid specificity. Proc Natl Acad Sci USA 1983;80:6056–6060.

57. Stewart PM, Wallace AM, Valentino R, Burt D, Shackleton CH, Edwards CR. Mineralocorticoid activity of liquorice: 11-beta-hydroxysteroid dehydrogenase deficiency comes of age. Lancet 1987;2:821–824.

58. Edwards CR, Stewart PM, Burt D, Brett L, McIntyre MA, Sutanto WS, de Kloet ER, et al. Localisation of 11 beta-hydroxysteroid dehydrogenase—tissue specific protector of the mineralocorticoid receptor. Lancet 1988;2:986–989.

59. Funder JW, Pearce PT, Smith R, Smith AI. Mineralocorticoid action: target tissue specificity is enzyme, not receptor, mediated. Science 1988;242:583–585.

60. Obeid J, White PC. Tyr-179 and Lys-183 are essential for enzymatic activity of 11 beta-hydroxysteroid dehydrogenase. Biochem Biophys Res Commun 1992;188:222–227.

61. Lakshmi V, Monder C. Purification and characterization of the corticosteroid 11 beta-dehydrogenase component of the rat liver 11 beta-hydroxysteroid dehydrogenase complex. Endocrinology 1988;123:2390–2398.

62. Tannin GM, Agarwal AK, Monder C, New MI, White PC. The human gene for 11 beta-hydroxysteroid dehydrogenase. Structure, tissue distribution, and chromosomal localization. J Biol Chem 1991;266:16,653–16,658.

63. Agarwal AK, Monder C, Eckstein B, White PC. Cloning and expression of rat cDNA encoding corticosteroid 11 beta-dehydrogenase. J Biol Chem 1989;264:18,939–18,943.

64. Mercer WR, Krozowski ZS. Localization of an 11 beta hydroxysteroid dehydrogenase activity to the distal nephron. Evidence for the existence of two species of dehydrogenase in the rat kidney. Endocrinology 1992;130:540–543.

65. Rusvai E, Naray-Fejes-Toth A. A new isoform of 11 beta-hydroxysteroid dehydrogenase in aldosterone target cells. J Biol Chem 1993;268:10,717–10,720.

66. Agarwal AK, Mune T, Monder C, White PC. NAD$^+$-dependent isoform of 11 beta hydroxysteroid dehydrogenase:cloning and characterization of cDNA from sheep kidney. J Biol Chem 1994; 269:25,959–25,962.

67. Albiston AL, Obeyesekere VR, Smith RE, Krozowski ZS. Cloning and tissue distribution of the human 11-HSD type 2 enzyme. Mol Cell Endocrinol 1994;105:R11–R17.

68. Agarwal AK, Rogerson FM, Mune T, White PC. Gene structure and chromosomal localization of the human HSD11K gene encoding the kidney (type 2) isozyme of 11β-hydroxysteroid dehydrogenase. Genomics 1995;29:195–199.

69. Ulick S, Levine LS, Gunczler P, Zanconato G, Ramirez LC, Rauh W, Rosler A, et al. A syndrome of apparent mineralocorticoid excess associated with defects in the peripheral metabolism of cortisol. J Clin Endocrinol Metab 1979;49:757–764.

70. Oberfield SE, Levine LS, Carey RM, Greig F, Ulick S, New MI. Metabolic and blood pressure responses to hydrocortisone in the syndrome of apparent mineralocorticoid excess. J Clin Endocrinol Metab 1983;56:332–339.

71. Shackleton CH, Rodriguez J, Arteaga E, Lopez JM, Winter JS. Congenital 11 beta-hydroxysteroid dehydrogenase deficiency associated with juvenile hypertension: corticosteroid metabolite profiles of four patients and their families. Clin Endocrinol (Oxf) 1985;22:701–712.

72. Monder C, Stewart PM, Lakshmi V, Valentino R, Burt D, Edwards CR. Licorice inhibits corticosteroid 11 beta-dehydrogenase of rat kidney and liver: in vivo and in vitro studies. Endocrinology 1989;125:1046–1053.

73. Mune T, Rogerson FM, Nikkila H, Agarwal AK, White PC. Human hypertension caused by mutations in the kidney isozyme of 11 beta-hydroxysteroid dehydrogenase. Nat Genet 1995;10:394–399.

74. Wilson RC, Krozowski ZS, Li K, Obeyesekere VR, Razzaghy-Azar M, Harbison MD, Wei JQ, et al. A mutation in the HSD11B2 gene in a family with apparent mineralocorticoid excess. J Clin Endocrinol Metab 1995;80:2263–2266.

75. Mune T, White PC. Apparent mineralocorticoid excess: genotype is correlated with biochemical phenotype. Hypertension 1996;27:1193–1199.

76. Lingrel JB, Kuntzweiler T. Na+,K(+)-ATPase. J Biol Chem 1994;269:19,659–19,662.

77. Lingrel JB, Van Huysse J, O'Brien W, Jewell-Motz E, Askew R, Schultheis P. Structure-function studies of the Na,K-ATPase. Kidney Int Suppl 1994;44:S32–S39.

78. Whorwood CB, Stewart PM. Transcriptional regulation of Na/K-ATPase by corticosteroids, glycyrrhetinic acid and second messenger pathways in rat kidney epithelial cells. J Mol Endocrinol 1995;15:93–103.

79. Coutry N, Farman N, Bonvalet JP, Blot-Chabaud M. Synergistic action of vasopressin and aldosterone on basolateral Na$^+$-K$^+$-ATPase in the cortical collecting duct. J Membr Biol 1995;145:99–106.

80. Kobayashi M, Kawakami K. ATF-1 CREB heterodimer is involved in constitutive expression of the housekeeping Na,K-ATPase α1 subunit gene. Nucleic Acids Res 1995;23:2848–2855.

81. Schoner W. Endogenous digitalis-like factors. Clin Exp Hypertens A 1992;14:767–814.

82. Hilton PJ, White RW, Lord GA, Garner GV, Gordon DB, Hilton MJ, Forni LG, et al. An inhibitor of the sodium pump obtained from human placenta. Lancet 1996;348:303–305.

83. Blaustein MP. Physiological effects of endogenous ouabain: control of intracellular Ca2+ stores and cell responsiveness. Am J Physiol 1993;264:C1367–C1387.

84. Canessa CM, Horisberger JD, Rossier BC. Epithelial sodium channel related to proteins involved in neurodegeneration. Nature 1993;361:467–470.

85. Canessa CM, Schild L, Buell G, Thorens B, Gautschi I, Horisberger JD, Rossier BC. Amiloride-sensitive epithelial Na+ channel is made of three homologous subunits. Nature 1994;367:463–467.

86. Rotin D, Bar-Sagi D, O'Brodovich H, Merilainen J, Lehto VP, Canessa CM, Rossier BC, et al. An SH3 binding region in the epithelial Na+ channel (alpha rENaC) mediates its localization at the apical membrane. EMBO J 1994;13:4440–4450.

87. Waldmann R, Champigny G, Bassilana F, Voilley N, Lazdunski M. Molecular cloning and functional expression of a novel amiloride-sensitive Na(+) channel. J Biol Chem 1995;270:27,411–27,414.

88. Bubien JK, Jope RS, Warnock DG. G-proteins modulate amiloride-sensitive sodium channels. J Biol Chem 1994;269:17,780–17,783.

89. Liddle GW, Bledsoe T, Coppage WS. A familial renal disorder simulating primary aldosteronism but with negligible aldosterone secretion. Trans Assoc Am Physicians 1963;76:199–213.

90. Botero-Velez M, Curtis JJ, Warnock DG. Brief report: Liddle's syndrome revisited—a disorder of sodium reabsorption in the distal tubule. N Engl J Med 1994;330:178–181.

91. Shimkets RA, Warnock DG, Bositis CM, Nelson-Williams C, Hansson JH, Schambelan M, Gill JR, Jr., et al. Liddle's syndrome: heritable human hypertension caused by mutations in the subunit of the epithelial sodium channel. Cell 1994;79:407–414.

92. Schild L, Canessa CM, Shimkets RA, Gautschi I, Lifton RP, Rossier BC. A mutation in the epithelial sodium channel causing Liddle disease increases channel activity in the Xenopus laevis oocyte expression system. Proc Natl Acad Sci USA 1995;92:5699–5703.

93. Hansson JH, Schild L, Lu Y, Wilson TA, Gautschi I, Shimkets R, Nelson-Williams C, et al. A de novo missense mutation of the beta subunit of the epithelial sodium channel causes hypertension and Liddle syndrome, identifying a proline-rich segment critical for regulation of channel activity. Proc Natl Acad Sci USA 1995;92:11,495–11,499.

94. Tamura H, Schild L, Enomoto N, Matsui N, Marumo F, Rossier BC. Liddle disease caused by a missense mutation of beta subunit of the epithelial sodium channel gene. J Clin Invest 1996;97:1780–1784.

95. Hansson JH, Nelson-Williams C, Suzuki H, Schild L, Shimkets R, Lu Y, Canessa C, et al. Hypertension caused by a truncated epithelial sodium channel gamma subunit: genetic heterogeneity of Liddle syndrome. Nat Genet 1995;11:76–82.

96. Kuhnle U, Hinkel GK, Akkurt HI, Krozowski Z. Familial pseudohypoaldosteronism: a review on the heterogeneity of the syndrome. Steroids 1995;60:157–160.

97. Armanini D, Karbowiak I, Zennaro CM, Zovato S, Pratesi C, De Lazzari P, Krozowski Z, et al. Pseudohypoaldosteronism: evaluation of type I receptors by radioreceptor assay and by antireceptor antibodies. Steroids 1995;60:161–163.

98. Komesaroff PA, Verity K, Fuller PJ. Pseudohypoaldosteronism: molecular characterization of the mineralocorticoid receptor. J Clin Endocrinol Metab 1994;79:27–31.

99. Zennaro MC, Borensztein P, Jeunemaitre X, Armanini D, Soubrier F. No alteration in the primary structure of the mineralocorticoid receptor in a family with pseudohypoaldosteronism. J Clin Endocrinol Metab 1994;79:32–38.

100. Arai K, Tsigos C, Suzuki Y, Listwak S, Zachman K, Zangeneh F, Rapaport R, et al. No apparent mineralocorticoid receptor defect in a series of sporadic cases of pseudohypoaldosteronism. J Clin Endocrinol Metab 1995;80:814–817.

101. Strautnieks SS, Thompson RJ, Hanukoglu A, Dillon MJ, Hanukoglu I, Kuhnle U, Seckl JR, et al. Localization of pseudohypoaldosteronism genes to chromosome 16p12.2–13.11 and 12p13.1-pter by homozygosity mapping. Hum Mol Genet 1996;5:293–299.

102. Chang SS, Grunder S, Hanukoglu A, Rosler A, Mathew PM, Hanukoglu I, Schild L, et al. Mutations in subunits of the epithelial sodium channel cause salt wasting with hyperkalaemic acidosis, pseudohypoaldosteronism type 1. Nat Genet 1996;2:248–253.

103. White PC. Disorders of aldosterone biosynthesis and action. N Engl J Med 1994;331:250–258.

14 Molecular Aspects of Pituitary Development

Philip S. Zeitler, MD, PhD
and Cheryl A. Pickett, MD, PhD

INTRODUCTION

The anterior pituitary is a well-characterized and accessible model for studying cell-specific gene activation and the process by which distinct cell-types develop within an organ *(1–3)*. Accordingly, the development of the pituitary gland has been a topic of particularly intense interest by molecular biologists and developmental biologists, as well as endocrinologists. Over the last few years, this activity has yielded remarkable progress in identifying crucial factors involved in anterior pituitary gene expression and development. However, there is an underlying dilemma in the study of pituitary development—namely, that the various pituitary cell types are currently recognizable only by the hormones they synthesize. Therefore, the distinction between factors that promote expression of the hormone gene (i.e., permit recognition of the cell type) and those which direct other facets of cell type differentiation is often blurred. In this chapter, we will review the current state of knowledge regarding the components required for normal development of the pituitary gland and its distinct cell types. Since the ontogeny of the pituitary has been most extensively examined in laboratory rodents, the data we present will be derived predominately from studies in the mouse and rat. However, the appearance of anatomical structures, hormones, and regulatory factors in the human appear to follow relatively similar patterns and where possible, we will include relevant information on human pituitary development and point out where differences are thought to exist.

From: *Molecular and Cellular Pediatric Endocrinology*
Edited by: S. Handwerger © Humana Press Inc., Totowa, NJ

ANATOMIC DEVELOPMENT OF THE ANTERIOR PITUITARY
AND ONTOGENY OF CELL TYPES

The anterior pituitary gland arises from Rathke's pouch, which first appears as an invagination of the oral ectoderm on $E_m8.5$ (mouse embryonic d 8.5) and E_r12 (rat embryonic d 12). By E_m12 and E_r14, Rathke's pouch becomes and independent structure, and shows asymmetric cellular proliferation leading to formation of the future pars distalis (anterior pituitary). During the same period, the infundibulum arises as an outpouching of the floor of the third ventricle and establishes direct contact with the developing anterior pituitary as early as E_m10, though even prior to direct contact only a few cell layers separate these two developing tissues. The lateral processes of Rathke's pouch proliferate and surround the enlarging infundibulum to form the pars tuberalis and eventually invest the tuber cinereum of the median eminence. The portion of the Rathke's pouch epithelium that is in close approximation to the infundibulum remains thin and represents the primordium of the pars intermedia. Subsequently, the infundibulum differentiates into a thin stalk and a round posterior lobe, the pars tuberalis fuses with the median eminence, and the residual lumen between the pars distalis and the pars intermedia narrows to form Rathke's cleft *(4–7)*.

Since the pituitary anlage and infundibulum are nearly contiguous throughout their development, the potential exists for paracrine interactions between these two tissues prior to vascular connection *(8,9)*. Furthermore, immature blood vessels in the developing pituitary are detectable at E_r14 on the surface of the median eminence and pars distalis *(4,10–12)*, providing a vascular link between the infundibular process and the pars distalis *(12,13)* prior to development of the true hypophyseal portal system. True vascularization of the interior pars distalis is evident at $E_m16–18$. At the same time, the first hypothalamic axon terminals can be demonstrated in the external zone of the median eminence and the initial expression of hypothalamic releasing/trophic factors is observed *(2,14–16)*. The portal vessels begin to develop at $E_m17–18$ and deep capillary loops invade the internal layer of the median eminence at PN1–2 (postnatal d 1–2). There is also evidence for direct arterial supply to the pituitary from the internal carotids as early as E_m16, providing the infrastructure for circulating hormones to reach the developing pituitary *(13)*.

The mature pituitary is composed of five phenotypically distinct hormone-producing cell types that develop from pluripotent progenitor cells in a stereotypical order *(7,17,18)*. The synthesis of the glycoprotein α-subunit (common to FSH, LH, and TSH) occurs in the anterior and ventral portion of the pituitary anlage by E_r12 *(2,7)*. However, the first distinct cell type to appear is the corticotroph; transcripts for the ACTH precursor, POMC, can be demonstrated on E_r14, followed shortly by the βTSH transcript. The gonadotropin (LH/FSH) transcripts appear on E_r16, followed by the appearance and rapid increase in GH expression $(E_r17–17.5)$. GH expression continues to increase rapidly during the postnatal period up through PN10 and then more slowly until adulthood (PN40). Expression of prolactin (PRL) transcripts first occurs soon after the appearance of GH $(E_r17.5)$, though neither PRL gene expression nor peptide content becomes significant until PN2 *(2,19,20)*. Ablation of thyrotroph and gonadotroph precursors by transgenic expression of diphtheria toxin driven by the glycoprotein α-subunit promoter resulted in normal development of somatotrophs, lactotrophs, and corticotrophs indicating that although thyrotrophs appear early in pituitary development, they are not obligate intermediates in the development pathway *(21)*. On the other hand, a variety of lines of evidence indicate that the somatotroph (GH-expressing) and lactotroph (PRL-expressing) lineages overlap significantly during developmental and suggest that lactotrophs develop from somatotrophs, either directly or through a separate mammosomatotroph entity *(22–26)*. Finally, a sixth nonhormone-secreting population of cells (folliculo-stellate cells) is found within the anterior pituitary and thought to be of neuroectoderm origin *(27)*.

Development of the human pituitary is less well understood. Rathke's pouch begins to form between the fourth and fifth week of gestation, at which time the anterior wall of the primordium contacts the diencephalon. Formation of the infundibular recess and loss of continuity between Rathke's pouch and the oral cavity begins at the sixth fetal week. The remaining processes of pituitary formation appear to parallel those seen in the mouse and rat and are essentially complete by the 14th week of gestation. In terms of specific pituitary cell-type development, ACTH is detectable at 8–9 wk of gestation, GH, PRL, and βLH at 8–13 wk, α-subunit at 9 wk, βTSH, and βFSH at 12–13 wk *(28–30)*.

AUTOCRINE AND PARACRINE CONTROL
OF PITUITARY DEVELOPMENT

Hypothalamic Neuropeptides

The hypothalamus and pituitary, despite arising from distinct ectodermal primordia, exhibit remarkable developmental coordination. Contact between the developing hypothalamus and Rathke's pouch is critical for proper determination and differentiation of both of these structures during the early stages of their development *(8,31–33)*. However, the nature of the signals exchanged during development is unknown. The hypothalamic neuropeptides, growth hormone-releasing hormone (GHRH), corticotrophin-releasing hormone (CRH), gonadotrophin-releasing hormone (GnRH), and thyrotropin-releasing hormone (TRH), are known to stimulate the synthesis and secretion of hormones from their respective target cells in the adult pituitary. These hypothalamic neuropeptides also promote expansion of populations of their target cells and in some cases act as mitogens.

GHRH

GHRH mediates activation of GH gene expression *(34,35)*, as well as promoting the expansion of populations of somatolactotrophs and somatotrophs *(36–41)* both in vitro and in transgenic mice overexpressing GHRH. In humans, overexpression of GHRH promotes development of pituitary somatotroph adenomas *(42,43)*. Agents that elevate intracellular cAMP mimic these actions and transgenic mice with chronic elevation of somatotroph cAMP resulting from GH promoter-coupled expression of diphtheria toxin develop GH excess accompanied by somatotroph hyperplasia *(40,44,45)*. Conversely, impairment of GHRH action, either with anti-GHRH antiserum *(58–60)* or by ablation of GHRH neurons with monosodium glutamate *(61)*, leads to somatotroph hypoplasia *(46–49)*. Similarly, GH-promoter driven overexpression of an inactive variant of the cAMP response element (CRE) binding protein (CREB) leads to somatotroph hypoplasia *(50)*.

The discovery and characterization of several spontaneously occurring dwarf rodent phenotypes with abnormalities in function of the GHRH receptor (GHRH-R) have helped define the role of GHRH in the differentiation of somatolactotrophs. Homozygous *little* (lit/lit), mice, and spontaneous dwarf *(dw/dw)* rats appear normal in size at birth, but demonstrate severe dwarfism within several weeks after birth. The *little* mouse, which is approximately two-thirds the size of normal and exhibits somatotroph hypoplasia and a profound decrease in pituitary GH mRNA and protein, results from a point mutation in the GHRH binding region of the GHRH-R gene *(51–55)*. These mice have an associated, but less severe, decrease in PRL synthesis. In the *dw* rat, a GHRH-R signal transduction defect of unknown type *(56–59)*, leads to a phenotype very similar to that of the *lit* mouse with severe GH deficiency and somatotroph hypoplasia. An examination of the fetal *dw* rat pituitary indicates that somatotroph hypoplasia is identifiable at the earliest stages of somatotroph development and suggests that GHRH-R dysfunction is associated with abnormal somatotroph differentiation, as well as impaired population expansion *(60)*. On the other hand, the observation that GHRH-R deficient rodents are not completely devoid of somatotrophs suggests that some somatotrophs may arise by a GHRH/GHRH-R independent mechanism *(3,52,61)*. In the Snell mouse, in which a defect impairs normal expression of the pituitary transcription factor *Pit-1 (see below)*, somatotrophs are expressed early in development though they fail to proliferate properly, suggesting that GHRH is not required for initial stem cell differentiation but becomes crucial for continued replication or cell survival. Similarly, GH secretion from human fetal pituitary cells in culture was detectable at 8–9 wk of gestation prior to GHRH responsiveness. At 12–13 wk, GHRH stimulated GH, suggesting that somatotroph commitment precedes GHRH responsiveness *(29)*. Taken together, these studies indicate that GHRH is necessary for normal development of pituitary somatotrophs and somatolactotrophs, though the details of the role of GHRH remain to be elucidated.

CRH

Corticotrophs increase in number after exposure to CRH both in vivo and in culture *(62–64)*, and CRH increases the mitotic activity of its target cells *(64)*. Basal and CRH stimulated secretion of POMC products (β-endorphin) occur in the fetal rat pituitary beginning at E_r15 *(65)*. However, CRH immunoreactivity itself was not detected in the fetal pituitary until $E_r19.5$ suggesting that the ability of the corticotrophs to respond to CRH was present before significant delivery of this factor to the anterior pituitary *(34)*. On the other hand, CRH responsiveness in cultured human fetal pituitary cells, like that of GHRH, lags behind the synthesis and secretion of ACTH *(29)*.

TRH AND GnRH

The role of TRH and GnRH on the development of their respective pituitary target cells has been more difficult to define. TRH appears has complex effects on somatolactotrophs, acting either to promote or to inhibit their proliferation depending upon the concentration of TRH administered *(66)*. However, little data is available as to the role of TRH during differentiation of thyrotrophs, though TRH does stimulate expression of αGSU, βTSH genes, and PRL genes *(67–69)*. As with GH and ACTH synthesis, αGSU, βLH, and βTSH immunoreactivity appear in human fetal pituitary cells in culture before the onset of responsiveness to their respective hypothalamic hormones *(29)*, suggesting that TRH and GnRH are not required for commitment of thyrotrophs and gonadotrophs in the human.

OTHER NEUROPEPTIDES

Other hypothalamic and pituitary factors may play a role in differentiation of the pituitary cell subtypes. These include vasopressin, which has been implicated in control of ACTH, β-endorphin and PRL *(70,71)*, and two inhibitory factors, dopamine and somatostatin, with important functions in regulating pituitary gene expression and/or secretion. Dopamine, the predominant inhibitor of PRL secretion, is present in high concentration in the human fetal hypothalamus by 15 wk of gestation *(72)*. Messenger RNA for all five receptor subtypes of the somatostatin (SRIH) receptor has been identified in the pituitary *(73,74)*, though only receptor types and II and V are expressed to a significant extent. It remains unclear whether negative regulation by dopamine or somatostatin is involved in promoting normal development of the pituitary.

Growth Factors

The developing pituitary is exposed to a variety of growth factors from contiguous mesenchymal tissue or synthesis within the pituitary. Potential roles for nerve growth factor (NGF), epidermal growth factor (EGF), the fibroblast growth factors (FGFs), and the transforming growth factors (TGFs), including activin and inhibin, have been suggested.

TGF

TGF-β1, a mesenchymal growth factor produced within anterior pituitary tissues *(75)*, exerts a potent inhibitory action on both basal and estrogen-induced secretion of PRL, on basal PRL mRNA levels, and on estrogen-induced proliferation of lactotrophs in primary culture *(75,76)*. Secretion of other pituitary hormones is not affected. These findings suggest that TGF-β is a specific negative regulator of lactotroph activity and may play a role in lactotroph differentiation. Activins and inhibins are additional members of the TGF-β family *(77)* that modulate activity of gonadotrophs and somatotrophs. Within the pituitary gland, both α- and β-subunits and activin receptors are synthesized, suggesting that these factors have autocrine effects on pituitary development and function *(78)*. Activin A stimulates growth and differentiation of gonadotroph cells and FSH secretion *(79)*. Activin also inhibits GHRH-stimulated cAMP synthesis, GH synthesis and secretion, and somatotroph proliferation *in vitro (80,81)*. Mice deficient in either activin βA- or both βA- and βB-subunit have multiple craniofacial abnormalities and die within 24 h. Exogenous activin A has antimitogenic effects on rat somatotroph cells in primary culture and AtT20 cells *(82,83)* and inhibits GH and ACTH secretion in somatotroph and corticotroph cell lines. These data suggest that activin plays an important role in development of the basal skull and associated structures (for review *see* ref. *84*), as well as modulating cell proliferation and pituitary hormone gene expression.

TGF-α, a factor structurally and functionally related to epidermal growth factor (EGF) that acts through the EGF receptor *(85)*, has been described in normal pituitary and pituitary tumors *(86–89)*. Expression within pituitary cell subtypes has been variable, with localization to somatotrophs and/or lactotrophs most consistent *(88–90)*. TGF-α to promotes growth and DNA synthesis in rat pituitary cells in culture *(91)* and transgenic rats overexpressing human TGF-α develop lactotroph hyperplasia and prolactinomas *(92)*.

NGF

Low levels of NGF mRNA have been detected in the pituitary and NGF-like immunoreactivity has been found within the hypothalamus and anterior pituitary. Both somatolactotroph and lactotroph cells express receptors for NGF *(93)*. NGF increases the number and rate at which mature lactotrophs appear in primary cultures of neonatal rat pituitary cells *(94)* and induces the differentiation of GH3 somatolactotrophs to a lactotroph phenotype *(95)*. The response of GH3 cells to NGF is analogous to that seen with EGF, including decreased cell proliferation, increased PRL synthesis, and decreased GH production. In addition, the NGF treated GH3 cells regained expression of the dopamine D-2 receptor. Finally, overexpression of NGF in lactotrophs of transgenic mice results in massive lactotroph hyperplasia and tumorigenesis *(96)*. Taken together these data implicate NGF as a potential regulator of lactotroph proliferation and differentiation.

EGF

Epidermal growth factor (EGF) receptors are present at low levels, on all subtypes of pituitary cells *(97,98)* and mRNA for EGF is present in somatotrophs, gonadotrophs *(97)*, and thyrotrophs *(98)*. In GH4/GH3 somatolactotroph cell lines, EGF induces alterations in morphology, growth rate, and relative transcription of the GH and PRL genes *(99,100)*. EGF also promotes proliferation of lactotrophs without affecting somatotroph proliferation in both GH3 and primary neonatal pituitary cultures *(101)*. EGF may also act as a mitogen for corticotrophs *(62,63)* and can increase expression of both POMC mRNA and ACTH secretion from corticotrophs *(102)*. EGF and EGF-R expression in pituitary tumors are extremely variable, with decreased EGF-R expression reported in most adenoma subtypes *(98,103,104)*, while marked overexpression has been observed in nonhormone secreting tumors and in tumors demonstrating a more aggressive phenotype *(98,104)*. Exposure of nonhormone secreting tumors to EGF resulted in an increased mitotic rate, upregulation of the EGF-R gene and suppression of hormone gene expression, suggesting a role for EGF in development and/or progression of these tumors *(98)*.

FGF

Basic fibroblast growth factor (bFGF or FGF-2) is found in high concentration in the adult anterior pituitary *(105)* and its temporal appearance during development (E_r15–16), particularly within gonadotrophs *(12)*, along with its minimal expression in the adult, has raised the possibility that bFGF may play a role in terminal differentiation. However, a recent study in human pituitaries demonstrated bFGF expression in both fetal and adult somatotrophs *(106)*. Exposure of neonatal rat pituitary cells in culture to bFGF results in specific enhancement of PRL-secreting cells without affecting the relative abundance of GH-secreting cells *(107)*. Recently, FGF-4, another member of the FGF family, encoded by the heparin-binding secretory transforming gene *(hst)*, has been implicated in pituitary tumorogenesis and induces a more aggressive phenotype in lactotroph tumors *(108)*. Since *hst* expression is restricted to early stages of development, FGF-4 may play a role in early differentiation and be extinguished as development proceeds.

LIF

Leukemia inhibitory factor, an immunoregulatory cytokine, is secreted by both adult and fetal pituitary cells in culture *(109)* and induces POMC gene expression and ACTH secretion *(110)*. Disruption of the LIF gene by homologous recombination results in an attenuated ACTH stress response *(111)*. Conversely, overexpression of LIF in transgenic mice results in a dwarf phenotype with markedly altered pituitary development *(112)*, consisting of increased corticotrophs and decreased somatotrophs and lactotrophs. Furthermore, cystic cavities, most likely representing Rathke's cleft cysts, were observed.

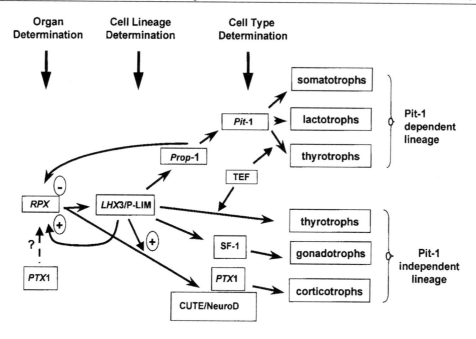

Figure 1. Transcription factor expression during pituitary otogeny.

TRANSCRIPTION FACTORS IN PITUITARY DEVELOPMENT

Cell phenotypes are determined by the sequential activation of a cascade of regulatory genes that control the pattern of expression of gene products *(113,114)*. In particular, considerable evidence suggests that tissue- and cell-specific factors are critical for the activation of genes that subsequently define cell type. These factors often exhibit spatially and/or temporally restricted distribution that allow for the activation of a unique combination of target genes and result in a stem cell entering a specific morphogenic pathway. Because the pituitary is so accessible and well-characterized, this gland has been a common model system in which to study developmental cascades and, accordingly, a great deal of progress has been made in understanding the molecular events involved in pituitary differentiation and gene regulation. Indeed, *Pit-1/GHF-1*, a transcription factor important in pituitary differentiation, was the first mammalian transcription factor directly shown to bind to DNA, lead to activation of specific genes, and regulate ontogeny of discrete cellular phenotypes (Fig. 1).

Homeobox Transcription Factors

THE POU DOMAIN FAMILY

The POU homeodomain transcription factors include P̲it-1, O̲ct-1, and Oct-2 and U̲nc-86. These factors share the novel POU-specific domain, upstream of the conserved homeodomain. The discovery that specific POU domain genes are expressed selectively during mammalian development suggests functions in early development (for review *see* ref. *115*).

Pit-1/GHF-1. Pit-1/GHF-1 was cloned based on knowledge of the sequence of critical regulatory regions of both the GH and PRL genes. In the anterior pituitary, Pit-1 protein is expressed exclusively in GH-, PRL-, and TSH-producing cells, though mRNA for *Pit-1* appears in gonadotrophs and corticotrophs *(2)* but is not translated. The exact timing of appearance of *Pit-1* transcripts is somewhat controversial. Simmons and coworkers *(2)* reported that *Pit-1* transcripts were undetectable on $E_r13.5$, but were present at $E_r15.5$ in the rat embryo, whereas Dolle and coworkers *(116)* were able to detect transcripts at $E_r13.5$ with a marked increase at E_r14 and 15. Both groups reported that Pit-1 protein could not be detected until E_r15. The relative expression of *Pit-1* mRNA increases progressively through PN10 *(2)*. Initiation of *Pit-1* expression correlated both spatially and temporally with activation of its distal target genes, hence, *Pit-1* was selectively activated in the caudomedial part of the developing gland, preceding activation of PRL, GH, and βTSH genes in this region *(2,116)*. The exception to this spatial correlation was the appearance of βTSH transcripts in the rostral tip of the developing pituitary in the absence of significant *Pit-1* expression *(2)*.

Several isoforms of Pit-1 have been described which result from alternative mRNA splicing. These include Pit-1β (also referred to as GHF-2) and Pit-1T *(117–120)*. Pit-1β selectively stimulates the GH promoter *(118,119)* and represses both basal and *ras*-activated PRL expression in pituitary cells *(121)*. Pit-1T selectively stimulates the βTSH promoter and specifically synergizes with Pit-1 on this target gene *(120)*. These findings suggest that distinct Pit-1 isoforms may further refine specificity of function within the cells in which the transcription factor is expressed.

The mechanisms involved in activation of the *Pit-1* gene provide intriguing insights into early steps in cell differentiation. The 5'-flanking sequence of the *Pit-1* gene contains an enhancer in which five Pit-1 binding sites are located, and the proximal promoter itself contains two Pit-1 binding sites *(122)*. At least three of the Pit-1 sites within the enhancer are important for activation of the gene, suggesting that Pit-1, like other developmentally important transcription factors, positively autoregulates its own expression *(123)*. In the Snell mouse, which lacks functional Pit-1 protein, the *Pit-1* gene is activated at the appropriate time during gestation and *Pit-1* expression is detectable in a subgroup of cells in the Snell mice until PN0 *(124)*. However, high-level expression of *Pit-1* and proliferation of Pit-1-dependent cell types does not occur. These data suggest that *Pit-1* autoregulation is not critical for initial activation and that alternate mechanisms dictate the initial pattern of expression of this transcription factor.

Recently, examination of the Ames dwarf mouse, identified *Prop-1* (prophet of *Pit-1*), a *paired*-like homeodomain transcription factor expressed early in pituitary development *(125)*. *Prop-1* appears to be critical for initial expression of *Pit-1* and its expression declines rapidly at the same time as the switch to *pit-1* autoregulation. Whereas the *Pit-1* early enhancer contains two sites that bind Prop-1 as a homodimer with high affinity, there is no activation of the *pit-1* transcript, suggesting that other factors and/or signals are required for Prop-1 function. The pituitary transcription factor *Rpx (see below)* forms heterodimers with Prop-1, however, this interaction appears to be antagonistic. As noted below, *Rpx* expression is abnormally prolonged in Ames dwarf mice, suggesting that *Prop-1* restricts *Rpx* expression as development proceeds.

Pit-1 plays multiple roles in specifying cell phenotype. Pit-1 activates the PRL, GH and βTSH genes in vitro. Conversely, the lack of expression of the PRL, GH, βTSH, and GHRH-R genes in Pit-1 defective mice and humans suggests that Pit-1 is also required for full expression of these genes in vivo. The failure of proliferation of thyrotroph, somatotroph and lactotroph cell types in the Snell dwarf indicates that Pit-1 is critical, either directly or indirectly, for proliferation and/or survival of these three cell types. The mechanisms by which Pit-1 functions as a morphogen remain unclear. Functional interactions between Pit-1 and other morphogenic signals, such as the retinoic acid receptor, have been demonstrated *(122)*.

Oct-1. *Oct-1*, another member of the POU-domain transcription factor family, is expressed in a wide variety of cell types, including the anterior pituitary. In the developing mouse it is expressed much earlier than Pit-1 $(E_m 8)$ *(126)*. Oct-1 can bind to the proximal Pit-1 binding element on the PRL promoter, as well as Pit-1 binding sites in other important pituitary genes including the *Pit-1* gene itself *(127)*. Coexpression of *Pit-1* and Oct-1 results in synergistic transcriptional effects on genes under control of either the native PRL promoter or a single Pit-1 response element *(128)*. These data suggest that a combinatorial pattern of heterodimeric and homodimeric interactions between these two members of the POU-domain gene family coexpressed in the developing pituitary, could regulate differential gene activation.

DISPERSED ANTERIOR HOMEOBOX GENES

Homeobox genes were originally identified as members of the homeotic gene clusters in *Drosophila* and play critical roles in the gene hierarchy governing the embryonic body plan of the fly. The vertebrate homologues, the *Hox* gene family, are structurally and functionally equivalent to their *Drosophila* counterparts and are critical in defining positional identity along the rostrocaudal axis *(129)*. However, the *Hox* genes are not expressed anterior to the hindbrain and distinct regulatory genes are responsible for determining the positioning of anterior brain structures. A number of murine homologs of *Drosophila* head homeobox genes have been identified and are promising candidates for cephalic regulatory genes, including the forebrain homeobox genes Otx1, Otx2, and goosecoid (gsc) *(130)*. However, these genes are not expressed in the developing anterior pituitary. Recently, murine homologs of *Drosophila* head homeobox genes have been identified that appear to have a specific role in pituitary development.

Lhx3. The LIM (Lin, Isl, Mec) homeodomain family of transcription factors has been shown to mediate crucial events in organogenesis and terminal differentiation. *Lhx3* (P-LIM) is selectively expressed in the pituitary *(131)* throughout development, but is highest at the early stage of development of Rathke's pouch, where it can be detected on $E_r 9$, and declines with time coincident with the differentiation of specific pituitary cell types and expression of terminal pituitary genes. *Lhx3* is expressed before discernible signal for both α-GSU and Pit-1 and activates the α-GSU promoter in vitro. When a targeted disruption of *Lhx3* was introduced into transgenic mice, the anterior and intermediate lobes of the pituitary were absent as a result of growth arrest after $E_m 10.5$ *(132)*, accompanied by absence of expression of GH, TSH, as well as α-GSU, and LH, suggesting that *Lhx3* expression is required for the cells of the pituitary primordium to commit to these pituitary lineages. On the other hand, initial POMC expression $(E_m 10.5)$ is normal in the mutant mice, though the eventual expression of POMC is drastically restricted to a small cohort of cells corresponding to the presumptive birthplace of early corticotrophs. Thus, the specification of initial corticotrophs occurred in the absence of *Lhx3* activity, supporting the suggestion that the corticotroph lineage is distinct and that its pathway departs from that of the other lineages at an early stage of pituitary development. Yet, without *Lhx3*, corticotrophs appear to be incapable of proliferating, suggesting that *Lhx3* may play a later role in the corticotroph lineage.

Rpx (Rathke's Pouch Homeobox). A screen for head homeobox genes in the mouse revealed a novel member of the paired homeodomain family *(129)*. Developmental analysis of the expression of the mRNA for this 185-amino acid peptide revealed that *Rpx* was initially detectable by E_m7 in the mesoderm underlying the prospective cephalic neural plate and becomes restricted to neuroectoderm of the developing prosencephalon. By E_m9, however, there is dramatic restriction of *Rpx* expression to the ectodermal cells that give rise to Rathke's pouch. *Rpx* expression continues throughout the pouch until approx E_m13, when downregulation of *Rpx* begins both spatially and temporally coincident with the differentiation of definitive pituitary cell types. Interestingly, in the *Lhx3* gene disruption *(see above) (132)* initial *Rpx* expression was intact, both spatially and temporally, suggesting that initial *Rpx* expression is independent of Lhx3 protein. However, *Rpx* expression disappeared abruptly by $E_m12.5$ in the *Lhx3* mutants, suggesting that continued expression of *Rpx* in the differentiating pituitary is directly or indirectly dependent on *Lhx3*. Similarly, in the Ames dwarf mouse, in which *Prop-1* is defective *(125)*, expression of *Rpx* was abnormally prolonged, suggesting that expression of *Prop-1* serves to restrict expression of *Rpx* as development progresses. Thus, *Rpx* is the earliest known gene expressed in the pituitary primordium and may be involved in both the positional identification and early commitment of the organ.

Ptx1 (Pituitary Homeobox 1). An expression library screen using an element of the POMC promoter that confers high-level, cell-specific expression revealed a novel member of the *bicoid* class of the *paired* homeobox family *(133)* closely related to the anterior homeobox genes *gsc* and *Otx-1* and *Otx-2*. This protein, Ptx1, was found to be a required, specific, and potent transcription factor that activates gene expression in a cell-specific manner and synergizes with the corticotroph specific helix-loop-helix transcription factor, CUTE, to promote POMC expression *(see below)*. *Ptx1* is expressed throughout the anterior lobe from E_m10 to E_m16, following which its expression becomes restricted to POMC positive cells. These results suggest that *Ptx1* may play an early role in formation of the pituitary anlage and later in development become specifically recruited as a regulator of corticotroph development.

bZIP Transcription Factors

The bZIP family of transcription factors is characterized by a conserved DNA-binding domain, containing clusters of basic amino acids, immediately adjacent to a conserved dimerization domain. This dimerization domain contains a leucine residue at every seventh position: the leucine zipper motif. These factors can form homodimers and heterodimers with other members of the bZIP family, which includes the Fos–Jun transcription factors, cAMP response element binding-activating transcription factor (CREB-ATF), the CCAAT/enhancer-binding protein (C/EBP), and the thyrotroph embryonic factor (TEF)/albumin D box-binding proteins (DBP) (for comprehensive review, *see* ref. *134*).

TEF. TEF was cloned based on its ability to bind to the proximal Pit-1 binding element of the PRL promoter, but may be more important in regulating βTSH expression *(135)*. *In situ* hybridization studies indicate that TEF transcripts first appear in the rostral part of the anterior pituitary gland on E_r14, corresponding both temporally and spatially to the pattern of βTSH gene expression. This restricted pattern of TEF gene expression is maintained through E_r16, though in the juvenile and adult rat TEF transcripts are observed in several tissues. The proximal βTSH promoter contains three independent binding domains for TEF and TEF is able to transactivate a reporter gene under the transcriptional control of the βTSH promoter. Because of the spatial and temporal pattern of TEF expression, and its relatively selective activation of the βTSH gene expression, TEF may functions alone or in concert with other factors to promote differentiation of the TSH cell.

CREB. In the human anterior pituitary, α-GSU transcription is regulated by cAMP through two tandem CREs *(136)*, though there is no evidence for this region conferring cAMP responsiveness in the rodent. *Pit-1/GHF-1* gene transcription is also regulated at least in part by two CRE sites within the promoter region *(137,138)*. Studies with transgenic mice overexpressing a dominant-negative (nonphosphorylatable) variant of CREB, indicate that the loss of functional CREB results in dwarfism and somatotroph hypoplasia *(50,137)*. Interestingly, targeting of the inactive CREB transgene to lactotrophs had no effect on the expansion of this cell population. Basal CREB activity is elevated by enhanced phosphorylation in GH secreting pituitary adenomas, some of which harbor an oncogenic Gαs mutation *(139)*. Whereas the ubiquitous nature of CRE makes it unlikely that these mechanisms control differentiation, several studies have suggested that other transcription factors may bind within the CRE region of the human α-GSU *(136,140,141)*. Hence, the CRE binding proteins may act in concert with other transcription factors to confer tissue specificity to these CRE regulated genes.

Helix-Loop-Helix Transcription Factors

The basic-helix-loop-helix (bHLH) transcriptional activators contain a conserved domain rich in basic amino acids, an amphipathic α-helix, a loop region, and then a second conserved α-helix. The basic region is necessary for DNA binding, whereas the HLH domain functions in dimerization, which is required for transcriptional activation. The ability to heterodimerize can regulate DNA-binding activity, by providing either activation or inhibition of transcription through the formation of functional or nonfunctional heterodimers.

CUTE. The proopiomelanocortin (POMC) promoter contains an E-box motif typical of binding sites for bHLH transcription factors and a cell specific E-box binding protein has been identified in nuclear extracts from the POMC-expressing corticotroph tumor cell line, AtT-20 cells *(142)*. This protein, named corticotroph upstream transcription element-binding protein (CUTE) appears to be specific to POMC-expressing cells and was not found in other pituitary cell lines tested. The temporal pattern of appearance of CUTE during pituitary development has not been examined, but this factor may be important in specifying differentiation of the corticotroph cell. Furthermore, CUTE may synergize with the homeobox transcription factor, *Ptx-1*, which is restricted to POMC-expressing cells during later stages of pituitary development *(see above) (133)*.

Zinc Finger Transcription Factors

Zn-15. The proximal GH promoter contains an unusually well conserved sequence between the proximal and distal Pit-1 binding sites (referred to as the GH-Z box) which when mutated resulted in markedly impaired GH expression *(143)*. A systematic search for factors binding this region in pituitary cells identified Zn-15, a factor possessing an unusual DNA-binding domain consisting of three Cys/His zinc fingers in the context of 12 other potential zinc fingers. In GC pituitary cells, endogenous Zn-15 complexes with the GH-Z region of the GH promoter in the GC cell and activates the GH promoter, whereas Pit-1 had little effect. Expression of both Zn-15 and Pit-1 simultaneously resulted in synergistic activation. These data suggest that functional interactions between Pit-1 and Zn-15 may be a critical component in the regulation of GH gene expression.

Nuclear Hormone Receptors. Nuclear hormone receptors represent one of the largest transcription factor families known (for review, *see* ref. *144*). These receptors mediate the signals of a broad variety of hormones including the steroid hormones, thyroid hormones and retinoids.

SF-1. The α-GSU gene contains a conserved element, termed the gonadotropin-specific element (GSE), that interacts with steroidogenic factor 1 (SF-1), a member of the nuclear hormone receptor superfamily *(145–148)*. SF-1 transcripts are found specifically in the gonadotrophin derived cell line, the αT3-1 cell, and not in cell lines derived from the hypothalamus or in other pituitary derived cell lines. In normal pituitary cells, the expression of SF-1 and gonadotroph-specific markers (α-GSU, βLH, βFSH) colocalize *(145)*. Mice with homozygous disruption of the *Ftz-F1* gene, which encodes SF-1, failed to express LH, FSH, or the GnRH receptor *(149)*. In contrast, TSH, GH, PRL, ACTH, and Pit-1 protein expression were comparable to that in normal mice. Furthermore, there were normal levels of POMC transcripts and low levels of α-GSU transcripts, whereas βLH and βFSH transcripts were absent.

SF-1 transcripts are initially detected at $E_m13.5$ and increase through $E_m17.5$ *(145)*. Thus, initial expression of SF-1 occurs after the onset of α-GSU expression (E12.5), and before the onset of βLH and βFSH (E16.5) *(2,150)*. In addition to interactions with the GSE to regulate α-GSU expression in gonadotrophs *(145)*, SF-1 can bind to a specific region of the βLH gene with sequence homology to the GSE *(151)*. Taken together these data suggest that SF-1 may regulate the expression of α-GSU, βLH and possibly βFSH during ontogeny of the gonadotroph phenotype.

Estrogen Receptor. Estrogen has important effects on the expression of gonadotrophins and prolactin and may play a role in cellular commitment. While many of the effects of estrogen on the pituitary are indirectly mediated through the hypothalamus, estradiol directly enhances βLH gene transcription *(152,153)*, and the PRL gene distal enhancer requires the ligand-activated estrogen receptor in combination with Pit-1 for full activation *(154)*. ER expression, is detectable in all cells of the normal adult pituitary and in pituitary tumors, but is highest in gonadotrophs and lactotrophs *(155,156)*. ER expression is absent in GH tumors but present in both PRL and GH/PRL producing tumors suggesting that divergence of somatotrophs and lactotrophs may involve regulation of the ER gene. Studies of ER expression during pituitary development are limited. In mice, functional ERs are detectable in neonates; increasing in number and responsiveness over the first several weeks of life *(157)*. Human fetal lactotrophs show a functional response to estrogen at 12 wk gestation *(29)*. The role of estradiol in pituitary development as opposed to gene expression remains unclear.

Glucocorticoid Receptor. The most thoroughly studied pituitary effect of glucocorticoids is the repression of the POMC gene. A glucocorticoid-dependent response element mediating GR repression of POMC gene transcription has been characterized *(158)*. The region of the promoter containing this GRE also contains binding sites for several nuclear transactivating factors that act synergistically in POMC gene expression. In the GH3 cell line, glucocorticoids decrease PRL mRNA expression while increasing GH mRNA *(137,159)*, and glucocorticoids are required for normal expression of the GHRH receptor. GR mRNA and immunoreactivity are present in developing fetal rat pituitary glands as early as E_r15 (the earliest time examined) *(160)*. In the fetus, GR ligand binding properties are similar to those in the adult, however, the biological activity of the GR and the role that GR plays in morphogenesis and initial cell commitment is unclear *(161)*.

Thyroid Hormone Receptor. In the rat, the ligand activated thyroid hormone receptor (TR) is an important negative regulator of both α and βTSH gene transcription *(162–165)*. Like ER and the GR, TR appears to exert its effect through interaction with other transactivating factors binding in the region of a specific TR element (TRE). In contrast to TSH, GH gene expression is activated by the TR, and a specific TRE has been identified in the GH promoter *(166–168)*. Detectable levels of TR have been demonstrated by *in situ* hybridization in the fetal rat pituitary by d 13.5 *(169)* and recent studies have demonstrated a differential pattern of expression of the four TR isoforms in developing rat brain *(170)*. These data suggest that thyroid hormone and its receptor isoforms may play an important role in early differentiation of thyrotrophs and somatotrophs.

THE ETS FAMILY OF TRANSCRIPTION FACTORS

The Ets superfamily is a novel structural class of transactivating phosphoproteins that have important roles in the control of growth and development *(171)*. Recent data suggest a synergistic interaction between Ets-1 and Pit-1 in mediating PRL promoter activity via a composite element consisting of an Ets-1 binding domain and the distal Pit-1 domain on the proximal rat PRL promoter *(172)*. Specific expression of Ets transcription factors in the anterior pituitary during embryogenesis has not been examined. However, *in situ* hybridization studies of the expression of Ets-1 and Ets-2 in the mouse suggest both tissue specific and temporally specific patterns of expression of both these genes beginning as early as E_m8 *(173)*.

SUMMARY

Significant progress has been made in identifying the molecular factors involved in differentiation, proliferation, and maintenance of pituitary cell types. Initial organ determination resulting from contact between the primordial ectoderm and the neuroepithelium is followed by the expression of a series of homeodomain factors in patterns that mirror the compartmentalized development of body segments dictated by the *Hox* genes. This cascade of gene expression appears to establish zones, both temporal and spatial, in which successive lineages of pituitary cells develop. Thus, specific patterns of temporal and spatial restriction, as well as regulation and modification of gene activation by autocrine, paracrine and endocrine factors, critical to pituitary cell-type specification. The similarity of this "compartmentalizing" cascade of gene expression to molecular events occurring in both body segment determination and development of the prosencephalon suggest that embryonically distinct tissues utilize parallel mechanisms for cell-type specification. Furthermore, this conservation means that the pituitary will remain an important model for the study of the mechanisms of tissue and organ differentiation.

REFERENCES

1. Ingraham H, Albert V, Chen R, Crenshaw E, Elsholtz H, He X, et al. A family of POU-domain and Pit-1 tissue-specific transcription factors in pituitary and neuroendocrine development. Ann Rev Physiol 1990;52:773–791.

2. Simmons DM, Voss JW, Ingraham HA, Holloway JM, Broide RS, Rosenfeld MG, Swanson LW. Pituitary cell phenotypes involve cell-specific Pit-1 mRNA translation and synergistic interactions with other classes of transcription factors. Genes Dev 1990;4:695–711.

3. Li S, Crenshaw E, Rawson E, Simmons D, Swanson L, Rosenfeld M. Dwarf locus mutants lacking three pituitary cell types result from mutations in the POU-domain gene pit-1. Nature 1990;347:528–533.

4. Dearden NM, Holmes RL. Cyto-differentiation and portal vascular development in the mouse adeno-hypophysis. J Anat 1976;121:551–569.

5. Kaufman MH. The Atlas of Mouse Development. Academic, London, 1992.

6. Rugh R. The Mouse: Its Reproduction and Development. Burgess Minneapolis, MN, 1968.

7. Watanabe YD, Daikoku S. An immunohistochemical study on the cytogenesis of adenohypophysial cells in fetal rats. Dev Biol 1979;68:559–567.

8. Daikoku S, Chikamori M, Adachi T, Maki Y. Effect of the basal diencephalon on the development of Rathke's pouch in rats: a study in combined organ cultures. Dev Biol 1982;90:198–202.

9. Chatelain A, Dupuoy JP, Dubois MP. Ontogenesis of cells producing polypeptide hormones (ACTH, MSH, LPH, GH, prolactin) in the fetal hypophysis of the rat: influence of the hypothalamus. Cell Tissue Res 1979;196:409–427.

10. Daikoku S, Kawano H, Abe K, Yoshinga K. Topographical appearance of adenohypophysial cells with special reference to the development of the portal system. Arch Histol Jap 1981;44:103–116.

11. Fink G, Smith GC. Ultrastructural features of the developing hypothalamo-phypophysial axis in the rat. Z Zellforsch 1971;119:208–226.

12. Schechter JE, Patgtison A, Pattison T. Development of the vasculature of the anterior pituitary: ontogeny of basic fibroblast growth factor. Develop Dynam 1993;197:81–93.

13. Dearden NM, Holmes RL. Cyto-differentiation and portal vascular development in the mouse adeno-hypophysis. J Anat 1976;121:551–569.

14. Jansson J, Ishikawa K, Katakami H, Frohman L. Pre- and postnatal developmental changes in hypo-thalamic content of rat growth hormone-releasing factor. Endocrinology 1987;120:525–530.

15. Daikoku S, Kawano H, Noguchi M, Nakanishi J, Tokuzen M, Chihara K, et al. Ontogenetic appearance of immunoreactive GRF-containing neurons in the rat hypothalamus. Cell Tissue Res 1985;242:511–518.

16. Ishikawa K, Katakami H, Jansson J, Frohman LA. Ontogenesis of growth hormone-releasing hormone neurons in the rat hypothalamus. Neuroendocrinology 1986;43:537–542.

17. Nemeskeri A, Setalo G, Halasz B. Ontogenesis of the three parts of the fetal rat adenohypophysis. Neuroendocrinology 1988;48:534–543.

18. Nemeskeri A, Setalo G, Halasz B. Ontogenesis of the three parts of the fetal rat adenohypophysis: a detailed immunohistochemical analysis. Neuroendocrinology 1988;48:534–543.

19. Kineman RD, Faught WJ, Frawley LS. The ontogenic and functional relationships between growth hormone- and prolactin-releasing cells during the development of the bovine pituitary. J Endocrinol 1992;134:91–96.

20. Hoeffler JP, Boockfor FR, Frawley LS. Ontogeny of prolactin cells in neonatal rats: initial prolactin secretors also release growth hormone. Endocrinology 1985;117:187–195.

21. Burrows HL, Birkmeier TS, Seasholtz AF, Camper SA. Targeted ablation of cells in the pituitary primorida of transgenic mice. Mol Endocrinol 1996;10:1467–1477.

22. Kineman RD, Faught WJ, Frawley LS. Steroids can modulate transdifferentiation of prolactin and growth hormone cells in bovine pituitary cultures. Endocrinology 1992;130:3289–3294.

23. Borrelli E, Hayman RA, Arias C, Sawchenko PE, Evans RM. Transgenic mice with inducible dwarf-ism. Nature 1989;339:538–541.

24. Behringer RR, Mathews LS, Palmiter RD, Brinster RL. Dwarf mice produced by genetic ablation of growth hormone-expressing cells. Genes Dev 1988;2:453–461.

25. Frawley LS, Boockfor FR, Hoeffler JP. Identification by plaque assays of a pituitary cell type that secretes both growth hormone and prolactin. Endocrinology 1985;116:734–737.

26. Frawley LS, Boockfor FR. Mammosomatotrophs: presence and functions in normal and neoplastic pituitary tissue. Endocr Rev 1991;12:337–355.

27. Coates PJ, Doniach I. Development of folliculo-stellate cells in the human pituitary. Acta Endocrinol (Copenh) 1988;119:16–20.

28. Asa SL, Kovacs K, Lazlo FA, Domokos I, Ezrin C. Human fetal adenohypophysis: histologic and immunocytochemical analysis. Neuroendocrinology 1986;43:308–316.

29. Asa SL, Kovacs K, Singer W. Human fetal adenohypophysis: morphologic and functional analysis in vitro. Neuroendocrinology 1991;53:562–572.

30. Ikeda H, Suzuki J, Sasano N, Niizuma H. The development and morphogenesis of the human pituitary gland. Anat Embryol 1988;178:327–336.

31. Kikuyama S, Inaco H, Jenks BG, Kawamura K. Development of the ectopically transplanted primordium of epithelial hypophysis (anterior neural ridge) in Bufo japonicus embryos. J Exp Zool 1993;266:216–220.

32. Daikoku S, Chikamori M, Adachi T, Okamura Y, Nishiyama T, Tsuruo Y. Ontogenesis of hypothalamic immunoreactive ACTH cells in vivo and in vitro: role of Rathke's pouch. Dev Biol 1983;97: 81–88.

33. Kawamura K, Kikuyama S. Induction from posterior hypothalamus is essential for the development of the pituitary proopiomelanocortin (POMC) cells of the toad (Bufo japonicus). Cell Tissue Res 1995;279:233–239.

34. Barinaga M, Yamamoto G, Rivier C, Vale WW, Evans RM, Rosenfeld MG. Transcriptional regulation of growth hormone gene expression by growth hormone-releasing factor. Nature 1983;306:84,85.

35. Gick GG, Zeytin FN, Ling NC, Esch FS, Bancroft C, Brazeau P. Growth hormone-releasing factor regulates growth hormone mRNA in primary cultures of rat pituitary cells. Proc Natl Acad Sci USA 1984;81:1553–1555.

36. Lloyd RV, Jin L, Chang A, Kulig E, Camper SA, Ross BD, et al. Morphologic effects of hGHRH gene expression on the pituitary, liver, and pancreas of MT-hGRH transgenic mice: an in situ hybridization analysis. Am J Pathol 1992;141:895–906.

37. Asa SL, Kovacs K, Stefaneanu L, Horvath E, Billestrup N, Gonzalez-Manchon C, Vale W. Pituitary adenomas in mice transgenic for growth hormone-releasing hormone. Endocrinology 1992;131: 2083–2089.

38. Mayo K, Hammer RE, Swanson LW, Brinster RL, Rosenfeld MG, Evans RM. Dramatic pituitary hyperplasia in transgenic mice expressing a human growth hormone-releasing factor gene. Mol Endocrinol 1988;2:606–612.

39. Stefaneanu L, Kovacs K, Horvath E, Asa SL, Losinski NE, Billestrup N, et al. Adenohypophysial changes in mice transgenic for human growth hormone-releasing factor (hGRF): a histological, immunocytochemical and electron microscopic investigation. Endocrinology 1989;125:2710–2718.

40. Billestrup N, Swanson LW, Vale W. Growth hormone-releasing factor stimulates proliferation of somatotrophs in vitro. Proc Natl Acad Sci USA 1986;83:6854–6857.

41. Barinaga M, Bilezikjian LM, Vale W, Rosenfeld MG, Evans RM. Independent effects of growth hormone-releasing factor on growth hormone release and gene transcription. Nature 1985;314: 279–281.

42. Asa SL, Scheithauer BW, Bilbao JM, Horvath E, Ryan N, Kovacs K, et al. A case for hypothalamic acromegaly: a clinicopathological study of six patients with hypothalamic gangliocytomas producing growth hormone-releasing factor. J Clin Endocrinol Metab 1984;58:796–803.

43. Frohman LA, Szabo M, Berelowitz M, Stachura ME. Partial purification and characterization of a peptide with growth hormone-releasing activity from extrapituitary tumors in patients with acromegaly. J Clin Invest 1980;65:43–54.

44. Billestrup N, Mitchell RL, Vale W, Verma IM. Growth hormone-releasing factor induces c-fos expression in cultured primary pituitary cells. Mol Endocrinol 1987;1:300–305.

45. Burton F, Hasel K, Bloom F, Sutcliffe J. Pituitary hyperplasia and gigantism in mice caused by a cholera toxin transgene. Nature 1991;350:74–77.

46. Wehrenberg WB, Voltz DM, Cella SG, Müller EE, Gaillard RC. Long-term failure of compensatory growth in rats following acute neonatal passive immunization against growth hormone-releasing hormone. Neuroendocrinology 1992;56:509–515.

47. Wehrenberg WB, Bloch B, Phillips BJ. Antibodies to growth hormone-releasing factor inhibit somatic growth. Endocrinology 1984;115:1218–1220.

48. Cella SG, Locatelli V, Mennini T, Zanini A, Bendotti C, Forloni GL, et al. Deprivation of growth hormone-releasing hormone early in the rat's neonatal life permanently affects somatotropic function. Endocrinology 1990;127:1625–1634.

49. Maiter D, Underwood LE, Martin JB, Koenig JI. Neonatal treatment with monosodium glutamate: effects of prolonged growth-hormone (GH)-releasing hormone deficiency on pulsatile GH secretion and growth in female rats. Endocrinology 1991;128:1100–1106.

50. Struthers RS, Vale WW, Arias C, Sawchenko PE, Montminy MR. Somatotroph hypoplasia and dwarfism in transgenic mice expressing a non-phosphorylatable CREB mutant. Nature 1991;350: 622–624.

51. Cheng T, Beamer W, Phillips J, Bartke A, Mallonee R. Etiology of growth hormone deficiency in Little, Ames, and Snell dwarf mice. Endocrinology 1983;113:1669–1678.

52. Lin S-C, Lin CR, Gukovsky I, Lusis AJ, Sawchenko PE, Rosenfeld MG. Molecular basis of the *little* mouse phenotype and implications for cell type-specific growth. Nature 1993;364:208–213.

53. Chua SC, Hennessey K, Zeitler P, Leibel RL. The little *(lit)* mutation cosegregates with the growth hormone releasing factor receptor on mouse Chromosome 6. Mammal Genome 1993;4:555–559.

54. Jansson J-O, Downs TR, Beamer WG, Frohman LA. Receptor-associated resistance to growth hormone-releasing factor in dwarf "little" mice. Science 1986;232:511,512.

55. Godfrey P, Rahal JO, Beamer WG, Copeland NG, Jenkins NA, Mayo KE. GHRH receptor of *little* mice contains a missense mutation in the extracellular domain that disrupts receptor function. Nature Genetics 1993;4:227–232.

56. Charlton HM, Clark RG, Robinson ICAF, Porter-Goff AEP, Cox BS, Bugnon C, Bloch BA. Growth hormone-deficient dwarfism in the rat: a new mutation. J Endocrinol 1988;119:51–58.

57. Downs TR, Frohman LA. Evidence for a defect in growth hormone-releasing factor signal transduction in the dwarf *(dw/dw)* rat pituitary. Endocrinology 1991;129:58–67.

58. Brain CE, Chomczynski P, Downs TR, Frohman LA. Impaired generation of cyclic adenosine 3',5'-monophosphate in a somatomammotroph cell line derived from dwarf *(dw)* rat anterior pituitaries. Endocrinology 1991;129:3410–3416.

59. Zeitler P, Downs TR, Frohman LA. Impaired growth hormone-releasing hormone signal transduction in the dwarf *(dw)* rat is independent of a defect in the stimulatory G protein subunit. Endocrinology 1993;133:2782–2786.

60. Zeitler P, Downs TR, Frohman LA. Development of pituitary cell types in the spontaneous dwarf *(dw)* rat: evidence for an isolated defect in somatotroph differentiation. Endocrine 1994;2:729–733.

61. Gage PJ, Lossie AC, Scarlett LM, Lloyd RV, Camper SA. Ames dwarf mice exhibit somatotroph commitment but lack growth hormone-releasing hormone response. Endocrinology 1995;136: 1161–1167.

62. Asa SL, Kovacs K, Hammer GD, Liu B, Roos BA, Low MJ. Pituitary corticotroph hyperplasia in rats implanted with a medullary thyroid carcinoma cell line transfected with a corticotropin-releasing hormone complementary deoxyribonucleic acid expression vector. Endocrinology 1992;131: 715–720.

63. Gertz BJ, Contreras LH, McComb KI, Kivacs JB, Tyrrel JB, Dallman M. Chronic administration of corticotropin-releasing factor increases pituitary corticotroph number. Endocrinology 1987;120: 381–388.

64. Childs GV, Rougeau D, Unabia G. Corticotropin-releasing hormone and epidermal growth factor: mitogens for anterior pituitary corticotrophs. Endocrinology 1995;136:1595–1602.

65. Hotta M, Shibasaki T, Masuda R, Imaki T, Demura H, Ohno H, et al. Ontogeny of pituitary responsiveness to corticotropin-releasing hormone in rat. Regul Peptides 1988;21:245–252.

66. Ramsdell JS. Thyrotropin-releasing hormone inhibits GH4 pituitary cell proliferation by blocking entry into S phase. Endocrinology 1990;126:472–479.

67. Murakami M, Muri M, Kato Y, Kobayashi I. Hypothalamic thyrotropin-releasing hormone regulates pituitary β- and α-subunit mRNA levels in the rat. Neuroendocrinology 1991;53:276–280.

68. Shupnik MA, Greenspan SL, Ridgeway EC. Transcriptional regulation of thyrotropin subunit genes by thyrotropin-releasing hormone and dopamine in pituitary cells. J Biol Chem 1986;261:12,675–12,679.

69. Tashjian AH, Barowsky NJ, Jensen DK. Thyrotropin-releasing hormone: direct evidence for stimulation of prolactin production by pituitary cells in culture. Biochem Biophys Res Commun 1971;43:516–523.

70. Matthews SG, Parrott RF. Centrally administered vasopressin modifies stress hormone (cortisol, prolactin) secretion in sheep under basal conditions, during restrain, and following intravenous corticotrophin-releasing hormone. Europ J Endocrinol 1994;130:297–301.

71. Aguilera G. Regulation of pituitary ACTH secretion during chronic stress. Frontiers Neuroendocrinol 1994;15:321–350.

72. Hyyppa M. Hypothalamic monoamines in human fetuses. Neuroendocrinology 1972;9:257–266.

73. Bruno J, Xu Y, Song J, Berelowitz M. Tissue distribution of somatostatin receptor subtype messenger ribonucleic acid in the rat. Endocrinology 1993;133:2561–2567.

74. Wulfsen I, Meyerhof W, Fehr S, Richter D. Expression patterns of rat somatostatin receptor genes in pre- and post-natal brain and pituitary. J Neurochem 1993;61:1549–1552.

75. Sarkar DK, Kim KH, Minami S. Transforming growth factor-beta1 messenger RNA and protein expression in the pituitary gland: its action on prolactin secretion and lactotropic growth. Mol Endocrinol 1992;6:1825–1833.

76. Delidow BC, Billis WM, Agarwal P, White BA. Inhibition of prolactin gene expression by transforming growth factor-B in GH3 cells. Mol Endocrinol 1991;5:1716–1722.

77. Massague J. The TGF-beta family of growth and differentiation factors. Cell 1987;49:437,438.

78. Roberts VJ, Barth SL. Expression of messenger ribonucleic acids encoding the inhibin/activin system during mid-and late-gestation rat embryogenesis. Endocrinology 1994;134:914–923.

79. Katayama T, Shioto K, Takahashi M. Activin A increase the number of follicle-stimulating hormone cells in anterior pituitary cultures. Mol Cell Endocrinol 1990;69:179–185.

80. Billestrup N, Gonzalez-Manchon C, Potter E, Vale W. Inhibition of somatotroph growth and growth hormone biosynthesis by activin in vitro. Mol Endocrinol 1990;4:356–362.

81. Bilezikjian LM, Corrigan AZ, Vale W. Activin-A modulates growth hormone secretion from cultures of rat anterior pituitary cells. Endocrinology 1990;126:2369–2376.

82. Billestrup N, González-Manchón C, Potter E, Vale W. Inhibition of somatotroph growth and growth hormone biosynthesis by activin in vitro. Mol Endocrinol 1990;4:356–362.

83. Bilezikjian LM, Blount AL, Camper SA, Gonzalez-Manchon C, Vale W. Activin A inhibits proopiomelanocortin messenger RNA accumulation and adrenocorticotropin secretion in AtT20 cells. Mol Endocrinol 1991;5:1389–1395.

84. Matzuk MM, Kumar TR, Shou W, Coerver KA, Lau AL, Behringer RR, Finegold MJ. Transgenic models to study the roles of inhibins and activins in reproduction, oncogenesis, and development. Rec Prog Horm Res 1996;51:123–154.

85. Marquardt H, Hunkapiller MW, Hoodk LE, Todaro G. Rat transforming growth factor type 1: structure and relation to epidermal growth factor. Science 1984;223:1079–1082.

86. Samsoondar J, Kobrin MS, Kudlow JE. A-transforming growth factor secreted by untransformed bovine anterior pituitary cells in culture. J Biol Chem 1986;261:14,408–14,413.

87. Finley E, Ramsdell JS. A transforming growth factor-a pathway is expressed in GHCl rat pituitary tumors and appears necessary for tumor formation. Endocrinology 1994;135:416–422.

88. Finley EL, King JS, Ramsdell JS. Human pituitary somatotropes express transforming growth factor-a and its receptor. J Endocrinol 1994;141:547–554.

89. Ezzat S, Walpola IA, Ramjar L, Smyth HS, Asa SL. Membrane-anchored expression of transforming growth factor a in human pituitary adenoma cells. J Clin Endocrinol Metab 1995;80:534–539.

90. Kobrin MS, Asa SL, Samsoondar J, Kudlow JE. a-transforming growth factor in the bovine anterior pituitary gland: secretion by dispersed cells and immunohistochemical localization. Endocrinology 1987;121:1412–1416.

91. Renner U, Mojto J, Arzt E, Lange M, Stalla J, Muller OA, Stalla GK. Secretion of polypeptide growth factors by human nonfunctioning pituitary adenoma cells in culture. Neuroendocrinology 1993; 57:825–834.

92. McAndrew J, Paterson AJ, Asa SL, McCarthy KJ, Kudlow JE. Targeting of transforming growth factor-α expression to pituitary lactotrophs in transgenic mice results in selective lactotroph proliferation and adenomas. Endocrinology 1995;136:4479–4488.

93. Patterson JC, Childs GV. Nerve growth factor and its receptor in the anterior pituitary. Endocrinology 1994;135:1689–1696.

94. Missale C, Boroni F, Frassine M, Caruso A, Spano P. Nerve growth factor promotes the differentiation of pituitary mammotroph cells in vitro. Endocrinology 1995;136:1205–1213.

95. Missale C, Boroni F, Sigala S, Zanellato A, DalToso R, Balsari A, Spano P. Nerve growth factor directs differentiation of the bipotential cell line GH3 into the mammotroph phenotype. Endocrinology 1994;135:290–298.

96. Borelli E, Sawchenko PE, Evans RM. Pituitary hyperplasia induced by ectopic expression of nerve growth factor. Proc Natl Acad Sci USA 1992;89:2764–2768.

97. Fan X, Childs GV. Epidermal growth factor and transforming growth factor-a messenger ribonucleic acids and their receptors in the rat anterior pituitary: localization and regulation. Endocrinology 1995;136:2284–2293.

98. Chaidarun SS, Eggo MC, Sheppard MC, Stewart PM. Expression of epidermal growth factor (EGF), its receptor, and related oncoprotein (erbB-2) in human pituitary tumors and response to EGF in vitro. Endocrinology 1994;135:2012–2021.

99. Murdoch GH, Potter E, Nicolaisen AK, Evans RM, Rosenfeld MG. Epidermal growth factor rapidly stimulates prolactin gene transcription. Nature 1982;300:192–194.

100. Johnson L, Baxter J, Vlodavsky I, Gospodorowicz D. Epidermal growth factor and expression of specific genes: effects on cultured rat pituitary cells are dissociable from the mitogenic response. Proc Natl Acad Sci USA 1980;77:394–398.

101. Felix R, Meza U, Cota G. Induction of classical lactotropes by epidermal growth factor in rat pituitary cell cultures. Endocrinology 1995;136:939–946.

102. Childs GV. Epidermal growth factor enhances ACTH secretion and expression of POMC mRNA by corticotropes in mixed and enriched cultures. Mol Cell Neurosci 1991;2:235–241.

103. Birman P, Michard M, Li JY, Peillon F, Bression D. Epidermal growth factor binding sites, present in normal human and rat pituitaries, are absent in human pituitary adenomas. J Clin Endocrinol Metab 1987;65:275–281.

104. LeRiche VK, Asa SL, Ezzat S. Epidermal growth factor and its receptor (EGF-R) in human pituitary adenomas: EGF-R correlates with tumor aggressiveness. J Clin Endocrinol Metab 1996;81:656–662.

105. Gospodorowicz D, Ferrara N. Fibroblast growth factor and the control of pituitary and gonad development and function. Steroid Biochem 1989;32:183–191.

106. Marin F, Boya J. Immunocytochemical localization of basic fibroblast growth factor in the human pituitary gland. Neuroendocrinology 1995;62:523–529.

107. Porter TE, Wiles CD, Frawley L. Stimulation of lactotrope differentiation in vitro by fibroblast growth factor. Endocrinology 1994;134:164–168.

108. Shimon I, Huttner A, Said J, Spirina OM, Melmed S. Heparin-binding secretory transforming gene (hst) facilitates rat lactotrope cell tumorigenesis and induces prolactin gene transcription. J Clin Invest 1996;97:187–195.

109. Ferrara N, Winer J, Henzel WJ. Pituitary follicular cells secrete an inhibitor of aortic endothelial cell growth; identification as leukemia inhibitory factor. Proc Natl Acad Sci USA 1992;89:698–702.

110. Ray DW, Ren S-G, Melmed S. Leukemia inhibitory factor (LIF) stimulates proopiomelanocortin (POMC) expression in a corticotroph cell line-role of STAT pathway. J Clin Invest 1996;97:1852–1859.

111. Akita S, Malkin J, Melmed S. Disrupted murine leukemia inhibitory factor (LIF) gene attenuates adrenocorticotropic hormone (ACTH) secretion. Endocrinology 1996;137:3140–3143.

112. Akita S, Readhead C, Stefaneanu L, Fine J, Malkin J, Said J, et al. Transgenic overexpression of pituitary-directed leukemia inhibitory factor: novel dwarf phenotype. Program Int Soc Endocrinol 1996, OR39-8, p. 120.

113. Davidson EH. How embryos work: a comparative view of diverse modes of cell fate specification. Development 1990;108:365–389.

114. Gehring WJ. Homeoboxes in the study of development. Science 1987;236:1245–1252.

115. Rosenfeld MG. POU-domain transcript factors: pou-er-ful developmental regulators. Genes Dev 1991;5:897–907.

116. Dolle P, Castrillo J, Theill LE, Deerinck T, Ellisman M, Karin M. Expression of GHF-1 protein in mouse pituitaries correlates both temporally and spatially with the onset of growth hormone gene activity. Cell 1990;60:809–820.

117. Theill LE, Hattori K, Lazzaro D, Castrillo J-L, Karin M. Differential splicing of the GHF1 primary transcript gives rise to two functionally distinct homeodomain proteins. EMBO J 1992;11:2261–2269.

118. Morris AE, Kloss B, McChesney RE, Bancroft C, Chasin LA. An alternatively spliced Pit-1 isoform altered in its ability to trans-activate. Nucleic Acids Res 1992;20:1355–1361.

119. Konzak KE, Moore DD. Functional isoforms of Pit-1 generated by alternative mRNA splicing. Mol Endocrinol 1992;6:241–247.

120. Haugen BR, Gordon DF, Nelson AR, Wood WM, Ridgway EC. The combination of Pit-1 and Pit-1T has a synergistic stimulatory effect on the thyrotropin β-subunit promoter but not the growth hormone or prolactin promoters. Mol Endocrinol 1994;8:1574–1582.

121. Diamond S, Gutierrez-Hartman A. A 26-amino acid insertion domain defines a functional transcription switch motif in Pit-1 beta. J Biol Chem 1996;271:28,925–28,932.

122. Rhodes SJ, Chen R, DiMattia GE, Scully KM, Kalla KA, Lin S, et al. A tissue-specific enhancer confers Pit-1 dependent morphogen inducibility and autoregulation on the pit-1 gene. Genes Dev 1993;7:913–932.

123. Chen R, Ingraham H, Treacy MN, Aalbert V, Wilson L, Rosenfeld M. Autoregulation of pit-1 gene expression mediated by two cis-active promoter elements. Nature 1990;346:583–586.

124. Lin S, Li S, Drolet DW, Rosenfeld MG. Pituitary ontogeny of the Snell dwarf mouse reveals Pit-1-independent and Pit-1-dependent origins of the thyrotrope. Development 1994;120:515–522.

125. Sornson MW, Wu W, Dasen J, Flynn S, Norman DJ, O'Connell SM, et al. Pituitary lineage determination by the prophet of Pit-1 homeodomain factor defective in Ames dwarfism. Nature 1996; 384:327–333.

126. He X, Treacy MM, Simmons DM, Ingraham HA, Swanson LW, Rosenfeld MG. Expression of a large family of POU-domain regulatory genes in mammalian brain development. Nature 1989;340:35–42.

127. Chen C, Ingraham HA, Treacy MM, Albert VA, Wilson L, Rosenfeld MG. The pituitary POU-domain protein Pit-1 positively and negatively regulates transcription of its own promoter. Nature 1991;346:583–586.

128. Voss JW, Wilson L, Rosenfeld MG. POU-domain proteins Pit-1 and Oct-1 interact to form a heteromeric complex and can cooperate to induce expression of the prolactin promoter. Genes Dev 1991;5:1309–1320.

129. Hermesz E, Mackem S, Mahon KA. Rpx: a novel anterior restricted homeobox gene progressively activated in the prechordal plate, anterior neural plate and rathke's pouch of the mouse embryo. Development 1996;122:41–52.

130. Blum M, Gaunt SJ, Cho KWY, Steinbeisser H, Blumberg B, Bittner D, DeRobertis EM. Gastrulation in the mouse: the role of the homeobox gene goosecoid. Cell 1992;69:1097–1106.

131. Bach I, Rhodes SJ, Pearse RV, Heinzel T, Gloss B, Scully KM, et al. P-Lim, a LIM homeodomain factor, is expressed during pituitary organ and cell commitment and synergizes with Pit-1. Proc Natl Acad Sci USA 1995;92:2720–2724.

132. Sheng HZ, Zhadonov AB, Mosinger B, Giji T, Bertuzzi S, Grinberg A, et al. Specification of pituitary cell lineages by the LIM homeobox gene lhx3. Science 1996;272:1004–1007.

133. Lamonerie T, Tremblay JJ, Lanctot C, Therrien M, Gauthier Y, Drouin J. Ptx1, a bicoid-related homeobox transcription factor involved in transcription of the proopiomelanocortin gene. Genes Dev 1996;10:1284–1295.

134. Busch SJ, Sassone-Corsi P. Dimers, leucine zippers and DNA-binding domains. Trends in Genetics 1990;6:36–40.

135. Drolet DW, Scully KM, Simmons DM, Wegner M, Chu KT, et al. TEF, a transcription factor expressed specifically in the anterior pituitary during embryogenesis, defines a new class of leucine zipper proteins. Genes Dev 1991;5:1739–1753.

136. Delegeane AM, Ferland LH, Mellon PL. Tissue specific enhance of the human glycoprotein hormone a subunit gene: dependence on cAMP inducible elements. Mol Cell Biol 1987;7:3994–4002.

137. Theill LE, Karin M. Transcriptional control of GH expression and anterior pituitary development. Endocr Rev 1993;14:670–689.

138. McCormick A, Brady H, Theill LE, Karin M. Regulation of the pituitary specific homeobox gene GHF-1 by cell-autonomous and environmental cues. Nature 1990;345:829–832.

139. Bertherat J, Chanson P, Montminy M. The cyclic adenosine 3',5'-monophosphate responsive factor CREB is constitutively activated in human somatotroph adenomas. Mol Endocrinol 1995;9:777–783.

140. Schoderbek WE, Kim KE, Ridgway EC, Mellon PL, Maurer RA. Analysis of DNA sequences required for pituitary-specific expression of the glycoprotein hormone a-subunit gene. Mol Endocrinol 1992;6:893–903.

141. Akerblom IE, Slater EP, Becto M, Baxter JD, Mellon PL. Negative regulation by glucocorticoids through interference with a cAMP responsive enhancer. Science 1988;241:350–353.

142. Therrien M, Drouin J. Cell-specific helix-loop-helix factor required for pituitary expression of the pro-opiomelanocortin gene. Mol Cell Biol 1993;13:2342–2353.

143. Lipkin SM, Naar AM, Kalla KA, Sack RA, Rosenfeld MG. Identification of a novel zinc finger protein binding a conserved element critical for Pit-1 dependent growth hormone gene expression. Genes Dev 1993;7:1674–1687.

144. Mangelsdorf DJ, Thummel C, Beato M, Herrlich P, Schutz G, Umesono K, et al. The nuclear receptor superfamily: the second decade. Cell 1995;3:835–839.

145. Horn F, Windle JJ, Barnhart KM, Mellon PL. Tissue specific gene expression in the pituitary: the glycoprotein hormone α-subunit gene is regulated by a gonadotrope-specific protein. Mol Cell Biol 1992;12:2143–2153.

146. Ingraham HA, Lala DS, Ikeda Y, Luo X, Shen W, Nachtigal MW, et al. The nuclear receptor steroidogenic factor 1 acts at multiple levels of the reproductive axis. Genes Dev 1994;8:2302–2312.

147. Honda S, Morohashi K, Nomura M, Takeya H, Kitajima M, Omura T. Ad4BP regulating steroidogenic P-450 gene is a member of the steroid hormone receptor superfamily. J Biol Chem 1993;268: 7494–7502.

148. Lala DS, Rice DA, Parker KL. Steroidogenic factor 1, a key regulator of steroidogenic enzyme expression, is the mouse homolog of gushi tarazu-factor 1. Mol Endocrinol 1993;6:1249–1258.

149. Shinoda K, Lei H, Yoshii H, Nomura M, Nagano M, Shiba H, et al. Developmental defects of the ventromedial hypothalamic nucleus and pituitary gonadotrophs in the Ftz-F1 disrupted mice. Development Dynam 1995;24:22–29.

150. Japon MG, Rubenstein M, Low MJ. In situ hybridization analysis of anterior pituitary hormone gene expression during fetal mouse development. J Histochem Cytochem 1994;42:1117–1125.

151. Shupnik MA, Fallest PC. Endo Soc Annual Meeting P1–521 1995 (abstract).

152. Shupnik MA, Weinmann CM, Notides AC, Chin WW. An upstream region of the rat luteinizing hormone β gene binds estrogen receptor and confers estrogen responsiveness. J Biol Chem 1989;264:80–86.

153. Shupnik MA, Rosenzweigk BA. Identification of an estrogen-responsive element in the rat LHb gene. J Biol Chem 1991;266:17,084–17,091.

154. Day RN, Koikw a, Sakai M, Murumatsu M, Maurer RA. Both Pit-1 and the estrogen receptor are required for estrogen responsiveness of the rat prolactin gene. Mol Endocrinol 1990;4:1964–1971.

155. Stefaneanu L, Kovacs K, Horvath E, Lloyd RV, Buchfelder M, Fahlbusch R, Smyth H. *In situ* hybridization study of estrogen receptor messenger ribonucleic acid in human adenohypophysial cells and pituitary adenomas. J Clin Endocrinol Metab 1994;78:83–88.

156. Friend KE, Chiou Y-K, Lopes MBS, Laws ER, Jr., Hughes KM, Shupnik MA. Estrogen receptor expression in human pituitary: correlation with immunohistochemistry in normal tissue, and immunohistochemistry and morphology in macroadenomas. J Clin Endocrinol Metab 1994;78: 1497–1504.

157. Slabaugh MB, Lieberman ME, Rutledge JJ, Gorski J. Ontogeny of growth hormone and prolactin gene expression in mice. Endocrinology 1982;110:1489–1497.

158. Drouin J, Trifiro MA, Plante RK, Nemer M, Eriksson P, Wrange O. Glucocorticoid receptor binding to a specific DNA sequence is required for hormone-dependent repression of proopiomelanocortin gene transcription. Mol Cell Biol 1989;9:5303–5314.

159. Elsholtz HP. Molecular biology of prolactin: cell-specific and endocrine regulators of the prolactin gene. Seminars in Reproduct Endocrinol 1992;10:183–195.

160. Cintra A, Solfrini V, Bunnemann B, Okret S, Bortolotti F, Gustafsson J, Fuxe K. Prenatal development of glucocorticoid receptor gene expression and immunoreactivity in the rat brain and pituitary gland: a combined *in situ* hybridization and immunocytochemical analysis. Neuroendocrinology 1993; 57:1133–1147.

161. Meaney MJ, Sapolsky RM, McEwen BS. The development of the glucocorticoid receptor system in the rat limbic brain. I. Ontogeny and autoregulation. Dev Brain Res 1985;18:159–164.

162. Wondisford FE, Farr EA, Radovick S, Steinfelder HJ, Moates JM, McClaskey JH, Weintraub BD. Thyroid hormone inhibition of human thyrotropin β-subunit gene expression is mediated by a cis-acting element located in the first exon. J Biol Chem 1989;264:14,601–14,604.

163. Chatterjee VKK, Lee J, Tentoumis A, Jameson JL. Negative regulation of the thyroid-stimulating hormone a gene by thyroid hormone: receptor interaction adjacent to the TAT box. Proc Natl Acad Sci USA 1989;86:9114–9118.

164. Carr RE, Burnside J, Chin WW. Thyroid hormones regulate rat thyrotropin b gene promoter activity expressed in GH3 cells. Mol Endocrinol 1989;3:709–716.

165. Burnside J, Darling DS, Carr FE, Chin WW. Thyroid hormone regulation of the rat glycoprotein hormone α-subunit gene promoter activity. J Biol Chem 1989;2645:6886–6891.

166. Glass CK, Franco R, Weinberger C, Albert VR, Evans RM, Rosenfeld MG. A c-erbA binding site in rat growth hormone gene mediates trans-activation by thyroid hormone. Nature 1987;329:738–741.

167. Brent GA, Harney JW, Chen Y, Warne RG, Moore DD, Larsen PR. Mutations of the rat growth hormone promoter which increase and decrease response to thyroid hormone define a consensus thyroid hormone response element. Mol Endocrinol 1989;3:1996–2007.

168. Sven C, Chin WW. Ligand-dependent, Pit-1/Growth hormone factor-1 (GHF)-independent transcriptional stimulation of rat growth hormone gene expression by thyroid hormone receptors in vitro. Mol Cell Biol 1993;13:1719–1727.

169. Bradley DJ, Towle JC, Young WS, III. Spatial and temporal expression of α and β-thyroid hormone receptor mRNA's including the B2 subtype, in the developing mammalian system. J Neuroscience 1992;12:2288–2302.

170. Rodriguez-Garcia M, Jolin T, Santos A, Perez-Castillo A. Effect of perinatal hypothyroidism on the developmental regulation of rat pituitary growth hormone and thyrotropin genes. Endocrinology 1995;136:4339–4350.

171. Wasylyk B, Hahn SH, Giovane A. The Ets family of transcription factors. Eur J Biochem 1993; 211:7–18.

172. Bradford AP, Conrad KE, Wasylyk C, Wasylyk B, Gutierrez-Hartmann A. Functional interaction of c-Ets-1 and GHF-1/Pit-1 mediates Ras activation of pituitary-specific gene expression: mapping of the essential c-Ets-1 domain. Mol Cell Biol 1995;15:2849–2857.

173. Maroulakou IG, Papas TS, Green JE. Differential expression of ets-1 and ets-2 protooncogenes during murine embryogenesis. Oncogene 1994;9:1551–1565.

15

Physiology and Molecular Biology of Placental Lactogen in Human Pregnancy

Randall G. Richards, PhD
and Stuart Handwerger, MD

CONTENTS

INTRODUCTION

Human placental lactogen (hPL) is a protein hormone that has striking homologies in its chemical and biological properties to human growth hormone (hGH) and human prolactin (hPRL) *(1,2)*. In this chapter, we will briefly discuss the role of hPL in the regulation of fetal growth and the regulation of hPL secretion in normal and pathologic pregnancies. We will then focus on recent advances in the regulation of hPL gene expression, giving particular attention to roles of nuclear hormone receptors and cytokines in transactivation of the hPL promoter.

hPL AS A FETAL GROWTH HORMONE

Early studies of the biological properties of hPL indicated that the hormone has growth-promoting and lactogenic activities in vivo and in vitro. Because of its growth-promoting activities and the marked increase observed in its plasma concentration during gestation,

From: *Molecular and Cellular Pediatric Endocrinology*
Edited by: S. Handwerger © Humana Press Inc., Totowa, NJ

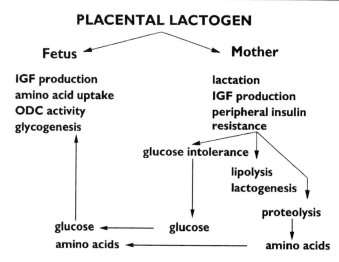

PLACENTAL LACTOGEN

Fig. 1. Placental lactogen has opposite, but complementary, actions in the maternal and fetal compartments. Fetal growth and metabolism is regulated by increasing the availability of maternal substrates to the fetal compartment, and by increasing the utilization of substrates by the fetus.

Grumbach et al. *(3)* many years ago presented a cogent argument for a major role of hPL as a maternal "growth hormone" of the second half of pregnancy. They suggested that hPL acts as an antagonist of insulin action in the mother, inducing glucose tolerance, lipolysis and proteolysis and promoting the transfer of glucose and amino acids to the fetus (Fig. 1). Considerable evidence now strongly supports this hypothesis *(4)*. More recent experiments indicate that hPL also affects fetal growth by acting directly on fetal tissues to stimulate ornithine decarboxylase activity, amino acid transport, glycogen synthesis, DNA synthesis and insulin-like growth factor (IGF) production *(4)*. Placental lactogen therefore regulates fetal growth and metabolism by increasing the availability of maternal substrates to the fetus and the utilization of fetal substrates, and by stimulating fetal IGF production. Growth hormone, which is critical in the regulation of postnatal growth, has little or no biological activities in human fetal tissues due to an absence or markedly reduced number of cell surface receptors *(5)*. Human fetuses born with growth hormone deficiency reach normal birth size and maintain normal plasma IGF concentrations *(6)*. Furthermore, transgenic mouse fetuses that overexpress growth hormone *in utero* are also normal size at birth and do not demonstrate excessive growth until about 3 wk of age *(7)*.

Placental lactogens have been detected in several subprimate species, but the chemical and biological properties and the molecular genetics of these placental lactogens are markedly different than those of hPL *(8)*. For example, the mouse and rat synthesize and secrete two different placental lactogens, one at midpregnancy and one in late pregnancy, that are products of separate genes. The two placental lactogens appear to have different biological properties and are regulated by different factors. The fundamental biological differences between human and subprimate placental lactogens prohibits the use of subprimate animal models in studies of hPL biology.

THE RELEASE OF hPL BY NORMAL AND PATHOLOGIC PLACENTAS

hPL is synthesized and secreted by the syncytiotrophoblast cells of the placenta and is first detected in maternal plasma at about 6 wk of gestation. Its concentration then increases linearly until about wk 30, when peak concentrations of 5000–7000 ng/mL are reached *(3)*. The plasma concentration in the mother during pregnancy is positively correlated with placental mass and is greater in multiple than in singleton gestations *(9,10)*. Near term, the secretion rate of hPL is about 1.0 g/d, a rate that is considerably greater than that of any other protein hormone during pregnancy *(11)*.

Although there have been many in vivo and in vitro studies to delineate the factors that regulate hPL secretion, the specific hormonal and metabolic factors involved are still poorly understood. In clinical studies, depression or elevation of plasma free fatty acid concentrations by pharmacological agents *(12)* has no effect on hPL secretion, and arginine and dexamethasone *(13)* (which affect pituitary hGH secretion) are also without effect. Prolonged fasting causes a 30–40% increase in plasma hPL concentrations in women during wk 16–22 of gestation (prior to therapeutic abortion) *(14,15)*. The increase in hPL concentrations, however, is not caused by hypoglycemia since insulin-induced hypoglycemia (as well as the iv infusion of glucose) has no consistent effects on hPL release *(11,16)*.

In vitro studies of placental lactogen release using placental explants and primary trophoblast cell cultures have shown no consistent effects of glucocorticoids, estrogens, oxytocin, prostaglandins, epinephrine, thyrotropin-releasing hormone, gonadotropin-releasing hormone or L-DOPA on the synthesis or secretion of hPL *(17–23)*. In addition, acute and chronic changes in extracellular glucose concentrations have been shown to have no consistent effects on hPL secretion in vitro *(24)*. Epidermal growth factor has been reported to stimulate the differentiation of cytotrophoblast cells to syncytiotrophoblast cells with a resultant increase in hPL release *(25)*. The increase in hPL release in response to EGF, however, does not appear to result from an increased rate of release but from the differentiation of hPL-producing cells. Angiotensin II *(26)* and IGF-I *(27)* have also been reported to stimulate hPL release.

Abnormalities of hPL secretion have been detected in many pathologic conditions of pregnancy associated with abnormal fetal growth, including diabetes mellitus, pre-eclampsia, erythroblastosis, and intrauterine growth retardation *(28–32)*. In one large series of patients, a single hPL concentration below 4 μg/mL in the last 5 wk of pregnancy was associated with 30% risk of fetal distress or neonatal asphyxia *(33)*. Low hPL concentrations on two separate occasions during the last 5 wk were associated with a fetal risk of 50% and low concentrations on three occasions with a risk of 71%. In another series of patients, hPL concentrations below 4 μg/mL were detected in 47 of 98 pre-eclamptic patients *(25)*. Perinatal mortality in the neonates born to the mothers with low hPL concentrations was 13% and intrauterine growth retardation was noted in 57% of the neonates.

REGULATION OF hPL RELEASE BY APOLIPOPROTEIN A-I

Studies performed by our laboratory have demonstrated that high density lipoproteins (HDL) at physiologic concentrations stimulates a dose-dependent acute increase in hPL release from cultured trophoblast cells *(34)*, with maximal stimulation six- to tenfold greater than basal levels (Fig. 2). In addition, the iv infusion of ovine HDL into pregnant ewes in late gestation was shown to stimulate a four- to sixfold increase in plasma placental lactogen concentrations (Fig. 3) *(35)*. Since plasma apolipoprotein A-I (apo A-I) and hPL concentrations increase concomitantly during pregnancy and the patterns of

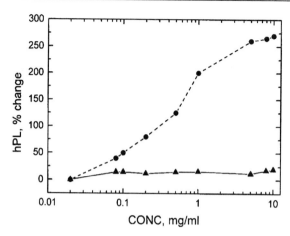

Fig. 2. In vitro effects of HDL on placental lactogen release. A 1-h exposure to HDL stimulated hPL release from human placental explants in a dose-dependent manner (circles). In contrast, LDL (triangles) had no effect on hPL release. Apo A-I, the predominant protein constituent of HDL, was subsequently shown to be the active component of HDL responsible for stimulating hPL release.

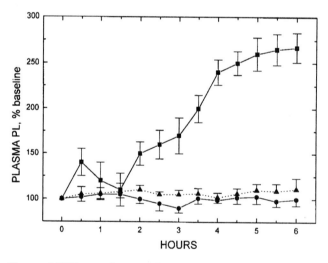

Fig. 3. In vivo effects of HDL on placental lactogen release. The effects of HDL (squares), lipoprotein-free plasma proteins (triangles), and saline (circles) on plasma PL concentrations were determined in pregnant ewes. The plasma PL concentrations are expressed as a percentage of the baseline (time 0) concentrations. The response to HDL represents the mean ± SEM of six experiments. The response to lipoprotein-free plasma proteins and to saline represents the results from four and six experiments, respectively.

plasma apo A-I and hPL concentrations during pregnancy are nearly identical *(36,37)*, these findings strongly suggest a novel physiologic role for HDL in the regulation of hPL secretion. As indicated below, abnormally low maternal plasma apo A-I concentrations have been detected in many women with pathologic conditions of pregnancy associated with growth failure.

Subsequent studies of the mechanism(s) by which apo A-I stimulates hPL release demonstrated that the stimulation is not caused by the lipid constituents of HDL since

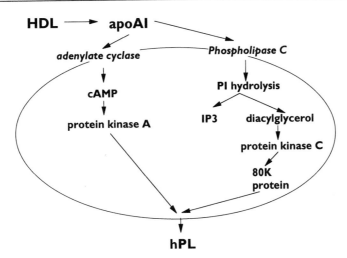

Fig. 4. The effects of Apo A-I are mediated through the cAMP and phosphoinositide signal transduction pathways.

complete delipidation of HDL did not decrease stimulatory activity and delipidated plasma apo A-I and recombinant apo A-I were potent stimuli to hPL release. In contrast, other lipoprotein particles and apolipoproteins not associated with HDL did not affect hPL release *(34)*. The effect of apo A-I was specific for hPL release since apo A-I did not stimulate the release of hCG and had no effect on the release of growth hormone, prolactin and other pituitary hormones from human pituitary cell cultures.

Studies using derivatives of HDL and synthetic amphipathic peptides demonstrated that the effect of HDL on hPL release is not mediated by the binding of HDL to the high-affinity binding sites for HDL present on trophoblast cells but to an interaction of HDL with membrane phospholipids *(38)*. In the later studies, synthetic amphipathic peptides that closely mimic the tertiary structure of apo A-I were found to stimulate hPL release. The magnitude of the stimulation correlated with the ability of the peptides to displace apolipoproteins from HDL and with other measures of phospholipid binding affinity, such as the increase in alpha-helicity and the size of complexes formed between the peptide and phospholipid *(39)*. Subsequent investigations indicated that both the cAMP *(40)* and phosphoinositide signal transduction pathways *(41)* act as second messengers in apo A-I-mediated hPL release (Fig. 4).

In addition to stimulating an acute increase in hPL release, apo A-I was also noted to stimulate a secondary increase in hPL release beginning about 6 h after exposure to apo A-I *(42)*. The initial acute release results from the release of preformed hormone from intracellular stores, whereas the delayed increase results from the stimulation of hPL gene expression and the release of newly synthesized hormone.

Since the initial observation that apo A-I has biological actions that are unrelated to lipid metabolism, apo A-I has been shown to have many other nonlipid-dependent biological actions, including the stimulation of endothelial cell proliferation *(43)*, the stimulation of endothelin-1 production by renal tubular cells *(44)*, and the inhibition of degranulation and superoxide dismutase activity in neutrophils *(45)*. In each instance, the effect of apo A-I occurred at physiological concentrations. Studies of the mechanisms involved in the stimulation of renal endothelin production by apo A-I also demonstrated that HDL binding sites in the kidney are not essential for biological action and that multiple signal transduction pathways are stimulated in response to apo A-I. Taken together, these studies indicate that apo A-I functions in many cell types as a novel secretagog and mitogen.

The observation that apo A-I regulates hPL gene expression may have implications for the pathophysiology of some disorders of pregnancy. Although it is probable that many factors contribute to the abnormal hPL concentrations observed in pathologic conditions of pregnancy, several studies suggest that abnormal apo A-I concentrations may contribute to the aberrations in hPL concentrations. In an earlier study, Rosing et al. *(46)* noted decreased plasma apo A-I concentrations in preeclampsia, a pathologic condition of pregnancy characterized by low hPL concentrations. Kaaja et al. *(47)* also noted decreased apo A-I concentrations in women with pregnancy-induced hypertension, and Knopp et al. *(48)* noted lower than normal apo A-I concentrations in pregnant women with insulin-dependent diabetes mellitus. In the women with diabetes, apo A-I concentration did not increase from 12 to 28 wk of gestation, whereas apo A-I concentrations in normal women increased by nearly twofold.

MOLECULAR BIOLOGY OF THE hPL/hGH GENE CLUSTER

Molecular studies strongly suggest that the hGH, hPL, and hPRL genes evolved from a common ancestral precursor in which the five genes of the hPL/hGH gene cluster arose from recombination events involving moderately repeated sequences *(49,50)*. The hGH/hPL and hPRL precursor genes then segregated onto two different chromosomes, with the hGH/hPL genes on chromosome 17 (q22–q24) and the hPRL gene on chromosome 6 *(51)*. The hGH/hPL locus contains five structurally related genes spanning 47 kb that are all organized in the same transcriptional orientation and are each composed of five exons and four introns *(52)*. The genes from 5' to 3' are hGH-N, hPL-L, hPL-A, hGH-V, and hPL-B (Fig. 5). The entire cluster and about 19.8 kb of flanking DNA have been sequenced. The genes are expressed in two mutually exclusive tissue specific patterns, with the hGH-N gene expressed solely in the pituitary and the other genes expressed solely in the syncytiotrophoblast layer of the placenta. The hGH-N gene encodes two alternatively spliced mRNAs that are translated into 22 and 20 kDa GH proteins. The placental genes hPL-A and hGH-V are alternatively spliced and encode 22 and 26 kDa gene products, whereas hPL-B encodes a single 22-kDa protein product. The expression of the hPL-L protein product(s) has not as yet been identified in maternal blood, although the gene produces several alternatively spliced mRNA transcripts with leader sequences. The members of the gene family share 91–99% sequence identity throughout the coding regions and within a 500 bp region immediately upstream of the genes. Although the hPL-A, hPL-B, and hPL-L genes also share 95% homology in an enhancer region located approx 2 kb downstream from each of the respective genes, the hPL-B gene enhancer is considerably more active *(53)*. The hPL-A and hPL-B mRNAs are 98% homologous and encode identical mature proteins, but have one amino acid difference in the signal peptides. The mRNAs for hPL-A and hPL-B comprise approx 3.5% of the total placental mRNA. During normal pregnancies, the hPL-A gene is expressed three to six times more than the hPL-B gene, probably due to differences in stability of the two mRNAs. Several pregnancies have been reported in which no radioimmunoassayable hPL was detected in the mother due to a homozygous deletion of the hPL-A, hPL-B and hGH-V genes *(52)*.

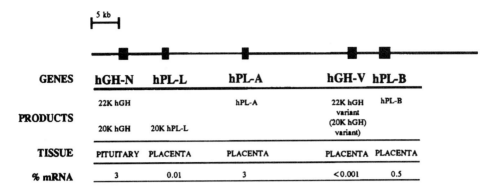

GENES	hGH-N	hPL-L	hPL-A	hGH-V	hPL-B
PRODUCTS	22K hGH		hPL-A	22K hGH variant	hPL-B
	20K hGH	20K hPL-L		(20K hGH) variant)	
TISSUE	PITUITARY	PLACENTA	PLACENTA	PLACENTA	PLACENTA
% mRNA	3	0.01	3	<0.001	0.5

Fig. 5. Structure of the hGH/hPL gene cluster. The gene assignment, the proteins produced by the genes, and the tissues in which the mRNAs are expressed are shown below the gene map. (Modified with permission from Chen et al. *[50]*).

However, a novel hGH-hPL hybrid protein was detected in maternal plasma that was probably a product of the hPL-L gene that compensated for the loss of the other gene products.

REGULATION OF TROPHOBLAST DIFFERENTIATION AND hPL GENE EXPRESSION

Placental lactogen is synthesized and secreted from the multinuclear syncytiotrophoblast layer of the placenta which is in direct contact with maternal serum. Earlier studies utilizing [^{3}H]thymidine incorporation, immunohistochemistry, and electron microscopy of placental tissue sections *(54–56)* had strongly suggested that the syncytiotrophoblast was formed by fusion of mononuclear cytotrophoblast cells that underly the syncytiotrophoblast layer. More recent in vitro studies have confirmed that trophoblast differentiation involves cytotrophoblast cell fusion, which initiates a series of biochemical events leading to the synthesis and release of hCG, and then to the synthesis and release of hPL *(57–60)*. Maternal serum supplemented medium is a highly efficient promoter of trophoblast differentiation in vitro *(60)*. Specific factors, such as IGF-1, CSF-1, GM-CSF-1, EGF, TGF-β, hCG, and cyclic AMP, have also been shown to stimulate trophoblast differentiation in vitro, but their mechanisms of action and their contribution to the regulation of trophoblast differentiation in vivo are unclear *(61–67)*.

Dual tissue specificity of the hGH/hPL gene cluster appears to be regulated by a locus control region located approx 23 kb upstream *(68)*. However, specific expression of the individual genes in the pituitary (hGH-N) or in the placenta (hGH-V, hPL-A, -B, -L) may be regulated by more proximal elements. Promoter activity for hPL has been identified in a 1200 bp region of 5'-DNA flanking each of the respective hPL genes, and studies are currently in progress to identify transcription factors and DNA elements involved in the regulation of hPL gene expression during trophoblast differentiation and in the fully differentiated syncytiotrophoblast cell. The transcription factor pit-1, which is critical for expression of the hGH-N gene in the pituitary, binds to the hPL-B promoter, but mutations within the pit-1 binding sites have no effect on hPL promoter activity *(69)*. Transient transfection of hPL-B promoter deletion constructs (from –1200/+1 to –77/+1) into JEG-3 choriocarcinoma cells indicated that the region between –142 bp and –129 bp, which

Table 1
Protein-Binding Regions Within the hPL Enhancer

Walker et al.[a]	Lytras and Catinni[b]	Jiang and Eberhardt[c]	Jacquemin et al.[d]
		+3745/+3774 (DF1)	
		+3808/+3835 (DF2)	
	+3899/+3920 (RF1)		+3889/+3912 (FP1)
	+3940/+3960 (DF1)	+3934/+3973 (DF3)	+3953/+3968 (FP2)
+4003/+4023 (TEF1)[e]	+4003/+4023 (TEF1)	+3989/+4024 (DF4)	+4000/+4025 (FP3)
			+4031/+4050 (FP4)
			+4080/+4125 (FP5)

[a]Ref. 72; DNase I footprinting using nuclear extracts from placental tissue or HeLa cells.
[b]Ref. 74; Gel mobility shift assay using nuclear extracts from JEG-3, BeWo, or HeLa cells.
[c]Ref. 73; DNase I footprinting using nuclear extracts from JEG-3, BeWo, HeLa, or GC cells.
[d]Ref. 75; DNase I footprinting using nuclear extracts from placental or HeLa cells.
[e]Basepairs from hPL-B initiation start site. Individual laboratory designations given in parenthesis.

binds the ubiquitous transcription factor Sp1, is important for basal promoter activity (70), and more recent studies have indicated that full basal and enhancer activity are dependent on the cooperative interaction of Sp1 with the TATA box and an initiator element (InrE) located between nt −15 and +1 of the hPL promoter (69). In experiments recently performed in our laboratory, transient transfection of hPL promoter deletion constructs into primary cultures of cytotrophoblast and syncytiotrophoblast cells suggest that upregulation of hPL expression during trophoblast differentiation is caused, in part, by the downregulation or neutralization of inhibitory factors acting at multiple sites on the hPL promoter (71). To date, no placental-specific transcription factors have been identified that act at the level of the hPL promoter.

Tissue-specific expression of hPL appears to be regulated by an enhancer element that is located 2 kb downstream from the 3' end of the hPL-B gene (72) and shares several DNA-binding motifs in common with the SV40 enhancer (73). Because the hPL enhancer increases the activity of several promoters, including hPL, hGH, SV40, RSV, and thymidine kinase (53,72,73), it has been suggested that elements of the enhancer interact with ubiquitous transcription factors of the transcription initiation complex rather than with promoter-specific factors (69). DNase I protection experiments with nuclear extracts have identified multiple sites of protein binding within the enhancer DNA region (Table 1). Initial experiments of Walker et al. (72) identified a 22 bp region overlapping a transcription enhancer factor (TEF)-1 binding site within 138 bp of enhancer DNA. This observation was then extended by Catinni et al. (74), who identified 240 bp of DNA containing a repressor site (RF-1) and a derepressor site (DF-1), in addition to the TEF-1 site. More recently, Jiang and Eberhardt have reported two additional footprints within this same region of DNA (73). Jacquemin et al. (75) have also studied the hPL-B enhancer. They reported four footprints (DF-1, DF-2, DF-3, and DF-4) within 300 bp of DNA that overlaps the 240 bp region defined by Catinni et al., and three of these sites contained the TEF-1 consensus motif. The DF-1 and TEF-1 sites reported by Catinni et al. correspond to the DF-3 and DF-4 sites reported by Jacquemin et al., and essentially all of the enhancer activity resides in the synergistic interaction of these two sites (53). Mutations in the DF-3 region have been shown to account for the decreased activity of the hPL-A and hPL-L enhancers (53). Tissue-specific expression appears to involve a placental form of

TEF-1 *(76,77)*, which would more readily account for the fact that TEF-1 protein is found in several cell types that do not express hPL including cervical carcinoma (Hela) cells *(78)*, keratinocytes *(79)*, and cardiac and skeletal muscle *(80)*. Surprisingly, TEF-1, itself, appears to act as a negative modulator of hPL-B enhancer activity *(76)*. In recent studies performed in our laboratory, transfection of expression plasmids for several members of the MAP kinase pathway upregulated hPL and SV40 enhancer activity in cytotrophoblast cells *(81)*, suggesting that the phosphorylation of a transcription factor common to both enhancers is an important requirement for the induction of hPL expression during trophoblast differentiation.

STUDIES OF NUCLEAR HORMONE RECEPTORS AND hPL GENE EXPRESSION

Retinoid receptors (RARs and RXRs), thyroid hormone receptors (TRs) and the vitamin D_3 receptor (VDR) belong to the superfamily of nuclear hormone receptor transcription factors. Both the retinoic acid and thyroid hormone receptors exist in multiple forms. Two distinct groups of retinoid receptors modulate the actions of retinoic acid, the RAR, and RXR receptors. The RAR group consists of three receptors, RARα, RARβ and RARγ. These receptors are coded by different genes and bind all-*trans* retinoic acid with high affinity. The RXR group consists of three receptors, RXRα, RXRβ and RXRγ. These receptors bind 9-cis-retinoic acid with high affinity. The thyroid hormone receptor exists in two forms, TRα and TRβ, which are also expressed by two different genes. Each of the forms exists as multiple isoforms. The levels of retinoid receptors increase during trophoblast differentiation and parallel the increase in hPL expression *(82)*.

Since these receptors have been shown to play a critical role in the regulation of hormone gene expression in many endocrine cells (such as pituitary cells) and since trophoblast cells express RAR, TR and VDRs, studies were performed to determine whether these nuclear hormone receptors are also involved in the regulation of human placental lactogen gene expression *(83,84)*. We observed that trophoblast cells from term placentas exposed to retinoic acid, triiodothyronine or 1,25-dihydroxyvitamin D_3 release five- to sixfold more hPL than control cells. The stimulation by RA, T_3, and vitamin D_3 was dose-dependent and was accompanied by stimulation of hPL mRNA levels. Retinoic acid, thyroid hormone and 1,25 dihydroxyvitamin D_3 had no significant effects on trophoblast differentiation suggesting that the effects of the vitamin are mediated directly at the transcriptional level.

These investigations are of interest since earlier studies had demonstrated that 1,25 dihydroxyvitamin D_3 is synthesized by the placenta and decidua. 1,25 dihydroxyvitamin D_3 is important in the regulation of cell growth, differentiation, immune function, and mineral metabolism *(85,86)*. During pregnancy, the placenta synthesizes 1,25 dihydroxyvitamin D_3 and the receptor for 1,25 dihydroxyvitamin D_3 is also detected in the placenta *(87,88)*. These observations suggest a possible autocrine/paracrine role for 1,25 dihydroxyvitamin D_3 in placental function. In an earlier study, Maruo et al. *(89)* also observed that T_3 stimulates the release of hPL, hCG, progesterone, and 17β-estradiol from first trimester placentas and suggested that the frequent occurrence of spontaneous abortion in early pregnancies in women with hypothyroidism or hyperthyroidism may result from the "inadequate thyroid hormone availability at the level of placental trophoblasts, followed by diminished expression of trophoblast endocrine function."

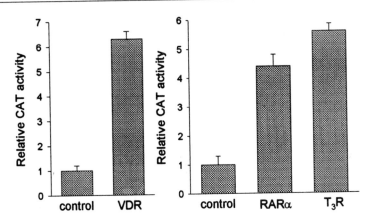

Fig. 6. The effect of VDR, RARα, and T₃R (TR) on hPL gene expression. BeWo choriocarcinoma cells were cotransfected for 48 h with a vector containing 1.1 kb of the hPL promoter (−1078/+2) coupled to a CAT reporter gene and an expression vector for VDR, RARα, or T₃R. The amount of CAT activity is expressed relative to that for β-galactosidase and represents the triplicate mean ± SEM.

In transient transfection studies, RARα, TRβ, and VDR, in the presence of their respective ligands, stimulated chloramphenicol acetyltransferase (CAT) activity in BeWo choriocarcinoma cells transfected transiently with a 2.3 kb fragment of the hPL promoter (−2300 to +2 bp) coupled to a CAT reporter gene, indicating that the stimulatory effect of the steroids is likely caused by stimulation of hPL gene expression (Fig. 6). The effects of RARα and TRβ on hPL promoter activity were enhanced when the cells were cotransfected with an expression vector for RXRβ, a member of the nuclear hormone receptor family that forms a heterodimer with RARα and TRβ and enhances transactivation by these nuclear hormone receptors in other cell types. In contrast, the stimulatory effects of RARα and TRβ were completely inhibited when the cells were cotransfected with an expression vector for apolipoprotein repressor protein-1 (ARP-1), an orphan member of the nuclear hormone receptor family homologous to COUP-TF2 that is known to inhibit transcription by RARα and TRβ *(90)*.

Deletion analysis of the hPL promoter indicated that the retinoic acid, T_3, and vitamin D_3 responsive elements (RARE, TRE, and VDRE) are localized from −0.5 to −1.1 kb upstream from the transcriptional start site (+1). Although a TR-binding site between −290 and −129 of the hPL promoter was previously reported by Barlow et al. *(91)*, T_3 failed to transactivate the −0.5 kb hPL proximal promoter. Earlier studies from many laboratories indicated that DNA response elements for the retinoic acid receptors, TRβ and VDR contain two copies of the half-site AG(G/T)T(C/G)A and that the number, spacing, and orientation of these motifs determine the specificity and affinity of the response elements *(92)*. Specificity of the response elements appeared to be determined in part by base-pair spacing between the half-site repeats, with spacing of 3, 4, and 5 nucleotides favoring a vitamin D response element (VDRE), thyroid hormone response element (TRE) or a retinoic acid responsive element (RARE), respectively. This rule, however, is not invariant and some promoters do not follow the 3-4-5 rule. The presence of composite response elements for VDR and RAR within the human osteocalcin

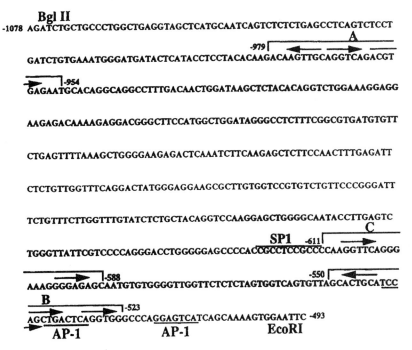

Fig. 7. Three regions (**A**, **B**, and **C**) between −493 and −1078 of the hPL promoter contain putative half-site motifs (indicated by the arrows) for the nuclear steroid hormone receptors, thyroid hormone, all-*trans* retinoic acid, and vitamin D_3. Also indicated are AP-1 and SP-1 sites.

promoter *(93)* and composite response elements for TR and RAR within the rat oxytocin promoter *(94)* suggests that other features of the response element may dictate receptor binding.

Computer analysis of the hPL promoter reveals three regions of the hPL promoter (−493 to −1078 bp) that contain several half-site motifs that closely resemble the responsive elements for thyroid hormone, all-*trans* retinoic acid and vitamin D_3 but with unusual spacing between the half-site repeats *(95)* (Fig. 7). Site A (−979 to −954 bp) consists of three putative half-site motifs that are arranged as direct repeats with 1 nucleotide spacing (DR 1). This arrangement is similar to the DR1 arrangement for the RXR element on the promoter of cytoplasmic retinoic acid binding protein II, a high-affinity binding site for homodimeric RXR that binds 9-*cis* retinoic acid as ligand *(96)*. Site B (−550 to −523 bp) has four possible half-site motifs, one set arranged as inverted palindromes with a spacing of 0. The other possible arrangements include a DR 3, which is a vitamin D_3 response element (VDRE), and an inverted repeat with a spacing of three nucleotides (IR3). A putative AP1 site *(97)* is "embedded" within the half-sites of region B. Site C (−611 to −588 bp) contains a DR 7 and also a putative Sp1 site adjacent to one of the half-site motifs. Transfection studies in BeWo choriocarcinoma cells indicated that site A is responsive to RARα, but not TRβ, site B is responsive to TRβ, RARα, and VDR, and site C is not responsive to RARα, TRβ, or VDR. Electrophoretic mobility shift assays using nuclear extracts from BeWo cells overexpressing RARα, TRβ, or VDR demonstrated specific gel retardation of ^{32}P-labeled site B by each of the nuclear extracts. These findings, together with the observation that placental cells express RARs, TRs, and VDR, suggest a novel role for these receptors in the regulation of the hPL gene. To date, site B is the only known composite site to confer transactivation by RARα, TRβ, and VDR.

An AP-1 site has been reported to be present within the VDRE/RARE of the human osteocalcin promoter (98). It has been suggested that these elements may be important in regulating cell proliferation and differentiation. The role of the AP-1 site in site B is unknown, but several lines of evidence suggest that the AP-1 site may be important in regulation of placental lactogen gene expression. Protein kinase C activators such as phorbol esters stimulate the synthesis and release of hPL from cultured trophoblast cells (99). Activation of protein kinase C in many cell types is known to increase expression of the proto oncogenes C-Fos and C-Jun that form homodimers or heterodimers that bind to promoters of genes containing AP-1 sites. Since phorbol esters stimulate a time and dose-dependant increase in hPL synthesis, the AP-1 site embedded within site B may be important in the regulation of hPL promoter activity. Previous studies have shown that Fos and Jun proteins antagonize the effects mediated by RARs and TRs, thereby inhibiting the transactivation potential of these transcription factors on promoter activity (100,101). This inhibitory effect may involve protein interactions between Fos and Jun with RARs and TRs. At present it is unknown whether the binding of RAR, TR, and VDR to site B of the hPL promoter are antagonized by Fos and Jun.

The Sp1 protein controls the gene expression of several proteins (102), and in recent studies (103,104) several promoters have been reported to contain a functional Sp1 site adjacent to a steroid hormone response element. This latter finding has led to the proposition that Sp1 may act as an auxiliary factor in stabilizing the interaction of the steroid hormone receptor complex with its DNA binding site. Although an Sp1 site downstream from site C (−142 to −129 bp) has been shown to play a role in the basal expression of hPL (52), at present, it is unknown whether the Sp1 site adjacent to site C is functional.

Using enzymatically dispersed trophoblast cells as a model system, we studied the ontogeny of nuclear hormone receptors and other transcription factors during trophoblast differentiation. Our initial studies, using reverse transcription polymerase chain reaction (RT-PCR) analysis of trophoblast RNA, demonstrated that RARα, RARβ, and RXRα mRNA levels increase during trophoblast differentiation, whereas the levels of RARγ mRNA remain relatively constant (82). The increase in retinoid receptor mRNA expression in each instance preceded the increase in the release of hPL. The levels of cellular retinoic acid binding protein II (CRBP-II) mRNA increased progressively after d 5, reaching a peak on d 13 that was 2.2-fold greater than that on d 1. Mobility shift assays using nuclear extracts from trophoblast cells and a labeled synthetic double stranded DNA probe containing a retinoic acid responsive element (RARE) demonstrated the presence of a specific retarded band on d 5 of culture when the cells had fused into a syncytium. However, no band was detected after 1 d of culture when the cells were mononuclear cytotrophoblast cells and did not release hPL. In more recent studies, using competitive PCR, we found that vitamin D receptor (VDR) and TRβ mRNAs increase during differentiation with a pattern similar to that of hPL expression (105). The finding that retinoic acid, thyroid hormone and vitamin D₃ stimulate hPL expression, together with the present data indicating upregulation of retinoid, TRβ, and VDR receptor mRNAs prior to the upregulation of hPL gene expression, suggests a possible role for these receptors in the regulation of hPL expression during placental differentiation.

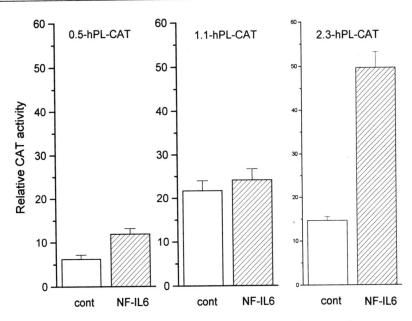

Fig. 8. NF-IL6 activates hPL promoter activity. BeWo choriocarcinoma cells were cotransfected with a 0.5, 1.1, or 2.3 kb fragment of the hPL promoter coupled to a CAT reporter gene and a NF-IL6 expression vector. CAT activity was normalized to that of β-galactosidase. Each bar represents the mean ± SEM of triplicate wells.

STUDIES OF CYTOKINES AND hPL GENE EXPRESSION

IL-6, which is known to stimulate hormone release from pituitary and other endocrine cells, was shown to stimulate the synthesis and release of hPL from primary cultures of normal trophoblast cells and to stimulate hPL promoter activity in BeWo cells *(106)*. Transfection of BeWo cells with an expression vector for NF-IL6, one of the transcription factors that mediates the action of IL-6 in other cell types, also stimulated the activity of the −2.3 kb hPL promoter, but did not stimulate the activity of the −1.1 or −0.5 kb hPL promoters (Fig. 8). Since the hPL promoter contains 3 NF-IL6 response elements between −1.3 to −1.1 kb, these results strongly suggest that the action of IL-6 on hPL gene expression is mediated at least in part, by NF-IL6 *(107)*. The synthesis and release of IL-6 by placental macrophages and syncytiotrophoblast cells *(108,109)* further suggests that the action of IL-6 in the regulation of hPL release may occur by an autocrine/paracrine mechanism involving NF-IL6.

Studies of the ontogeny of the cytokine receptor mRNAs during trophoblast differentiation indicate that expression of the mRNAs for the cytokines IL-1α, IL-1β, and IL-6, in contrast to the expression of the nuclear hormone receptor mRNAs, decrease markedly during differentiation *(110)*. Exogenous IL-6 had differential effects on cytokine mRNA expression during differentiation. Prior to differentiation to syncytiotrophoblast cells, IL-6 markedly inhibited IL-6, IL-1α, and IL-1β mRNA expression. However, following differentiation, IL-6 stimulated IL-1α, and IL-1β mRNA expression. Taken together, these results indicate that IL-1 and IL-6 mRNA expression decreases markedly during cytotrophoblast differentiation in vitro and that the regulation of trophoblast cytokine mRNA levels changes during differentiation.

SUMMARY

Investigations from many laboratories strongly suggest a role for hPL in the regulation of fetal growth. Although hPL has striking similarities in its chemical and biological properties to hGH and hPRL and is a member of the same gene family of these pituitary hormones, the regulation of hPL expression is markedly different. Several studies indicate that hPL expression is regulated by transcription factors that bind to the hPL promoter, however, tissue-specific expression appears to be regulated through an enhancer DNA element approx 2 kb downstream from the hPL-B gene. Recent studies strongly suggest a novel role for apo A-I, the major apolipoprotein constituent of HDL, in the regulation of hPL expression. Other studies of hPL expression also suggest that hPL synthesis and release is mediated by steroid hormones and IL-6. The effects of retinoic acid, thyroid hormone, and 1,25-dihydroxyvitamin D_3 are mediated by nuclear hormone receptors and the effect of IL-6 is mediated, at least in part, by the transcription factor NF-IL6. A better understanding of the hormones and other factors that regulate hPL expression may lead to the development of strategies to modulate hPL concentration in patients with pathologic conditions associated with aberrations in hPL secretion.

REFERENCES

1. Josimovich JB, McLaren JA. Presence in the human placenta and term serum of a highly lactogenic substance immunologically related to pituitary growth hormone. Endocrinology 1962;71:209–220.
2. Sherwood LS, Handwerger S, McLaurin WE, Lanner M. Amino acid sequence of human placental lactogen. Nature New Biol 1971;233:59–61.
3. Grumbach MM, Kaplan SL. On the placental origin and purification of chorionic "growth hormone-prolactin" and its immunoassay in pregnancy. Trans New York Acad Sci 1964;27:167–188.
4. Handwerger S. Clinical counterpoint: The physiology of placental lactogen in human pregnancy. Endocrine Rev 1991;12:329–336.
5. Freemark M, Comer M, Handwerger S. Placental lactogen and growth hormone receptors in sheep liver: Striking differences in ontogeny and function. Am J Physiol 1986;251:E328–E333.
6. Browne CA, Thornburn GD. Endocrine control of fetal growth. Biol Neonate 1989;55:331–346.
7. Palmiter RD, Norstedt G, Gelinas RE, Hammer RE, Brinster RL. Metallothionein-human GH fusion genes stimulate growth of mice. Science 1983;222:809–814.
8. Talamantes F, Ogren L. The placenta as an endocrine organ: polypeptides. In: Knobil E, Neill J, et al., eds. The physiology of reproduction. Raven, New York, 1988; pp. 2093–2144.
9. Tyson JE. Human chorionic somatomammotropin. Obstet Gynecol Ann 1972;1:421–452.
10. Saxena B, Emerson K, Selenkow H. Serum placental lactogen levels as an index of placental function. N Engl J Med 1969;281:225–231.
11. Grumbach MM, Kaplan SL, Sciarra JJ, Burr IM. Chorionic growth hormone-prolactin (CGP): Secretion, disposition, biologic activity in man, and postulated function as the "growth hormone" of the second half of pregnancy. Ann New York Acad Sci 1968;148:501–531.
12. Morris HHB, Vinik AI, Mulvihal M. Effects of acute alterations in maternal free fatty acid concentration on human chorionic somatomammotropin secretion. Am J Obstet Gynecol 1974;119:224–229.
13. Ylikorkala O, Kauppila A. Effect of dexamethasone on serum levels of human placental lactogen during the last trimester of pregnancy. J Obstet Gynecol Br Common 1974;81:368–370.
14. Kim YJ, Felig P. Plasma chorionic somatomammotropin levels during starvation in mid-pregnancy. J Clin Endocrinol Metab 1972;32:864–867.
15. Tyson JE, Austin KL, Farinholt JW. Prolonged nutritional deprivation in pregnancy: Changes in human chorionic somatomammotropin and growth hormone secretion. Amer J Obstet Gynecol 1971;109:1080–1082.
16. Ajabor LM, Yen SSC. Effect of sustained hyperglycemia on the levels of human chorionic somatomammotropin in mid-pregnancy. Am J Obstet Gynecol 1972;112:908–911.
17. Suwa S, Friesen HG. Biosynthesis of human placental proteins and human placental lactogen (hPL) in vitro. II. Dynamic studies of normal term placentas. Endocrinology 1969;85:1037–1045.

18. Desole E, Springolo E, Dichiari F, Franzolini L, Tosolini GC. Human placental lactogen production *in vitro*. I. Dynamic studies of normal-term placentas after stimulation with 17-á-oestrodiol. In: Salvadori B, ed. Therapy of Feto-Placental Insufficiency. Springer-Verlag, Berlin, 1975; p. 313.

19. Niven PAR, Buhi WC, Spellacy WN. The effect of intravenous oestrogen injections on plasma human placental lactogen levels. J Obstet Gynecol Brit Commonwealth 1974;81:466–468.

20. Belleville F, Lasbennes A, Nabet P, Paysant P. Etude des substances pouvant intervenir dans la regulation de la secretion de la somatomammotrophine chorionique (hCS) in vitro par le placenta en culture. Compte Rendu des Seances de la Societe de Biologie et de Ses Fliales (Paris) 1974;168: 1057–1062.

21. Handwerger S, Barrett J, Tyrey L, Schomberg D. Differential effect of cyclic adenosine monophosphate on the secretion of human placental lactogen and human chorionic gonadotropin. J Clin Endocrin Metab 1973;36:1268–1270.

22. Hershman JM, Kojima A, Friesen HG. Effect of thyrotropin-releasing hormone on human pituitary thyrotropin, prolactin, placental lactogen and chorionic thyrotropin. J Clin Endocrin Metab 1973;36:497–501.

23. Pujoi-Amat P, Gamessans O, Cabero L, Perez-Lopez PP, Benito E, Calaf J, Robyn C. In: Salvadori B, ed. Therapy of Feto-Placental Insufficiency. Springer-Verlag, Berlin, 1975, p. 246–249.

24. Handwerger S, Barrett J, Tyrey L. Unpublished observations.

25. Wilson EA, Jawad MJ, Vernon MW. Effect of epidermal growth factor on hormone secretion by term placenta in organ culture. Am J Obstet Gynecol 1984;149:579,580.

26. Petit A, Guillon G, Tence M, Jard S, Gallo-Payet N, Bellabarba D, et al. Angiotensin II stimulates both inositol phosphate production and human placental lactogen release from human trophoblastic cells. J Clin Endocrin Metab 1989;69:280–286.

27. Bhaumick B, Dawson EP, Bala RM. The effects of insulin-like growth factor-I and insulin on placental lactogen production by human term placental explants. Biochem Biophys Res Comm 1987;144:674–682.

28. Singer W, Desjardins P, Friesen HG. Human placental lactogen: an index of placental function. Obstet Gynecol 1970;36:222–232.

29. Ursell W, Brudenell M, Chard T. Placental lactogen levels in diabetic pregnancy. Brit Med J 1973;2: 80–82.

30. Josimovich JB, Kosar B, Boccella L, Mintz DH, Hutchinson DL. Placental lactogen in maternal serum as an index of fetal health. Obstet Gynecol 1970;36:244–250.

31. Lindberg BS, Nilsson BA. Human placental lactogen (HPL) levels in abnormal pregnancies. J Obstet Gynecol Br Common 1973;80:1046–1053.

32. Kelly AM, England P, Lorrimer JD, Ferguson JC. An evaluation of human placental lactogen levels in hypertension of pregnancy. Brit J Obstet Gynecol 1975;82:272–277.

33. Letchworth AT, Chard T. Placental lactogen levels as a screening test for fetal distress and neonatal asphyxia. Lancet 1972;1:704–706.

34. Handwerger S, Quarfordt S, Barrett J, Harman I. Apolipoproteins AI, AII, and CI stimulate placental lactogen release from human placental tissue: a novel action of HDL apolipoproteins. J Clin Invest 1987;79:625–628.

35. Grandis A, Jorgensen V, Kodack L, Quarfordt S, Handwerger S. High density lipoproteins (HDL) stimulate placental lactogen secretion in pregnant ewes: further evidence for a role of HDL in placental lactogen secretion during pregnancy. J Endocrinol 1989;120:423–427.

36. Desoye G, Schweditsch MO, Pfeiffer KP, Zechner R, Kostner GM. Correlation of hormones with lipid and lipoprotein levels during normal pregnancy and postpartum. J Clin Endocrin Metab 1987;64: 704–712.

37. Handwerger S, Richards RG, Myers S. Novel regulation of the synthesis and release of human placental lactogen by high density lipoproteins [Review]. Trophoblast Res 1994;8:339–354.

38. Jorgensen EV, Gwynne JT, Handwerger S. High density lipoprotein 3 binding and biological action: high affinity binding is not necessary for stimulation of placental lactogen release from trophoblast cells. Endocrinology 1989;125:2915–2921.

39. Jorgensen EV, Anantharamaiah GM, Segrest JP, Gwynne JT, Handwerger S. Synthetic amphipathic peptides resembling apolipoproteins stimulate the release of human placental lactogen. J Biol Chem 1989;264:9215–9219.

40. Wu YQ, Jorgensen EV, Handwerger S. High density lipoproteins stimulate placental lactogen release and adenosine 3',5'-cyclic monophosphate production in human trophoblast cells: evidence for cyclic AMP as a second messenger in hPL release. Endocrinology 1988;123:1879–1884.

41. Wu YQ, Handwerger S. High density lipoproteins stimulate Mr 80K protein phosphorylation in human trophoblast cells: Evidence for a protein kinase C-dependent pathway in human placental lactogen release. Endocrinology 1992;131:2935–2940.

42. Handwerger S, Myers S, Richards RG, Richardson B, Turzai L, Moeykins C, et al. Apolipoprotein A-I stimulates placental lactogen expression by human trophoblast cells. Endocrinology 1995; 136:5555–5560.

43. Darbon JM, Tournier JF, Tauber JP, Bayard F. Possible role of protein phosphorylation in the mitogenic effect of high density lipoproteins on cultured vascular endothelial cells. J Biol Chem 1986;261:8002–8008.

44. Ong AC, Jowett TP, Moorhead JF, Owen JS. Human high density lipoproteins stimulate endothelin-1 release by cultured human renal proximal cells. Kidney Int 1994;46:1315–1321.

45. Blackburn WD, Jr., Dohlman JG, Venkatachalapathi YV, Pillion DJ, Koopman WJ, Segrest JP, Anantharamaiah GM. Apolipoprotein A-I decreases neutrophil degranulation and superoxide production. J Lipid Res 1991;32:1911–1918.

46. Rosing U, Samsioe G, Olund A, Johansson B, Kallner A. Serum levels of apolipoprotein A-I, A-II and HDL-cholesterol in second half of normal pregnancy and in pregnancy complicated by preeclampsia. Hormone Metab Res 1989;21:376–382.

47. Kaaja R, Tikkanen MJ, Viinikka L, Ylikorkala O. Serum lipoproteins, insulin, and urinary prostanoid metabolites in normal and hypertensive pregnant women. Obstet Gynecol 1995;85:353–356.

48. Knopp RH, Van Allen MI, McNeely M, Walden CE, Plovie B, Shiota K. Effect of insulin-dependent diabetes on plasma lipoproteins in diabetic pregnancy. J Reproduct Med 1993;38:703–710.

49. Barsh GS, Seeburg PH, Gelinas RE. The human growth hormone gene family: Structure and evolution of the chromosomal locus. Nucleic Acids Res 1983;11:3939–3958.

50. Chen EY, Liao YC, Smith DH, Barrera-Saldana HA, Gelinas RE, Seeburg PH. The human growth hormone locus nucleotide sequence, biology, and evolution. Genomics 1997;4:479–497.

51. Owerbach D, Rutter W, Martial J, Baxter JD, Shows TB. Genes for growth hormone, chorionic somatomammotropin, and growth hormone-like genes on chromosome 17 in humans. Science 1980;209:289–292.

52. Walker WH, Fitzpatrick SL, Barrera-Saldana HA, Resendez-Perez D, Saunders GF. The human placental lactogen genes: Structure, function, evolution and transcriptional regulation. Endocrine Rev 1991;12:316–328.

53. Jacquemin P, Alsat E, Oury C, Belayew A, Muller M, Evain-Brion D, Martial JA. The enhancers of the human placental lactogen B, A, and L genes: Progressive activation during in vitro trophoblast differentiation and importance of the DF-3 element in determining their respective activities. DNA Cell Biol 1996;15:845–854.

54. Midgley AR, Jr., Pierce GB, Deneau GA, Gosling JRG. Morphogenesis of syncytiotrophoblast in vivo: an autoradiographic demonstration. Science 1963;141:349,350.

55. Midgley AR, Jr., Pierce GB. Immunohistochemical localization of human chorionic gonadotropin. J Exp Med 1962;115:289–294.

56. Pierce GB, Midgley AR, Jr. The origin and function of human syncytiotrophoblastic giant cells. Amer J Pathol 1963;43:153–171.

57. Kliman HJ, Nestler JE, Sermasi E, Sanger JM, Strauss JF, III. Purification, characterization and in vitro differentiation of cytotrophoblasts from human term placentae. Endocrinology 1986;118:1567–1582.

58. Douglas GC, King BF. Differentiation of human trophoblast cells in vitro as revealed by immunocytochemical staining of desmoplakin and nuclei. J Cell Sci 1990;96:131–141.

59. Boime I. Human placental hormone production is linked to the stage of trophoblast differentiation. In: Miller RK, Thiede HA, eds. Trophoblast Research. Verav Medical, Rochester, NY, 1991, pp. 57–60.

60. Richards RG, Hartman SM, Handwerger S. Human cytotrophoblast cells cultured in maternal serum progress to a differentiated syncytial phenotype expressing both human chorionic gonadotropin and human placental lactogen. Endocrinology 1994;135:321–329.

61. Cross JC, Werb Z, Fisher SJ. Implantation and the placenta: Key pieces of the development puzzle. Science 1994;266:1508–1517.

62. Shi QJ, Lei ZM, Rao CV, Lin J. Novel role of human chorionic gonadotropin in differentiation of human cytotrophoblasts. Endocrinology 1993;132:1387–1395.

63. Garcia-Lloret MI, Morrish DW, Wegmann TG, Honore L, Turner AR, Guilbert LJ. Demonstration of functional cytokine-placental interactions: CSF-1 and GM-CSF stimulate human cytotrophoblast differentiation and peptide hormone secretion. Exper Cell Res 1994;214:46–54.

64. Millio LA, Hu J, Douglas GC. Binding of insulin-like growth factor I to human trophoblast cells during differentiation *in vitro*. Placenta 1994;15:641–651.

65. Wice B, Menton D, Geuze H, Schwartz AL. Modulators of cyclic AMP metabolism induce syncytiotrophoblast formation *in vitro*. Exper Cell Res 1990;186:306–316.

66. Strauss JF, III, Kido S, Sayegh R, Sakuragi N, Gafvels ME. The cAMP signalling system and human trophoblast function [Review]. Placenta 1992;13:389–403.

67. Amemiya K, Kurachi H, Adachi H, Morishige KI, Adachi K, Imai T, Miuake A. Involvement of epidermal growth factor (EGF)/EGF receptor autocrine and paracrine mechanism in human trophoblast cells: Functional differentiation *in vitro*. J Endocrinol 1994;143:291–301.

68. Jones BK, Monks BR, Liebhaber SA, Cooke NE. The human growth hormone gene is regulated by a multicomponent locus control region. Mol Cellular Biol 1995;15:7010–7021.

69. Jiang S, Shepard AR, Eberhardt NL. An initiator element is required for maximal human chorionic somatomammotropin gene promoter and enhancer function. J Biol Chem 1995;270:3683–3692.

70. Fitzpatrick SL, Walker WH, Saunders GF. DNA sequences involved in the transcriptional activation of a human placental lactogen gene. Mol Endocrinol 1990;4:1815.

71. Richards RG, Richardson BR, Schmidt CM, Handwerger S. Inhibitory elements within the human placental lactogen (hPL) promoter prevent hPL gene expression in cytotrophoblast cells. The 79th Ann Meet Endocrine Society (June 11–14, 1997), Minneapolis, MN, abstr P3–541.

72. Walker WH, Fitzpatrick SL, Saunders GF. Human placental lactogen transcriptional enhancer: Tissue specificity and binding with specific proteins. J Biol Chem 1990;265:12,940–12,948.

73. Jiang S, Eberhardt NL. The human chorionic somatomammotropin gene enhancer is composed of multiple DNA elements that are homologous to several SV40 enhansons. J Biol Chem 1994;269:10,384–10,392.

74. Lytras A, Cattini PA. Human chorionic somatomammotropin gene enhancer activity is dependent on the blockade of a repressor mechanism. Mol Endocrinol 1994;8:478–489.

75. Jacquemin P, Oury C, Peers B, Morin A, Belayew A, Martial JA. Characterization of a single strong tissue-specific enhancer downstream from the three human genes encoding placental lactogen. Mol Cell Biol 1994;14:93–103.

76. Jiang S, Eberhardt NL. Involvement of a protein distinct from transcription enhancer factor-1 (TEF-1) in mediating human chorionic somatomammotropin gene enhancer function through the GT-IIC enhanson in choriocarcinoma and COS cells. J Biol Chem 1995;270:13,906–13,915.

77. Jacquemin P, Martial JA, Davidson I. Human TEF-5 is preferentially expressed in placenta and binds to multiple functional elements of the human chorionic somatomammotropin-B gene enhancer. J Biol Chem 1997;272:12,928–12,937.

78. Davidson I, Xiao JH, Rosales R, Staub A, Chambon P. The HeLa cell protein TEF-1 binds specifically and cooperatively to two SV40 enhancer motifs of unrelated sequence. Cell 1988;54:931–942.

79. Ishiji T, Lace MJ, Parkkinen S, Anderson RD, Haugen TH, Cripe TP, et al. Transcriptional enhancer factor (TEF)-1 and its cell-specific co-activator activate human papillomavirus-16 E6 and E7 oncogene transcription in keratinocytes and cervical carcinoma cells. EMBO J 1992;11:2271–2281.

80. Stewart AF, Larkin SB, Farrance IK, Mar JH, Hall DE, Ordahl CP. Muscle-enriched TEF-1 isoforms bind M-CAT elements from muscle-specific promoters and differentially activate transcription. J Biol Chem 1994;269:3147–3150.

81. Richards RG, Kanda Y, Handwerger S. Overexpression of MAP kinase in term placental cytotrophoblast cells activates transcription of the human placental lactogen promoter. The 79th Ann Meet Endocrine Society (June 11–14, 1997), Minneapolis, MN, abstr P3–540.

82. Stephanou A, Sarlis NJ, Richards RG, Handwerger S. Expression of retinoic acid receptor subtypes and cellular retinoic acid binding protein-II mRNAs during differentiation of human trophoblast cells. Biochem Biophys Res Comm 1994;202:772–780.

83. Stephanou A, Ross R, Handwerger S. Regulation of human placental lactogen expression by 1,25-dihydroxyvitamin D. Endocrinology 1994;135:2651–2656.

84. Stephanou A, Handwerger S. Retinoic acid and thyroid hormone regulate placental lactogen expression in human trophoblast cells. Endocrinology 1995;136:933–938.

85. Bikle DD, Pillai S. Vitamin D, calcium, and epidermal differentiation. Endocrine Rev 1993;14:3–19.

86. Holloran BP. Is 1,25-dihydroxyvitamin D required for reproduction. Proc Soc Exp Biol Med 1989;191:227–232.

87. Weisman Y, Harell A, Endelstein S, David M, Spirer Z, Gollander A. 1,25-Dihydroxyvitamin D3 and 24,25-dihydroxyvitamin D3 *in vitro* synthesis by human decidua and placenta. Nature 1979;281: 317–319.

88. Ross R, Florer J, Halbert K, McIntyre L. Characterization of 1,25-dihydroxyvitamin D3 receptors and *in vivo* targeting of 3H-1,25(OH)2D3. Placenta 1989;10:553–567.

89. Maruo T, Matsuo H, Mochizuki M. Thyroid hormone as a biological marker of differentiated trophoblast in early pregnancy. Acta Endocrinol (Copenh) 1991;125:58–66.

90. Stephanou A, Handwerger S. The ARP-1 orphan receptor represses basal and steroid-mediated stimulation of human placental gene expression. J Mol Endocrinol 1996;16:221–227.

91. Barlow JW, Voz MLJ, Eliard PH, Mathy-Hartert M, De Nayer P, Economidis IV, et al. Thyroid hormone receptors bind to defined regions of the growth hormone and placental lactogen genes. Proc Natl Acad Sci USA 1986;83:9021–9025.

92. Umesono K, Murakami KK, Thompson CC, Evans RM. Direct repeats as selective response elements for the thyroid hormone, retinoic acid, and vitamin D3 receptors. Cell 1991;65:1256–1266.

93. Schule R, Umesono K, Mangelsdorf DJ, Bolado J, Pike JW, Evan RM. Jun-Fos and receptors for vitamin A and D recognize a common response element in the human osteocalcin gene. Cell 1990;61:497–504.

94. Adan RA, Cox JJ, Beischlag TV, Burbach JP. A composite hormone response element mediates transactivation of the rat oxytocin gene by different classes of nuclear hormone receptors. Molec Endocrinol 1993;7:47–57.

95. Stephanou A, Handwerger S. Identification of a composite steroid hormone response element on the human placental lactogen promoter. Molec Cell Endocrinol 1995;112:123–129.

96. Durand B, Saunders M, Leroy P, Leid M, Chambon P. All-trans and 9-cis retinoic acid induction of CRABPII transcription is mediated by RAR-RXR heterodimers bound to DR1 and DR2 repeated motifs. Cell 1992;71:73–85.

97. Lee W, Mitchell P, Tjian R. Purified transcription factor AP-1 interacts with TPA-inducible enhancer elements. Cell 1987;49:741–752.

98. Owen TA, Bortell R, Yocum SA, et al. Coordinate occupancy of AP-1 sites in the vitamin D-responsive and CCAAT box elements by Fos-Jun in the osteocalcin gene: model for phenotype suppression of transcription. Proc Natl Acad Sci USA 1990;87:9990–9994.

99. Harman I, Zeitler P, Ganong B, Bell RM, Handwerger S. Sn-1,2-diacylglycerols and phorbol esters stimulate the synthesis and release of human placental lactogen from placental cells: a role for protein kinase C. Endocrinology 1986;119:1239–1244.

100. Schule R, Rangarajan P, Yang N, Kliewer S, Ransone LJ, Bolado J, et al. Retinoic acid is a negative regulator of AP-1-responsive genes. Proc Natl Acad Sci USA 1991;88:6092–6096.

101. Schmidt ED, Cramer SJ, Offringa R. The thyroid hormone receptor interferes with transcriptional activation via the AP-1 complex. Biochem Biophys Res Comm 1993;192:151–160.

102. Kadonaga JT, Jones KA, Tjian R. Promoter-specific activation of RNA polymerase II transcription by Sp1. Trends Biochem Sci 1986;11:20–32.

103. Leone TC, Cresci S, Carter ME, Zhang Z, Lala DS, Strauss AW, Kelly DP. The human medium chain Acyl-CoA dehydrogenase gene promoter consists of a complex arrangement of nuclear receptor response elements and Sp1 binding sites. J Biol Chem 1995;270:16,308–16,314.

104. Sylvester I, Scholer HR. Regulation of the Oct-4 gene by nuclear receptors. Nucleic Acids Res 1994;22:901–911.

105. Shah M, Handwerger S. Upregulation of vitamin D receptor (VDR) during human trophoblast differentiation. The Ann Meet Amer Pediatric Soc and Soc Pediatric Res (May 1996), Washington, DC, abstr 33558.

106. Stephanou A, Handwerger S. Interleukin-6 stimulates placental lactogen expression by human trophoblast cells. Endocrinology 1994;135:719–723.

107. Stephanou A, Handwerger S. The nuclear factor NF-IL-6 activates human placental lactogen gene expression. Biochem Biophys Res Comm 1994;206:215–222.

108. Kameda T, Matsuzuki N, Sawai K. Production of interleukin 6 by normal trophoblast cells. Placenta 1990;11:205–213.

109. Paulesu L, King A, Loke YW, Cintorino M, Bellizzi E, Boraschi D. Immunohistochemical localization of IL-1 alpha and IL-1 beta in normal human placenta. Lymphokine Cytokine Res 1991;10:443–448.

110. Stephanou A, Myatt L, Eis ALW, Handwerger S. Ontogeny of the expression and regulation of interleukin-6 (IL-6) and IL-1 mRNAs by human trophoblast cells during differentiation *in vitro*. J Endocrinol 1995;147:487–496.

16 Molecular and Cellular Basis of Immune-Mediated (Type 1) Diabetes

Regis Coutant, MD and Noel K. MacLaren, MD

INTRODUCTION

Immune-mediated (type I) diabetes (IMD), a multifactorial autoimmune disease, is determined by both environmental and genetic factors *(1)*. Lymphocytic infiltration of pancreatic islets (insulitis) is the hallmark of the disease *(2,3)*. The infiltration of islets proceeds slowly and has most times been present for years before the clinical diagnosis *(4–6)*. Studies suggest that the autoimmune process that leads to IMD often begins during the first few years of life *(7,8)*. The inflammatory infiltrate of islets consists mostly of CD8+ T cells plus variable numbers of CD4+ T cells, B-lymphocytes, macrophages, and natural killer cells *(3)*. Massive β cell destruction by infiltrating cells, however, could be a late event in the process, which results in symptomatic diabetes only when at least 80% of the volume of beta cells have been destroyed *(3)*. The destruction is mainly mediated by T cells. However, it is accompanied by circulating marker, islet cell autoantibodies (ICA) to pancreatic β-cells proteins *(9,10)*, which can be used to predict the disease.

IMD is sometimes familial. First degree relatives of patients with IMD are at about 15-fold increased risk of developing diabetes themselves, and more so in already multiplex families *(4,11)*. There appears to be a gene dose effect in the susceptibility to IMD, which involves as many as 10–20 separate and possibly interacting genes (epistasis) *(12,13)*. Penetrance of the disease might be enhanced by gene dose effects interacting with the environment.

From: *Molecular and Cellular Pediatric Endocrinology*
Edited by: S. Handwerger © Humana Press Inc., Totowa, NJ

Table 1
Lifelong Risks of Immune-Mediated Diabetes

Group	Absolute risk, %
Normal subjects	0.4
Nondiabetic relatives of patients	
with immune-mediated diabetes	
Parent	3
Offspring	6
Of an affected father	8
Of an affected mother	3
Sibling	
Identical twin	30–50
Other	5

Environmental triggers appear to be required, since the incidence of diabetes has increased over the last three decades, with temporal variations *(14)*. The concordance rate in monozygotic twins is only 34–50% *(15,16)*, whereas 90% of patients with newly diagnosed IMD do not have an affected relative *(17)*. Hence, combined genetic and epidemiological evidence suggested that unknown environmental factors may play a role in either inducing the autoimmunity and/or shaping its course in genetically susceptible individuals. Viral infections and dietary factors have been suggested to be important in this respect *(18)*.

We will review in this chapter the genetics of susceptibility to the IMD, the putative environmental events triggering and precipitating the disease, the immunological processes that lead to the destruction of pancreatic β cells and ultimately diabetes, and the metabolic alterations that precede clinical onset of diabetes.

GENETIC SUSCEPTIBILITY OF THE DISEASE

Genetic Analysis

Marked differences in risk have been found according to the familial relationship to the diabetic proband (Table 1) *(17,19)*. Clustering of diabetes in families can be caused by both genetic and environmental factors. The pattern of clustering of the disease in families, however, is not compatible with a simple recessive or dominant Mendelian inheritance, but is compatible with one that involves several genes. It is generally assumed that allelic variants of multiple genes, which affect their expressions or functions, combine to produce a susceptible genetic background. Each one of these genetic variants may have subtle quantitative effects (quantitative trait loci or QTL), which are difficult to distinguish individually. Only the epistasis, or the interaction between the multiple gene products involved, will produce the autoimmune phenotype. Several approaches have been used to determine which genes at which loci are associated with inherited susceptibility to IMD. The candidate gene approach, studying genes possibly involved in pathogenesis of the disease, permitted linkage between the major histocompatibility complex (MHC) and the insulin (INS) genomic regions to risk of diabetes to be established. Whole genome scans, however, using maps of microsatellite markers that cover the entire human genomes, have been completed on families with several affected (multiplex) siblings

Table 2
High Risk and Protective HLA DR/DQ Genes

DR/DQ	Effect		
	Highly susceptible, RR 5–30[a]	Suceptible, RR 4–10	Highly protective, RR 0.2
DRB1	0405	0401	0403–0406
	0402		1501
	301		1301
DQA1	0301	0501	
DQB1	0302		0602–0603
	0201		

[a]RR: relative risk.

(linkage analysis in affected sib-pairs). The aim was to identify the chromosomal regions (genomic intervals) that are inherited by affected progeny more often than expected from random Mendelian chance. These studies confirmed the MHC locus as harboring the major genes associated with inherited susceptibility to IMD. The insulin gene region has been identified as the second one. As many as 20 other loci have also been implicated as possible sites of genes influencing risk of IMD (12,13). However, linkage studies often give false positive results, as expected from a statistical viewpoint, corresponding to random patient ascertainment errors. All the loci so far implicated have thus to be confirmed in multiple independent data sets. Fine mapping, using denser microsatellite markers within a locus, have been carried out in multiplex as well as simplex families with one affected child. The aim was to reduce the genomic interval associated with susceptibility in order to identify the gene(s) truly involved (linkage disequilibrium mapping). These studies allowed circumscribing the insulin gene susceptibility region to the variable number of tandem repeats (VNTR) in the 5' flanking region of the human insulin gene. To date, the pathogenic mutations that lead to the predisposing allelic variants have only been determined for the HLA class II genes and for the insulin gene VNTR. These topics will be expanded below.

Major Histocompatibility (MHC) II Region

The HLA class II region of the major histocompatibility complex (MHC) on the short arm of chromosome 6 (IDDM 1) encodes the most important genetic factors, accounting for at least 30% of the familial aggregation seen in IMD. Susceptibility or resistance to the disease is associated with some HLA-DR and even more strongly with certain HLA-DQ molecules (20–24) (Table 2). These heterodimeric molecules are considered to be predisposing, or protective, when their frequency is significantly higher or lower respectively in diabetic patients than in ethnically matched normal controls. Islet cell antigens are processed into peptides by antigen-presenting cells (APCs) and antigenic peptides of 8–16 amino acids in length are presented on APCs by HLA class II molecules to CD4+ T lymphocytes. The recognition of the class II HLA-peptide complex by T lymphocyte receptors (TCR) triggers the activation and proliferation (clonal expansion) of those T lymphocytes. It is believed that susceptible HLA class II molecules affect the degree of immune responsiveness to a particular pancreatic β cell autoantigenic peptide (25,26), albeit an environmental antigen with molecular mimicry to an islet cell self protein could be involved.

These DR/DQ molecules comprise one A chain and one B chain, encoded by separate A and B chain genes, respectively. There is only one monomorphic DRA gene in all individuals, but there are several polymorphic DRB1, DRB3, DRB4, DRB5, as well as polymorphic DQA1 and DQB1 genes. DR molecules are determined by the product of the invariant DRA gene and the polymorphic DRB1 gene, carried by the homologous chromosome, although multiple other DR can be expressed also. Similarly, DQ molecules are determined by the product of the polymorphic DQA1 and DQB1 genes, through cis and trans complementations. Cis-dimers comprise A and B chains encoded by DQA1 and DQB1 genes of the same chromosome or haplotype, whereas trans-dimers are encoded by genes on both homologous chromosomes. Thus, there are two separate DR molecules that are products of DRA and DRB1 genes (other DR molecules are produced if the DRB3, DRB4, or DRB5 genes happen to be expressed) plus 4 DQ molecules expressed in all individuals, all of which act in concert to determine the overall HLA-encoded susceptibility to or protection from IMD (Fig. 1).

DQB1 alleles encoding an alanine at DQB residue 57 (DQB1*0201 and DQB1*0302) confer strong susceptibility to IMD in most races (23). Conversely, all DQB1 alleles coding for an aspartic acid at this position confer neutral (DQB1*0303) or often strongly protective (DQB1*0602, DQB1*0603) effects. The other susceptible or protective molecules are shown in Table 2. The nature of the amino acid at this position affects the shape and charge of the antigenic binding cleft of the DQ and thereby the peptide binding and T cell recognition. Generally, highly protective DR or DQ molecules act in a dominant manner, whereas most or all DR and DQ molecules expressed by any individual have to be susceptible factors in a predisposing HLA genotype. Thus, one protective molecule (such as DRB1*0403) can strongly counteract the predisposing effect of the DQB1*0201/ DQB1*0302 molecules if also present.

Apparent interracial discrepancies of HLA associations with IMD can be mainly explained by different DR-DQ linkage disequilibria and DQ-AB chain transcomplementation (24). In Caucasian populations, the genotype associated with the highest relative risk (RR 20–50) is DRB1*03-DQA1*0501-DQB1*0201 on one chromosome (haplotype), and DRB1*04-DQA1*0301-DQB1*0302 on the other. In this instance, transcomplementation leads only to susceptible DQ trans-dimers of DQA1*0301-DQB1*0201. In Blacks, the haplotype most associated with susceptibility is DRB1*07-DQA1*0301-DQB1*0201, leading to the same susceptible DQ molecules by cis-complementation (Fig. 1) (27). In addition, other genes within the MHC region, such as TNFα, could modulate the susceptibility or protection associated with the DR/DQ alleles (28). HLA-associated susceptibility or protection seems to be age-dependent, since adult-onset IMD patients show lower percentages of susceptible DRB1*03-DQB1*0201/DRB1*04-DQB1*0302 genotypes (29) and a higher percentage of protective DQB1*0602/0603 than those found in patients with childhood-onset diabetes.

Determination of HLA-DR and DQ haplotype sharing between a first-degree relative and a subject with type 1 diabetes greatly increases the ability to assess risk of IMD, with a maximum predictive value of 25% for those who share both susceptible HLA DR/DQ haplotypes (HLA DRB1*03-DQA1*0501-DQB1*0201 and DRB1*04-DQA1*0301-DQB1*0302) with a sibling affected by the disease. This percentage approaches that of

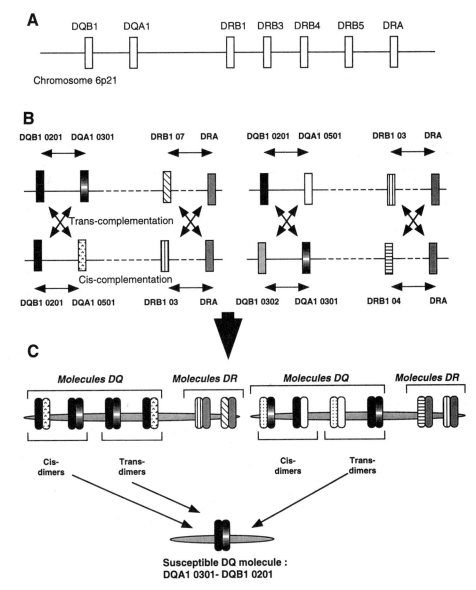

Fig. 1. (A) Major histocompatibility complex (chr 6p21). **(B)** Cis and transcomplementations of DQA1/DQB1 genes. **(C)** Susceptible DQA1 0301/DQB1 0201 cis dimer (Black population) or trans dimer (Caucasian population).

the one in three concordance in monozygotic twins who share all genes in common (Table 3) *(15,16)*. In general population, the absolute risk of individuals carrying the highest risk genotype (DRB1*03-DQA1*0501-DQB1*0201 and DRB1*04-DQA1*0301-DQB1*0302) is estimated to be about 5–10% (1:15) *(30,31)*.

Insulin (INS) Gene

The INS gene VNTR (IDDM 2) is also a strong genetic determinant of diabetes susceptibility *(32–34)*, accounting for about 15% of the familial aggregation of IMD. It

Table 3
Lifelong Risks of Immune-Mediated Diabetes,
According to HLA Phenotype

Group	Absolute risk %
Normal subjects	0.4
Nondiabetic relatives of patients with immune-mediated diabetes	
Sibling	5
HLA-identical	13
DR3/DR4 HLA-identical	25
HLA haploidentical	5
No HLA identity	1
Identical twins	30–50

is located on chromosome 11p15.5 in the 5' flanking region of the human insulin gene 365 bp from its transcription site. The VNTR corresponds to a repeat of a nucleotide motif. The short VNTR alleles (26–63 repeats) predispose to immune-mediated diabetes, whereas the long VNTR alleles (140–210 repeats) have dominant protective effects.

Whereas the class of the VNTR alleles only marginally affects the insulin mRNA levels transcribed by the human pancreas, this cannot explain diabetes susceptibility (35,36). However, the long (protective) VNTR-INS alleles have been associated with two- to threefold higher insulin mRNA levels than do the short (susceptible) alleles transcribed by the human fetal thymus (37,38). Thymic insulin mRNA is effectively translated into protein. This mechanism is thought to ensure immune tolerance by a central (intrathymic) deletion of autoreactive thymocytes (negative selection). The quantitative expression of self antigens in the thymus results in greater self immunological tolerance development, since thymocytes bearing TCRs capable of recognizing self-peptide-MHC complexes on APCs because of high affinity/avidity binding are negatively selected. This process has been shown to be dose-dependent because changes in the concentration of a selecting peptide in thymic organ cultures have quantitative effects on selection. The susceptible effect of the short VNTR allele may also depend on its maternal vs paternal transmission. It does not predispose to IMD if it is paternally inherited with the father's nontransmitted allele being a long VNTR allele. This suggests an imprinting of the transmitted INS allele, which occurs with an interaction between both VNTR alleles in the homologous chromosomes (39).

Other Loci

Many other loci (genomic intervals) associated with the disease have been reported. The contribution of these other possible genetic influences to susceptibility to the disease is less than the INS gene VNTR. Some contain genes involved in immunological regulation, such as IDDM 12, which contains CTLA-4 gene (40,41). CTLA-4 is a molecule expressed by activated T cells, which plays an important role in limiting the T cell proliferative response (clonal T cell expansion) after an antigenic stimulation. Therefore, a disruption of the immune regulation linked to a variant of the CTLA-4 could account for the effect of IDDM12, although the etiological mutations involved remain to be found. Three other loci, IDDM 4 on 11q13, IDDM5 on 6q25, and IDDM 8 on 6q27, have been

Table 4
Genetic Loci Associated with IMD Susceptibility

Locies		Main genes in the locus
6p21[a]	(IDDM1)	MHC II, TNFα
11p15.5	(IDDM2)	Insulin gene VNTR
15q26	(IDDM3)	
11q13	(IDDM4)	
6q25	(IDDM5)	
18q21	(IDDM6)	
2q31	(IDDM7)	
6q27	(IDDM8)	
10p11-10q11	(IDDM10)	
14q24.3-q31	(IDDM11)	
2q33	(IDDM12)	CTLA4/CD28
2q3–5	(IDDM13)	
6q	(IDDM15)	

[a]Confirmed loci are listed in boldface.

confirmed to be linked to IMD by multiple independent studies. No candidate gene within these regions has yet been discovered. The other loci require confirmation from independent studies (Table 4) *(40–50)*.

ENVIRONMENTAL EVENTS ASSOCIATED WITH AUTOIMMUNITY TO PANCREATIC B CELLS

Epidemiological, Clinical, and Experimental Studies

Viral infections, such as entero-virus *(51)*, congenital rubella *(52)*, or endogenous retrovirus infection *(53)*, and dietary factors, such as early exposure to cow's milk, have all been proposed to be important environmental factors in the development of diabetes, on the basis of epidemiological studies and clinical observations *(18)*. Several studies reported higher frequencies or higher titers of antibodies to Coxsackie B viruses in diabetic patients than in controls *(54,55)*. One study related the presence of such IgM antibodies to enteroviruses in pregnant women near delivery and the occurrence of diabetes in their offspring *(56)*. However, epidemiological studies did not always give consistent results *(57)*. Elsewhere, a variant of Coxsackie B4 virus was isolated from the pancreas of a patient with IMD at diagnosis, which was found to induce diabetes when transmitted to mice *(58)*. A Coxsackie B5 virus infection isolated from the feces of a newly diagnosed diabetic patient was also found to induce diabetes in certain susceptible strains of mice but not others *(59)*. Finally, a significant percentage of Coxsackie B3 and B4 sequences were detected by PCR in sera of young children at diagnosis of diabetes *(60)*, while a structural homology between the P2C protein of these viruses and an islet cell antigen (GAD$_{65}$) was identified (as discussed below). Patients with congenital rubella syndrome have a higher incidence of IMD than the general population. Some 10–20% of individuals with congenital rubella syndrome develop diabetes in 5–20 yr *(52)*.

A human endogenous retrovirus (HERV) was isolated in 2 IMD patients who died shortly after the onset of their disease, using a complex polymerase chain reaction strategy. This retrovirus, HERV K$_{1,2}$22, is related to the human endogenous retrovirus HERV-K10 family and to the mouse mammary tumor viruses (MMTV). Transcripts derived from the genome of this retrovirus were found in blood from all 10 diabetic patients tested, but not from nondiabetic controls. Furthermore, a protein with superantigenic activity was found within the envelope (env) protein, which stimulated T cells displaying TCR-comprising Vβ7 chains, but not those with other expressed variable genes *(53)*.

Epidemiological studies of infant feeding methods and milk protein consumption have shown correlations between ingestion of cow's milk protein and the risk of IMD in humans *(61–63)*. Antibodies to bovine serum albumin have been reported to be higher *(64)*, albeit not consistently *(65)*, in newly diabetic patients than in controls. It is therefore possible that human breast feeding may be protective rather than cow's milk harmful in respect to risk of IMD.

Environmental Events Implicated in Diabetes Pathogenesis: Mechanisms

Three mechanisms, not necessarily mutually exclusive, have been proposed to account for the activation of peripheral autoreactive T cells by environmental factors. First, an immune response against an exogenous protein that shares an amino acid sequence with a β cell protein could result in the appearance of T lymphocytes that react with the self protein. A striking "molecular mimicry" between the beta cell glutamate decarboxylase peptide GAD$_{65(250-273)}$ and Coxsackie B protein P2-C has been shown *(66)*. Furthermore, peripheral blood mononuclear cells of diabetic patients or patients at high risk of IMD are often found reactive to GAD$_{65}$ peptides that crossreact with the viral protein P2-C *(51)*. Homology among a peptide (ABBOS peptide) from BSA, a protein of cow's milk, and a 69 kDa protein of islet cells *(67)* has been suggested to explain a triggering role of cow's milk in the autoimmune process, although the structural homology between these antigens is trivial. Homology between Rubella virus capsid protein and a 52 kDa protein within islet cells has been also described *(68)*. Alternatively, an environmental insult of pancreatic β cells (infection with a β cell tropic virus) may generate cytokines and other inflammatory mediators that induce the expression of adhesion molecules in the vascular endothelium of the pancreatic islets or increase extravasation of circulating leukocytes and thereby the presentation of β cell antigens from the damaged β cells by infiltrating macrophages to T lymphocytes. Third, a viral or bacterial superantigen may trigger the polyclonal activation of a Vβ-restricted T cell subset, within which autoreactive T cells could initiate or accelerate organ-specific tissue destruction. The human endogenous retrovirus, HERV K$_{1,2}$22, has been reported to encode such a superantigen *(53)*. Whatever the role of the HERV in IMD pathogenesis, the factors that may lead to its expression are still undefined.

Conclusion

No environmental event has been unambiguously implicated as a trigger or precipitator of diabetes. Conversely, some environmental events could prevent rather than induce the disease. In the rodent models of the disease, a number of environmental events are clearly protective. The incidence rates in humans are the highest in the most fastidious Western countries and lowest in the developing world which tends to have lower hygiene standards. Several models, which are not necessarily mutually exclusive, may account for the influence of environmental events. Genetic susceptibility may confer a obligatory risk for the disease, which occurs only if specific environmental events are manifest at a precise time point. Alternatively, genetic susceptibility may confer a naturally very high risk for the disease, whereas most of the environmental events, such as nonspecific infections, could protect from the disease by modulating the immune system through promoting enhanced immunological tolerance to self.

AUTOIMMUNITY: ISLET CELL INFILTRATION AND DESTRUCTION

Immunological Analysis in Humans

Several β-cell autoantigens targeted by the immune process have been described. Studies first relied on the detection of reactive islet cell autoantibodies (ICA) in newly diabetic subjects. Islet cell autoantibodies (ICA) are detected by indirect immunofluorescence staining of frozen sections of human blood group "O" pancreas *(9)* in 70–80% of new onset IMD patients *(4,69,70)*. Results are expressed in JDF units using the international JDF reference serum *(71)*. Insulin autoantibodies (IAA) were subsequently discovered *(10)*. More recently, a series of islet cell proteins has been identified as targeted by the ICA in the disease, usually by immunoprecipitating them from islet lysates or by screening expression libraries with diabetic sera. These antibodies accompany the insulitis and appear several months, or years, before overt diabetes appears. Studies in children of diabetic mothers or fathers showed that autoantibodies appear as soon as the first or second year of life *(8)*. Therefore, their detection was also applied to relatives of diabetic subjects and children in the general population, and demonstrated ability to predict the disease. Although these antibodies are thought to be non-directly pathogenic, and pancreatic β cell destruction to be mainly mediated by T cells, they are likely to be directed against the same antigens as β cell-specific pathogenic T cells, although different epitopes are probably involved. More recently, several studies reported the detection of T cell responses to previously identified islet cell-proteins in persons with or at increased risk for IMD. Finally, the fine characterization of naturally processed T cell epitopes within these β cell antigens is progressing in several laboratories.

Autoantigens in Immune Mediated Diabetes

Autoantigen Targeted Antibodies

Several islet proteins have been identified as autoantigens in the disease. Insulin is targeted by insulin autoantibodies (IAA), usually determined by radioimmunoassay. They are detected in 30–50% of new onset immune-mediated diabetic patients, and more frequently (about 70%) in children younger than 5 yr *(72,73)*. Proinsulin autoantibodies have been also reported at a somewhat higher prevalence than IAA in new onset IMD subjects *(74)*.

Two proteins of the pancreatic β cell, glutamate decarboxylase GAD_{65} *(75–77)* and tyrosine phosphatase IA-2 *(78–82)*, are major autoantigens of β-cell that account for much of the reactivity of ICA *(79,83,84)*. Glutamate decarboxylase is a protein with two isoforms of molecular weight 65 and 67 kDa, located in islets and brain. GAD_{65}, encoded by a gene located on chromosome 10p11.2-p12, is the predominant form found in human islets *(85)*. GAD catalyses the formation of the inhibitory neurotransmitter GABA from glutamine. Within the islet, GAD may have a role in the inhibition of somatostatin and glucagon secretion, as well as regulating proinsulin biosynthesis and insulin secretion. GAD antibodies, best determined by radiobinding assay *(86)*, are detected in 70–80% of new onset IMD patients *(87)*. IA-2 and a separate but structurally homologous IA-2β antigen are both members of the transmembrane protein tyrosine phosphatase family, encoded by genes located on chromosomes 2q35 and 7q36, respectively (78–80,82,88). Both molecules are expressed in islet cells and brain tissue, and in cells of the neuroendocrine system (89). Their biological roles in islets are currently unknown, but they probably behave as receptors for an as yet unknown ligand. The intra cellular domains of IA-2 and IA-2β share 74% homology and carry virtually all of the epitopes targeted by autoantibodies (90). IA-2 and IA-2β autoantibodies are detected in about 70 and 45% of new onset IMD patients, respectively (79,81).

Several other β cell autoantigens have been reported inconsistently. These include carboxypeptidase H (91), a 52 kDa protein with homology to Rubella virus capsid protein (92), a 69 kDa protein with homology to bovine serum albumin (93,94), pancreatic glucose transporter GLUT-2 (95), a sialoglycolipid termed GM– ganglioside (96,97), and a membrane glycoprotein named Glima 38 (98). They are targeted by autoantibodies, although the prevalence of those in large-scale studies remains to be determined.

The detection of ICA, IAA, anti GAD_{65}, and anti IA2/IA-2β allow for the prediction of the disease in first degree relatives of diabetic probands, and also in children in the general population (4,99–104). They are detected in 2–4% of first degree relatives. The 5-yr risk for those with ICA-positive at titers ≥20 JDF U is about 40–50% (4,105,106). Risk factors for the development of IMD in ICA-positive relatives include younger age (107) and higher titers of ICA (108). Relatives positive for ICA (≥10 JDF U) and <10 yr old, or those with titers more than 40 JDF U, have a near 80% risk of contracting diabetes in the following 5 yr. The combined detection of antibodies, however, greatly improves their positive predictive values. The 5-yr risk of developing diabetes in first degree relatives rises to near 80–100% when three autoantibodies are identified (among ICA ≥10 JDF U, IAA, GAD_{65} or IA-2 antibodies) (105,106,109). The higher the titers of ICA, the more likely it is that these additional antibodies are present.

In the general school age population, ICA were found in 0.59–4% of children, higher than the expected prevalence of diabetes (110–118). However, children with high ICA titers usually also carry the predisposing HLA class II susceptibility alleles DR3/DQB1*0201 and/or DR4/DQB1*0302 haplotypes, and have been proven to be at high risk of developing diabetes. The 7-yr estimated risk of developing diabetes in ICA-positive (≥10 JDF U) children has been found to be 45%, which is as high as that in ICA-positive first degree relatives (110). Determination of additional immune markers greatly improve the prediction. Detection of at least two markers selected from GAD antibodies, IA-2, and/or ICA could give an estimated risk of about 70% (117,119,120). Conversely, those with ICA alone, especially if at low titers, have little risk of IMD over time. In these instances, the antigen that is reactive to ICA has not been identified.

T CELL REACTIVITY AGAINST AUTOANTIGENS

Since pancreatic β cells are thought to be destroyed by CD4+ and CD8+ T cells, T cell responses to islet cell-proteins were also looked for and detected in persons with or at increased risk for IMD. Evaluation of T cell autoreactivity is hampered by several factors. The precursor frequency of autoreactive T cells in peripheral blood is low, the presence of multiple HLA molecules in each individual makes the determination of MHC restriction elements difficult, T cell responses may be dependent on the disease stage, and T cell assays are not standardized (121).

Peripheral blood mononuclear cells have been found to have proliferative responses to islet cell extracts (122), insulin-secretory granules (123,124), GAD_{65} (125,126), insulin *(127)*, IA-2 *(128)*, the 69 kDa protein *(129)* and a 38 kDa islet autoantigen named Imogen 38 *(130)*. T cell responses to GAD_{65} peptides *(51,131–133)*, and to proinsulin peptides *(134)* have also been studied in order to determine immunodominant epitopes. To date, three independent studies have established that human GAD_{65} 270–285 peptide is a naturally processed T cell epitope that is presented in the context of HLA-DR 0401 molecules *(131,135,136)*.

It is believed that the autoimmune responses initially target few autoantigenic determinants, but they subsequently spread to a number of epitopes within a single antigen and to other autoantigens as well. However, the inciting antigen remains unidentified. One population study being conducted by Simell in Finland suggests that at the antibody level at least, initial autoimmunity appears to involve any of the above defined antigens.

Properties of T Cells from Diabetic Subjects

The primary abnormalities in the immune system that allow for the development of autoimmunity and IMD are largely unknown. CD4+ T cells are divided into Th1 and Th2 polarized subsets, whose functional properties are different. Th1 cells promote inflammatory cellular immune responses (delayed hypersensitivity) and secrete interferon-γ (IFN-γ) and IL-2. Th2 cells inhibit Th1 responses, induce humoral immunity, and secrete the interleukins IL-4, IL-5, IL-6, and IL-10 *(137)*. Lymphocyte cytokines in the development of IMD type 1 exhibits a bias toward the Th1 cytokine IFN-γ, but the cellular mechanisms that drive to Th1 or Th2 cell differentiation are poorly understood *(138)*. Furthermore, autoreactive T cells and autoantibodies in first degree relatives or identical twins who do not develop diabetes have also been only occasionally detected, suggesting that progression to disease is linked to changes within the autoreactive T cells. For instance, the HLA allele DQB–602 is associated with dominant protection from diabetes in ICA positive first degree relatives of patients with type 1 diabetes *(139)*. Quantitative and qualitative differences in a small "regulatory" subset of T cells between diabetic subjects and non progressor siblings or normal controls have been recently shown. Diabetic subjects had a lower percentage of circulating CD4- CD8- Vα24JαQ+ T cells than non progressor siblings and normal controls. Furthermore, CD4- CD8- Vα24JαQ+ T cell clones raised from these diabetic patients secreted only IFN-γ on stimulation, a cytokine associated with Th1 type inflammatory cellular immune responses. Conversely, similar T cell clones raised from at-risk nonprogressor or normal controls secreted both IFN-γ and IL-4, with IL-4 being a cytokine-inhibiting inflammatory cellular immune responses. This result supports a model in which T cell-mediated damage is initially regulated by Vα24JαQ T cells producing both cytokines, whereas the loss of their capacity to secrete IL-4 correlates with diabetes progression, and persistence of IL-4 secretion by these cells gives protection from the disease *(140)*.

Pathogenesis of Immune Mediated Diabetes from Animal Models

IMMUNOLOGICAL ANALYSIS IN ANIMALS

Animal studies have provided much of the knowledge of the pathogenesis of diabetes. The major models of genetically susceptible animals, the nonobese diabetic (NOD) mouse *(141)* and the Bio Breeding (BB) rat *(142)*, are close to human IMD disease, and thus have been much studied. Spontaneous immune-mediated diabetes usually develops between 3 and 6 mo in 70–90% of NOD female mice, and from about 4 mo in BB rats,

preceded by pancreatic β-cell inflammation (insulitis). In these animals, diabetes susceptibility is closely dependent on the MHC locus, and β-cell destruction is mediated by T
cells. These models allowed defining the natural history of the islet infiltrate and β cell
destruction, and the immune dysregulation underlying the process. T cell clones have been
derived from spleen, lymph nodes, and pancreatic infiltrates of NOD mice and are currently
in use for studying the respective roles of CD4+ and CD8+ T cell subsets, the antigenic
peptide specificities, and the mechanisms for autoimmunity development and β-cell
destruction *(143,144)*. Finally, animal models provide means for genetic (transgenic animals) and immunological manipulations that are unavailable in humans, and for evaluation
of various immunointervention procedure.

Several steps in immune recognition may be possibly involved in the development of
autoimmunity targeted to pancreatic β cells. Several inherent defects in the regulatory
immune responses have been described. However, whether these abnormalities are primary events driving the autoimmune process, or only reflect this process, remains to be
fully determined (Tables 5 and 6).

THYMUS DEFECT

Positive thymic selection of autoreactive T cells is a prerequisite for the development of diabetes. Immune manipulations involving the thymus in animals altered the
occurrence of the disease, asserting the role of the thymus in the autoimmune process
(145–149) (Table 6). The immune system has to discriminate between self and nonself, in order to eliminate non-self agents, such as infecting virus or bacteria, without
damage to self. The ontogeny of the immune system is a complex process involving
negative selection of T cells by the thymus, leading to the deletion of strongly
autoreactive T cells but persistance of only weakly or non-autoreactive T cells. Negative thymic selection depends on the efficient presentation of autoantigens in the thymus. However, the process is never absolute. Accordingly, even in normal persons,
some autoreactive T cells persist that are actively suppressed by peripheral immunoregulatory mechanisms. A large range of T cell specificities is required to combat most
of the nonself agents. The imbalance between allo-immune and autoimmune responses
may be genetically determined, with a propensity to autoimmunity appearing as a cost
of a strongly efficient immune system.

T CELL RESPONSES *(150–211)*

Respective Contribution of CD4+ and CD8+ T Cells. CD4+ T helper cells and
CD8+T cytotoxic cells are consistently present in pancreatic islets, although the respective contribution of each subtype is incompletely defined (Table 6). Activated CD4+ T
cells alone can destroy pancreatic β cells in the absence of CD8+ T cells *(200,201)*.
Conversely, CD8+T cells can not induce insulitis and diabetes by themselves in most of
the cases, as they are largely dependent on activated CD4+ T cells for the effects *(202,203)*.
Corecruitment of autoreactive CD4+ and CD8+ T cells into pancreatic islets appeared to
optimally lead to insulitis and diabetes, with a pre-eminent role for CD4+ T cells. However, some CD8+ T cells could be mandatory to initiate the lesions, but not as the insulitis
becomes established.

Defect in Activation/Regulation of T Cells. Optimal T cell activation requires signaling through the TCR-MHC II peptide complex as well as through the costimulatory
pathway. The latter involves interaction of constitutively expressed CD28 on T cells with

Table 5

Immune Manipulations Leading to Prevention or Acceleration of the Disease:
Insights into Pathogenesis of Diabetes (NOD Mice)

Immune manipulation	Interpretation
Thymus : selection of cells Neonatal thymectomy (145) : prevention Thymectomy at 3 weeks (146) : acceleration Intrathymic islet grafting (147) : prevention Transgenic mice expressing: -Proinsulin II in MHC class II cells (148) : prevention Thymus engraftment from NOD mice embryos to non diabetic prone newborn mice (149): insulitis -no diabetes	**Abnormal thymic selection = persistence of autoreactive T cells** -Interferes with thymic selection process -Tolerizes to islet (clonal deletion of autoreactive T cells or anergy) -Tolerizes to proinsulin (deletion of autoreactive T cells) Abnormal T cell repertoire selection by the NOD thymic epithelium induces autoimmunity.

Presentation of antigens
 	
Transgenic NOD mice expressing:
   MHC class II # from NOD (150) : prevention
 	
Monoclonal antibodies anti class II (151) : prevention
Administration of MHC class II binding peptides (152, 153)
 	
Transgenic NOD mice lacking:
   MHC class I (154): prevention
Monoclonal antibodies anti class I (155) : prevention
 	
Transfert of dendritic cells (156): prevention
 	
Transgenic NOD mice expressing MHC class II # from NOD together with diabetogenic Tcell receptor (TCR) on all CD4+T cells (157): prevention
	Interfering with antigen presentation prevents diabetes
	
	- MHC class II # from NOD provide dominant protection
	
	-Antigen presentation by MHC II to CD4+ T plays a role in pathogenesis
	
	-Antigen presentation by MHC I to CD8+ T plays a role in pathogenesis
	
	Dominant protection provided by MHC class II # from NOD is mediated by negative thymic selection of diabetogenic T cells or positive selection of T cells with modulating capabilities.

Recognition of antigens by T-cells Monoclonal antibodies anti CD3 (158), anti CD4 (159), anti CD8 (160), anti TCR (161) : prevention	**Interfering with antigen recognition by CD4+ and CD8+ T cells prevents diabetes**
Activation of T-cells Administration of Cyclosporin (162), Rapamycin, FK 506, anti lymphocyte serum (163), anti IL-2-R (164): prevention	**Interfering with T-cell activation prevents diabetes**
Monoclonal antibodies anti CD28, anti B7-2 (165): prevention Monoclonal antibodies anti B7-1 (165) : acceleration	**Interfering with T-cell co-stimulatory molecules prevents or accelerates diabetes**

its ligands B 7.1 and B 7.2 expressed on antigen-presenting cells. Interactions with the costimulatory pathway are important to the course of the insulitis and the disease, asserting the importance of this pathway in the pathogenic process *(165,179)*. It is interesting in this respect that the locus of the inducible CTLA4 gene, which is related to CD28, is associated with diabetes susceptibility in humans. In an active immune response, devel-

Table 6
Immune Manipulations Leading to Prevention or Acceleration of the Disease: Insights into Pathogenesis of Diabetes (NOD or NOD/Scid Mice)

Immune manipulation	Interpretation
Modification of Th1/Th2 imbalance (166)	**Th1 response accelerates diabetes** **Th2 response prevents diabetes**

Transgenic mice expressing:
   -Pancreatic IL 4 (167) : prevention
   -Pancreatic IL-10 (168): acceleration
	Cytokine promoting Th2 responses

-TNFα (169) : prevention -interferon γ (170): acceleration Antibodies anti γ interferon (171) anti TNFα (172) : prevention Administration of IL-12 (dendritic cell cytokine, 173): acceleration Administration of IL-2 (174), IL-4 (175), IL-10 (176) : prevention Administration of IL-1 (177), TNFα (178) : prevention	Cytokine promoting Th1 responses Target cytokines promoting Th1 responses
Stimulation of CD28 costimulatory receptors (179): prevention Administration of BCG (180) : prevention Administration of Vitamine D3 and analogs : prevention Antigen-specific immunotherapies: prevention (181)	↑ IL-4 production : Th2 responses Promoting Th2 responses Promoting Th2 responses **Promoting Th2 responses**
Administration of insulin, insulin B-chain, Insulin B: 9-23, GAD65, GAD 67, GAD peptides, Hsp65, Hsp65 peptides, Glucagon (182-199)	

Transfer of particular T-cells
   CD4+ T cells (200) or CD4+ T cells clones (201): acceleration
   CD8+ Tcells clones (202, 203): no effect or acceleration
   Th1 cells expressing a diabetogenic TCR (204): acceleration
   Th2 cells expressing a diabetogenic TCR (204): insulitis-no diabetes
	β-cell destruction mediated by CD4
	 β-cell destruction mediated by CD8
	 β-cell destruction mediated by Th1

Th2 cells to NOD/scid (205) : induction
   GAD-reactive CD4+Th1 cells obtained after GAD immunization (206): induction
   CD4 T cells (207, 208) : prevention
	Some Th2 cells can be harmful
	 Immunization may sometime promote diabetogenic Th1 responses
	 Some CD4 cells can be protective

Modification of cell migration Antibodies anti L-selectin, anti integrin α4 (209), anti ICAM-1 (210) : prevention	Interfering with homing to the pancreas prevents diabetes
Modification of effector cells Transgenic mice lacking: -Perforin (211) : prevention	β-cell destruction is mediated by perforin-dependent cytotoxicity
Modifications of target cells β cells deprivation-partial pancreatectomy (212): prevention	-Target cells are required for autoimmunity
Administration of Somatostatin (213)Diazoxide (214) : prevention	-Decreasing β-cell antigens exposure prevents diabetes?
Transgenic mice expressing: -pancreatic Fas ligand (215): acceleration	-β-cell destruction is mediated by Fas-Fas ligand interaction (apoptosis)

opment of expressed CTLA4 acts to inhibit or control the immune response. Thus, loss of this function would promote poorly controlled hyperimmune responsiveness and thereby autoimmunity. This has in fact been demonstrated in CTLA-4 gene knockout mice.

Defect in the Th1/Th2 Imbalance. It is generally recognized that the effector cells of diabetes are CD4+Th1 cells that secrete IL-2, IFN-γ, TNFα, and that the regulatory cells of importance in this process are CD4+Th2 cells that secrete IL-4, IL-5, IL-6, and IL-10 *(166)*. The functional imbalance between the two Th cell subsets, including an hyporesponsiveness of regulatory Th2 cells, may be a key determinant in pathogenesis. Many immune manipulations promoting Th1 activity induced or accelerated diabetes, whereas those promoting Th2 activity prevented the disease in mice *(167–199)*.

However, to view the regulation of the disease process strictly in terms of imbalance between Th1 and Th2 subsets is probably an oversimplification even in mice. The role of certain cytokines in diabetes pathogenesis is uncertain. IL-1, TNFα, and IL-10 may prevent or accelerate the disease *(168,169,176,178)*. Further, some Th1 autoreactive T cell clones have been established from NOD mice that can actually suppress diabetes *(207,208)*. Conversely, some Th2 cell lines failed to mitigate Th1-mediated target tissue destruction in adoptive transfer experiments in NOD mice *(204)*. Moreover, Th2 cells transfer in immunocompromised NOD.scid mice induced diabetes, suggesting that some Th2 cells may have deleterious rather than protective effects *(206)*. In conclusion, it is likely that pancreatic β cell destruction and T cell suppression of autoimmunity may each involve a more complex interplay between Th1 and Th2 cells than is currently conceived. For example, in humans, Th cells often display both Th1 and Th2 type cytokines.

Modulation of Th1-Th2 Cells Responses and Potential Immunotherapy. Specific antigen/peptides, such as insulin, insulin peptide, or GAD, may be used to induce selective immunomodulation. Antigen-specific tolerance is mediated by clonal anergy, deletion of autoreactive T cells, or induction of regulatory T cells in the periphery. The induction of antigen-specific regulatory Th2 T cells is thought to actively suppress the effects of nearby diabetogenic Th1 T cells through secretion of anti-inflammatory (Th2) cytokines IL-4, IL-10 and TGFb. The suppressive effect of the regulatory T cells is termed "antigen-driven bystander suppression" and has been said to be inducible even when the inciting antigen is unknown *(166,181)*. Intravenous, intrathymic, intraperitoneal, or subcutaneous injections of GAD_{65}, or intranasal administration of GAD_{65} peptides prevent diabetes in NOD mice *(191–196)*. Administration of subcutaneous insulin, subcutaneous immunization with metabolically inactive insulin B-chain, peptide B9–23, or B8–18, oral administration of insulin or insulin peptides, or intranasal administration of insulin peptide B9–23 protected NOD mice from diabetes *(182–189)*. The B9–23 peptide acts as a dominant epitope among insulin-specific CD4+ T cells isolated from islets of NOD mice. However, it is unclear whether it associates with class II molecule through the peptide-binding groove, or through a site outside the peptide-binding-groove of the MHC class II molecule, acting as a superantigen, as this peptide binds with all murine and probably most if not all human MHC class II molecules *(190)*.

However, the effects of antigen specific immunotherapies were not always consistent. Intrathymic administration of some GAD_{65} peptides actually accelerated diabetes onset in NOD mice *(196)*, while immunization of NOD mice by GAD_{65} could generate GAD-reactive CD4+ Th1 cells that could induce diabetes *(205)*.

DEFECT IN THE TARGET CELLS

The autoimmune response underlying IMD is antigen driven. T cells from NOD mice in which the pancreatic β cells have been ablated at an early age are no longer able to induce diabetes in adoptive T cell transfer experiments *(212)*. Insulin administration, like somatostatin *(213)* or diazoxide *(214)*, prevents diabetes in NOD mice or BB rats, through a putative inhibition of β-cell function and thereby decreased islet antigen expression.

Thus, the β cells with diminished expression of autoantigens may become "immunologically silent" and thus protected from destruction.

In NOD mice, insulin, GAD_{65} and GAD_{67} are the first known antigens toward which T cell reactivity is detectable *(191,192,217)*. Only a few antigens are targeted in the early stages. Subsequent autoreactivity develops to a number of epitopes within a single antigen and to other autoantigens *(218)*. Distinguishing antigens that play a primary role in initiating the autoimmune process from secondary antigens has not yet been achieved in the animal models or in humans. Apoptosis may be the major mechanism of destruction of pancreatic β cells *(219)*.

ALTERATION OF INSULIN SECRETION AND DIABETES

As a result of the autoimmunity, β cell function eventually becomes lost. Whereas the lymphocytic infiltration of the pancreas begins several years before the diagnosis of diabetes, the β cell destruction may not occur in parallel to the infiltration and could be a relatively late event in the process.

Insulin secretion has been evaluated at the prediabetic stage and at the onset of diabetes by iv glucose tolerance tests *(220)*. First phase insulin secretion (1+3 minute insulin level, FPIR) is extremely low in new onset IMD. In first degree relatives, low first phase insulin secretion, together with ICA positivity, is associated with a 70–90% risk of progressing toward diabetes in the next 3–5 yr *(221)*. In ICA-negative relatives who do not progress toward diabetes, FPIR has also been reported to be significantly lower than in normal children. If so, this could be related to a genetic defect of pancreatic β-cells, independent of the autoimmune process *(222)*.

CONCLUSION

Immune mediated (type I) diabetes is a complex but serious disease. Multiple genetic defects of immune regulation to self have been recognized as relevant to the pathogenesis. Natural history studies have indicated that pancreatic β cell autoimmunity begins in early life and despite the importance of class II MHC alleles to inherited susceptibility no one initiator or inductive self-antigen has been identified. The inductive events we believed are probably viral, although this contention remains unproved. Once established, islet cell autoimmunity progresses in a crescending manner, with induction of massive β cell apoptosis as a final step. Progression to diabetes depends on lack of IL-4 production from peripheral regulatory T cells (CD4- CD8- Vα24JαQ T cells), and is accompanied by determinant spreading of the underlying autoimmunity process. At least in mice, Th1 cells have been identified to be causal, whereas induction of the Th2 polarized subset directed to the same antigens are most often associated with protective responses. This and possibly other regulatory and protective mechanisms can be induced by a variety of interventions, especially variants of islet antigen administration. Of these, we are most interested in the potential of immunization by B chain 8–18 peptide as holding promise for human trials in the near future.

ACKNOWLEDGMENTS

Regis Coutant is supported by a fellowship from the Fondation pour la Recherche Medicale.

REFERENCES

1. Atkinson MA, Maclaren MK, The pathogenesis of insulin-dependent diabetes. N Engl J Med 1994;331:1428–1436.
2. Gepts W, DeMey J, Islet cell survival determined by morphology. An immunocytochemical study of the islets of Langerhans in juvenile diabetes mellitus. Diabetes 1978;27(suppl 1):251–261.
3. Foulis AK, Liddle CN, Farquharson MA, Richmond JA, Weir RS. The histopathology of the pancreas in type-1 (insulin-dependent) diabetes mellitus: a 25-year review of deaths in patients under 20 years of age in the United Kingdom. Diabetologia 1986;29:267–274.
4. Riley WJ, Maclaren NK, Krisher J, et al. A prospective study of the development of diabetes in relatives of patients with insulin-dependent diabetes. N Engl J Med 1990;323:116–172.
5. Tarn AC, Smith CP; Spencer KM; Bottazzo GF; Gale EA Type I (insulin dependent) diabetes: a disease of slow clinical onset? Br Med J 1987;294:342–345.
6. Srikanta S, Ganda OP, Soeldner JS, Eisenbarth GS. First degree relatives of patients with type I diabetes mellitus:islet cell antibodies and abnormal insulin secretion. N Engl J Med 1985;313: 461–464.
7. Ziegler AG, Hillebrand B; Rabl W, et al. On the appearance of islet associated autoimmunity in offspring of diabetic mothers: a prospective study from birth. Diabetologia 1993;36:402–408.
8. Roll U, Christie MR, Fuchtenbusch M, Payton MA, Hawkes CJ, Ziegler AG.Perinatal autoimmunity in offspring of diabetic parent: the German multi-center BABY-DIAB study: detection of humoral immune responses to islet antigens in early childhood. Diabetes 1996;45:967–973.
9. Bottazzo GF, Florin-Christensen A, Doniach D. Islet-cell antibodies in diabetes mellitus with autoimmune polyendocrine deficiencies. Lancet 1974 2:1279–1283.
10. Palmer JP, Asplin CM, Clemons P, et al. Insulin antibodies in insulin-dependent diabetics before insulin treatment. Science 1983;22:1337–1339.
11. Wagener DK, Sacks JM, LaPorte RE, Macgregor JM. The Pittsburgh study of insulin-dependent diabetes mellitus. Risk for diabetes among relatives of IDDM. Diabetes 1982;31:136–144.
12. Hashimoto L, Habita C, Beressi JP, et al. Genetic mapping of a susceptibility locus for insulin-dependent diabetes mellitus on chromosome 11q. Nature 1994;371:161–164.
13. Davies JL, Kawaguchi Y, Bennettt ST, et al. A genome wide search for human type 1 diabetes susceptibility genes. Nature 1994;371:130–136.
14. Karvonen M, Tuomilehto J, Libman I, LaPorte R. A review of the recent epidemiological data on the worldwide incidence of type 1 (insulin-dependent) diabetes. Diabetologia 1993;36:883–892.
15. Barnett AH, Eff C, Leslie RD, Pyke DA . Diabetes in identical twins. A study of 200 pairs. Diabetologia 1981;20:87–93.
16. Kyvik KO, Green A, Beck-Nielsen H. Concordance rates of insulin dependent diabetes mellitus: a population based study of young Danish twins. Br Med J 1995;311:913–917.
17. Chern MM, Anderson VE, Barbosa J. Empirical risk for insulin-dependent diabetes (IDD) in sibs. Further definition of genetic heterogeneity. Diabetes 1982;31:1111–1118.
18. Borch-Johnson K, Joner G, Mandrup-poulsen T, Christy M, Zachau-Christiansen B, Kastrup K, Nerup J. Relation between breast-feeding, incidence rates of insulin-dependent diabetes mellitus. Lancet 1984;2:1083–1086.
19. Warram JH, Krolewski AS, Gottlieb MS, Kahn CR. Differences in risk of insulin-dependent diabetes in offspring of diabeteic mothers and diabetic fathers. N Engl J Med 1984;311:14–52.
20. Thomson G, Robinson WP, Kuhner MK, et al. Genetic heterogeneity, modes of inheritance, and risk estimates for a joint study of caucasians with insulin-dependent diabetes mellitus. Am J Hum Genet 1988;43:799–816.
21. Baisch JM, Weeks T, Giles R, Hoover M, Stastny P, Capra JD. Analysis of HLA-DQ genotypes and susceptibility in insulin-dependent diabetes mellitus. N Engl J Med 1990;322:1836–1841.
22. Owerbach D, Lernmark A, Platz P, Ryder LP, Rask L, Peterson PA, Ludvigsson J. HLA-D region beta-chain DNA endonuclease fragments differ between HLA-DR identical healthy and insulin-dependent diabetic individuals. Nature 1983;303:815–817.
23. Todd JA, Bell JI, McDevitt HO. HLA-DQ beta gene contributes to susceptibility and resistance to insulin-dependent diabetes mellitus. Nature 1987;329:599–604.
24. She JX. Susceptibility to type I diabetes: HLA-DQ and DR revisited. Immunol Today 1996;17:323–329.
25. Nepom GT. A unified hypothsesis for the complex genetics of HLA association with IDDM. Diabetes 1990;39:1153–1157.

26. Sheehy MJ. HLA and insulin-dependent diabetes: a protective perspective. Diabetes 1992;41:123–129.

27. Nepom BS, Schwarz D, Palmer JP, Nepom GT. Transcomplementation of HLA genes in IDDM. HLA-DQ alpha- and beta-chains produce hybrid molecules in DR3/4 heterozygotes. Diabetes 1987;36:114–117.

28. Moghaddam PH, Zwinderman AH, de Knijff P, et al. TNFa microsatellite polymorphism modulates the risk of IDDM in caucasians with the high-risk genotype HLA DQA1 0501-DQB1 0201/DQA1 0301-DQB1 0302. Diabetes 1997;46:1514,1515.

29. Caillat-Zucman S, garchon HJ, Timsit J, Assan R, Boitard C, Djilali-Saiah I, Bougneres P, Bach JF. Age-dependent HLA genetic heterogeneity of type 1 insulin-dependent diabetes mellitus. J Clin Invest 1992;90:2242–2250.

30. Hagopian WA, Sanjeevi CB, Kockum I, et al. Glutamate decarboxylase-, insulin-, and islet cell-antibodies and HLA typing to detect diabetes in a general population-based study of swedish children. J Clin Invest 1995;95:1505–1511.

31. Rewers M, Bugawan TL, Norris JM, et al. Newborn screening for HLA markers associated with IDDM: diabetes autoimmunity study in the young (DAISY). Diabetologia 1996;39:807–812.

32. Julier C, Hyer RN, Davies J, Merlin F, Soularue P, Briant L, Cathelineau G, Deschamps I, Rotter JI, Froguel P, Boitard C, Bell JI, Lathrop GM. Insulin-IGF2 region on chromosome 11p encodes a gene implicated in HLA-DR4-dependent diabetes susceptibility. Nature 1991;354:155–159.

33. Bennett ST, Lucassen AM, Gough SCL, et al. Susceptibility to human type 1 diabetes at IDDM2 is determined by tandem repeat variation at the insulin gene minisatellite locus. Nat Genet 1995;9:284–292.

34. Lucassen AM, Julier C, Beressi JP, Boitard C, Froguel P, Lathrop M, Bell JI. Susceptibility to insulin dependent diabetes mellitus maps to a 4.1 kb segment of DNA spanning the insulin gene and associated VNTR. Nat Genet 1993;4:305–310.

35. Kennedy GC, German MS, Rutter WJ The minisatellite in the diabetes susceptibility locus IDDM2 regulates insulin transcription. Nat Genet 1995;9:293.

36. Lucassen AM, Screaton GR, Julier C, Elliottt TJ, Lathrop M, Bell JI. Regulation of insulin gene expression by the IDDM associated insulin locus haplotype. Hum Mol Genet 1995;4:501–506.

37. Vafiadis P, Bennett ST, Todd JA, et al. Insulin expression in human thymus is modulated by INS VNTR alleles at the IDDM2 locus. Nat Genet 1997;15:289–292.

38. Pugliese A, Zeller M, Fernandez Jr A, et al. The insulin gene is transcribed in the human thymus and transcription levels corrrelate with allelic variation at the INS VNTR-IDDM2 susceptibility locus for type 1 diabetes. Nat Genet 1997;15:293–297.

39. Bennett ST, Wilson AJ, Esposito L, Bouzekri N, Undlien DE, Cucca F, Nistico L, Buzzetti R, Bosi E, Pociot F, Nerup J, Cambon-Thomsen A, Pugliese A, Shield JP, McKinney PA, Bain SC, Polychronakos C, Todd JA. Insulin VNTR allele-specific effect in type 1 diabetes depends on identity of untransmitted paternal allele. The IMDIAB study. Nat Genet 1997;17:350–352.

40. Nistico L, Buzzetti R, Pritchard LE, et al. The CTLA4 gene region of chromosome 2q33 is linked to, and associated with, type I diabetes. Hum Mol Genet 1996;5:1075–1080.

41. Marron MP, Raffel LJ, Garchon HJ, et al. Insulin-dependent diabetes mellitus (IDDM) is associated with CTLA4 polymorphisms in multiple ethnic groups. Hum Mol Genet 1997;6:1275–1285.

42. Luo DF, Buzzetti R, Rotter JI, et al. Confirmation of three susceptibility genes to insulin-dependent diabetes mellitus: IDDM4, IDDM5, and IDDM8. Hum Mol Genet 1996;5:693–698.

43. Copeman JB, Cucca F, Hearne CM, et al. Linkage disequilibrium mapping of a type I diabetes susceptibility gene (IDDM7) to chromosome 2q3–3. Nat Genet 1995;9:80–85.

44. Merriman T, Twells R, Merriman M, et al. Evidence by allelic association-dependent methods for a type 1 diabetes polygene (IDDM6) on chromosome 18q21. Hum Mol Genet 1997;6:1003–1010.

45. Reed P, Cucca F, Jenkins S, et al. Evidence for a type I diabetes susceptibility locus (IDDM10) on human chromosome 10p11-q11. Hum Mol Genet 1997;6:1011–1016.

46. Field LL, Tobias R, Magnus T. A locus on chromosome 15q26 (IDDM3) produces susceptibility to insulin-dependent diabetes mellitus. Nature Genet 1995;8:189–194.

47. Davies LD, Cucca F, Goy JV, et al. Saturation multipoint linkage mapping of chromosome 6q in type 1 diabetes. Hum Mol Genet 1996;5:1071–1074.

48. Field LL, Tobias R, Thomson G, Plon S. Susceptibility to insulin-dependent diabetes mellitus maps to a locus (IDDM11) on human chromosome 14q24.3-q31. Genomics 1996;33:1–8.

49. Moharan G, Huang D, Tait BD, Colman PG, Harrison LC. Markers on distal chromosome 2q linked to insulin-dependent diabetes mellitus. Science 1996;272:1811–1813.

50. Delepine M, Pociot F, Habita C, et al. Evidence for a non-MHC susceptibility locus in type 1 diabetes linked to HLA on chromosome 6. Am J Hum Genet 1997;60:174–187.

51. Atkinson MA, Bowman MA, Campbell L, Darrow BL, Kaufman DL, Maclaren NK. Cellular immunity to a determinant common to glutamate decarboxylase, coxsackie virus in insulin-dependent diabetes. J Clin Invest 1994;94:2125–2129.
52. Patterson K, Chandra RS, Jenson AB. Congenital rubella, insulitis, and diabetes mellitus in an infant. Lancet 1981;i:1048, 1049.
53. Conrad B, Weissmahr RN, Boni Jurg, Arcari R, Schupbach J, Mach B. A human endogenous retroviral superantigen as candidate autoimmune gene in type I diabetes. Cell 1997;90:303–313.
54. Gamble DR, Kinsley ML, Fitzgerald MG, Bolton R, Taylor KW. Viral antibodies in diabetes mellitus. Br Med J 1969;3:627–630.
55. Banatvala JE, Bryant J, Schernthauer G, Borkenstein M, Schober E, Brown D, De Silva LM, Menser MA, Silink M. Coxsackie B, mumps, rubella, and cytomegalovirus specific IgM responses in patients with juvenile-onset insulin-dependent diabetes mellitus in Britain, Austria, and Australia. Lancet 1985;1:1409–1412.
56. Dahlquist GG, Ivarsson S, Lindberg B, Forsgren M. Maternal enteroviral infection during pregnancy as a risk factor for childhood IDDM. A population-based case-control study. Diabetes 1995;44:408–413.
57. Pagano G, Cavallo-perin P, Cavalot F, Dall'omo AM, Masciola P, Suriani R, Amoroso A, Curtoni SE, Borelli I, Lenti G. genetic, immunologic, and environmental heterogeneity of IDDM. Incidence and 12-mo follow-up of an Italian population. Diabetes 1987;36:859–863.
58. Yoon JW, Austin M, Onodera T, Notkins AL. Isolation of a virus from the pancreas of a child with diabetic ketoacidosis. N Engl J Med 1979;300:1173–1179.
59. Champsaur HF, Botazzo GF, Bertrans J, Assan R, Bach C. Virologic, immunologic, and genetic factors in insulin-dependent diabetes mellitus. J Pediatr 1982;100:15–20.
60. Clements GB, Galbraith DN, Taylor KW. Coxsackie B virus infection and onset of childhood diabetes. Lancet 1995;346: 221–223.
61. Borsch-Johnsen K, Mandrup-Poulsen T, Zachau-Christiansen B, Joner G, Christy M, Kastrup K, Nerup J. Relation between breast-feeding and incidence of IDDM. Lancet 1984;2:1083–1086.
62. Virtanen SM, Rasanen L, Ylonen K, et al. Early introduction of dairy products associated with increased risk of IDDM in Finnish children. Diabetes 1993;42:1786–1790.
63. Kostraba JN, Cruickhanks KJ, Lawler-Heavner J, et al. Early exposure to cow's milk, solid foods in infancy genetic predisposition, risk of IDDM. Diabetes 1993;42:288–295.
64. Karjalainen J, Martin JM, Knip M, et al. A bovine albumin peptide as a possible trigger of insulin-dependent diabetes mellitus. N Engl J Med 1992;327:302–307.
65. Atkinson MA, Bowman MA, Kao KJ, Campbell L, Dush PJ, Shah SC, Simell O, Maclaren NK. Lack of immune responsiveness to bovine serum albumin in insulin-dependent diabetes. N Engl J Med 1993;329:1853–1858.
66. Kaufman DL, Erlander MG, Clare-Salzler M, Atkinson MA, Maclaren NK, Tobin AJ. Autoimmunity to two forms of glutamate decarboxylase in insulin-dependent diabetes mellitus. J Clin Invest 1992;89:283–292.
67. Pietropaolo M, Castano L, Babu S, et al. Islet cell autoantigen 69 kD (ICA 69):molecular cloning and characterization of a novel diabetes-associated autoantigen. J Clin Invest 1993;92:359–371.
68. Karounos DG, Thomas JW. Recognition of common islet antigen by autoantibodies from NOD mice and humans with IDDM. Diabetes 1990;39:1085–1090.
69. Bruining GJ, Molenaar JL, Grobbee DE, et al. Ten-year follow-up study of islet-cell antibodies and childhood diabetes mellitus.Lancet 1989;1:1100–1103.
70. Landin-Olsson M, Karlsson A, Dahlquist G, Blom L, Lernmark A, Sundkvist. Islet cell and other organ-specific autoantibodies in all children developing type 1 (insulin-dependent) diabetes mellitus in Sweden during one year and in matched control children. Diabetologia 1989;32:387–395.
71. Gleichman H, Bottazzo GF. Progress toward standardization of cytoplasmic islet cell-antibody assay. Diabetes 1987;36:578–584.
72. Vardi P, Ziegler AG, Mathews JH, et al. Concentration of insulin autoantibodies at onset of type 1 diabetes: inverse log-linear correlation with age. Diabetes Care 1988;11:736–739.
73. Karjalainen J, Samala P, Ilonen J, Surcel HM, Knip M. A comparison of childhood and adult type I diabetes mellitus. N Engl J Med 1989;320:881–886.
74. Bohmer KH, Keilacker H, Kuglin B, Hübinger A, Bertrams J, Gries FA, Kolb H. Proinsulin autoantibodies are more closely associated with type 1 (insulin-dependent) diabetes mellitus than insulin autoantibodies. Diabetologia 1991;34:830–834.

75. Baekkeskov S, Aanstoot HJ, Christgau S, et al. Identification of the 64 K autoantigen in insulin-dependent diabetes is the GABA-synthesizing enzyme glutamic acid decarboxylase. Nature 1990;347:151–156.
76. Atkinson MA, Maclaren NK, Scharp DW, Lacy PE, Riley WJ. 64 000 Mr autoantibodies are predictive of insulin-dependent diabetes. Lancet 1990;335:1357–1360.
77. Solimena M, Folli F, Aparisi R, Pozzaq G, De Camilli P. Autoantibodies to GABA-ergic neurons and pancreatic beta cells in stiff-man syndrome. N Engl J Med 1990;322:1555–1560.
78. Lan MS, Lu J, Goto Y, Notkins AL. Molecular cloning and identification of a receptor-type protein tyrosine phosphatase IA-2, from human insulinoma. DNA Cell Biol 1994;13:505–514.
79. Lan MS, Wasserfall C, Maclaren NK, Notkins AL. IA-2, a transmembrane protein of the tyrosine phosphatase family, is a major autoantigen in insulin-dependent diabetes mellitus. Proc Natl Acad Sci USA 1996;93:6367–6370.
80. Lu J, Li Q, Xie H, et al. Identification of a second transmembrane protein tyrosine phosphatase, IA-2b, as an autoantigen in insulin-dependent diabetes mellitus: precursor of the 37-kDa tryptic fragment. Proc Natl Acad Sci USA 1996;93:2307–2311.
81. Li Q, Borovitskaya AE, deSilva MG, Wasserfall C, Maclaren NK, Notkins AL, Lan MS. Autoantigens in insulin-dependent diabetes mellitus: molecular cloning and characterization of human IA-2b. Proc Assoc Am Phys 1997;109:429–439.
82. Christie MR, Vohra G, Champagne P, Daneman D, Delovitch TL. Distinct antibody specificities to a 64-kD islet cell antigen in type 1 diabetes as revealed by trypsin treatment. J Exp Med 1990;172: 789–795.
83. Atkinson MA, Kaufman DL, Newman D, Tobin AJ, Maclaren NK. Islet cell cytoplasmic autoantibody reactivity to glutamate decarboxylase in insulin-dependent diabetes. J Clin Invest 1993;91:350–456.
84. Myers MA, Rabin DU, Rowley MJ. Pancreatic islet cell cytoplasmic antibody in diabetes is represented by antibodies to islet cell antigen 512 and glutamic acid decarboxylase. Diabetes 1995;44: 1290–1295.
85. Hagopian WA, Michelsen B, Karlsen AE, et al. Autoantibodies in IDDM primarily recognize the 65 000-Mr rather than the 67 000-Mr isoform glutamic acid decarboxylase. Diabetes 1993;42:631–636.
86. Schmidli RS, Colman PG, Bonifacio E, Participating laboratories. Disease sensitivity, specificity of 52 assays for glutamic acid decarboxylase antibodies. The second international GADAb wokshop. Diabetes 1995;44:636–640.
87. Baekkeskov S, Aanstoot HJ, Christgau S, et al. Identification of the 64 K autoantigen in insulin-dependent diabetes is the GABA-synthesizing enzyme glutamic acid decarboxylase. Nature 1990;347:151–156.
88. Payton MA, Hawkes CJ, Christie MR. Relationship of the 37 000-, 40 000-Mr tryptic fragments of islet antigens in insulin-dependent diabetes to the protein tyrosine phosphatase-like molecule IA-2 (ICA 512). J Clin Invest 1995;96:1506–1511.
89. Xie H, Notkins AL, Lan MS. IA-2, a transmembrane protein tyrosine phosphatase, is expressed in human lung cancer cell lines with neuroendocrine phenotype. Cancer Res 1996;56:2742–2744.
90. Zhang B, Lan MS, Notkins AL. Autoantibodies to IA-2 in IDDM. Location of major antigenic determinants. Diabetes 1997;46:40–43.
91. Castano L, Russo E, Zhou L, Lipes MA, Eisenbarth GS. Identification and cloning of a granule autoantigen (carboxypeptidase-H) associated with type I diabetes. J Clin Endocrinol Metab 1991;73:1197–1201.
92. Karounos DG, Thomas JW. Recognition of common islet antigen by autoantibodies from NOD mice and humans with IDDM. Diabetes 1990;39:1085–1090.
93. Pietropaolo M, Castano L, Babu S, et al. Islet cell autoantigen 69 kD (ICA 69):molecular cloning and characterization of a novel diabetes-associated autoantigen. J Clin Invest 1993;92:359–371.
94. Karjalainen J, Martin JM, Knip M, et al. A bovine albumin peptide as a possible trigger of insulin-dependent diabetes mellitus. N Engl J Med 1992;327:302–307.
95. Johnson TH, Crider BP, McCorkle K, Alford M, Unger RH. Inhibition of glucose transporter into rat islet cells by immunoglobulins from patients with new-onset insulin-dependent diabetes mellitus. N Engl J Med 1990;322:653–659.
96. Colman PJ, Nayak RC, Campbell IL, Eisenbarth GS. Binding of cytoplasmic islet cell antibodies is blocked by human pancreatic glycolipid extracts. Diabetes 1989;37:645–652.
97. Dotta F, Gianani R, Previti M, Lenti L, Dionisi S, D'Erme M, Eisenbarth GS, DiMario U. Autoimmunity to the GM– islet ganglioside before, and at the onset of type I diabetes. Diabetes 1996;45: 1193–1196.

98. Aanstoot HJ, Kang SM, Kim J, et al. Identification and characterization of Glima 38, a glycosylated islet cell membrane antigen, which together with GAD_{65} and IA2 marks the early phases of auto-immune response in type 1 diabetes. J Clin Invest 1996;97:2772–2783.

99. Tarn AC, Thomas JM, Dean BM, Ingram D, Schwartz G, Botazzo GF, Gale EAM. Predicting insulin-dependent diabetes. Lancet 1988;I: 845–850.

100. Ziegler AG, Dumont Herskowitz R, Jackson RA, Soeldner JS, Eisenbarth GS. Predicting type I diabetes. Diabetes Care 1990;13:762–775.

101. McCullough DK, Klaff LJ, Kahn SE, et al. Nonprogression of subclinical b-cell dysfunction among first degree relatives of IDDM patients. 5-yr follow-up of the Seattle family study. Diabetes 1990;39:549–556.

102. Chase HP, Voss MA. Diagnosis of pre type 1 diabetes. J Pediatr 1987;111:807–812.

103. Thivolet C, Beaufrere B, Geburher L, Chatelain P, Orgiazzi J, Francois R. Autoantibodies and genetic factors associated with the development of type I (insulin-dependent) diabetes mellitus in first degree relatives of diabetic patients. Diabetologia 1991;34:186–191.

104. Lesage C, Boitard C, Carel JC, Roger M, Chaussain JL, Bougneres PF. Results of 3 years of screening for preclinical phase of juvenile insulin-dependent diabetes mellitus. Arch Fr Pediatr 1990;47:709–713.

105. Bingley PJ, Christie MR, Bonifacio E, Bonfanti R, Shattock M, Fonte M, Bottazzo G, Gale EAM. Combined analysis of autoantibodies improves prediction of IDDM in islet cell antibody-positive relatives. Diabetes 1994;43:1304–1310.

106. Verge CF, Gianani R, Kawasaki E, Yu L, Pietropaolo M, Jackson RA, Chase HP, Eisenbarth GS. Prediction of type I diabetes in first degree relatives using a combination of insulin, GAD, and ICA512bdc/IA-2 autoantibodies. Diabetes 1996;45:926–933.

107. Cantor AB, Krisher JP, Cuthebertson DD, et al. Age and family relationship accentuate the risk of insulin-dependent diabetes mellitus (IDDM) in relatives of patients with IDDM. J Clin Endocrinol Metab 1995;80:3739–3743.

108. Krischer JP, Schatz D, Riley WJ, et al. Insulin and islet-cell autoantibodies as time dependent covariates in the development of insulin-dependent diabetes: a prospective study in relatives. J Clin Endocrinol Metab 1993;77:743–749.

109. Kulmala P, Savola K, Petersen JS, Vahasalo P, Karjalainen J, Lopponen T, Dyrberg T, Akerblom HK, Knip M, and the Childhood Diabetes in Finland Study Group. Prediction of insulin-dependent diabetes mellitus in siblings of children with diabetes. J Clin Invest 1998;101:327–336.

110. Schatz D, Krisher J, Horne G, Riley W, Spillar R, Silverstein J, Winter W, Muir A, Derovanesian D, Shah S, Malone J, Maclaren N. Islet cell antibodies predict insulin-dependent diabetes in United States school age children as powerfully as in unaffected relatives. J Clin Invest 1994;93:2403–2407.

111. Levy-Marchal C, Dubois F, Noel M, Tichet J, Czernichow P. Immunogentic determinants and prediction of IDDM in French Schoolchildren. Diabetes 1995;44:1029–1032.

112. Landin-Olsson M, Palmer JP, Lernmark A, Blom L, Sundkvist G, Nystrom L, Dahlquist G. Predicitve value of islet cell and insulin autoantibodies for type 1 diabetes mellitus in a population based study of newly diagnosed diabetic and matched control children. Diabetologia 1992;35:1068–1073.

113. Karjalainen JK. Islet cell antibodies as predictive markers for IDDM in children with high background incidence of disease. Diabetes 1990;39:1144–1150.

114. Bingley PJ, Bonifacio E, Gale EAM. Can we really predict IDDM? Diabetes 1993;42:213–220.

115. Boehm BO, Manfras B, Seibler J, et al. Epidemiology and immunogentic background of islet cell antibody-positive nondiabetic schoolchildren. Diabetes 1991;40:1435–1439.

116. Rowe R, Leech N, Nepom G, McCulloch D. High genetic risk for IDDM in the Pacific Northwest-first report from the Washington state diabetes prediction study. Diabetes 1994;43:87–94.

117. Hagopian WA, Sanjeevi CB, Kockum I, et al. Glutamate decarboxylase-, insulin-, and islet cell-antibodies and HLA typing to detect diabetes in a general population-based study of Swedish children. J Clin Invest 1995;95:1505–1511.

118. Bruining GJ, Molenaar JL, Grobbee DE, et al. Ten-year follow-up study of islet-cell antibodies and childhood diabetes mellitus. Lancet 1989;1:1100–1103.

119. Bingley PJ, Bonifacio E, Williams AJK, Genovese S, Bottazzo GF, Gale AM. Prediction of IDDM in the general population. Strategies based on combinations of autoantibody markers. Diabetes 1997;46:1701–1710.

120. Aanstoot HJ, Sigurdsson E, Jaffe M, et al. Value of antibodies to GAD_{65} combined with islet cell cytoplasmic antibodies for predictiong IDDM in a childhood population. Diabetologia 1994;37:917–924.

121. Roep BO, T-cell responses to autoantigens in IDDM. The search for the Holy Grail. Diabetes 1996;45:1147–1156.

122. Harrison LC, De Aizpurua H, Loudovaris T, Campbell IL, Cebon JS, Tait BD, Colman PG: reactivity to human islets and fetal pig proislets by peripheral blood mononuclear cells from subjects with preclinical and clinical insulin-dependent diabetes. Diabetes 1991;40:1128–1133.

123. Roep B, Arden SD, de Vries RR, Hutton JC. T-cell clones from a type-1 diabetes patient respond to insulin secretory granule protein in patients with recent onset type 1 diabetes. Nature 1990;345:632–634.

124. Chang JCC, Linarelli LG, Laxer JA, Froning KJ, Caralli LL, Brostoff SW, Carlo DJ. Insulin-secretory-granule specific T-cells clones in human IDDM. J Autoimmun 1995;8:221–234.

125. Atkinson MA, Kaufman DL, Campbell L, et al. Response of peripheral blood mononuclear cells to glutamate decarboxylase in insulin-dependent diabetes. Lancet 1992;339:458,459.

126. Harrison LC, Honeyman MC, DeAizpurua HJ, et al. Inverse relation between humoral and cellular immunity to glutamic acid decarboxylase in subjects at risk of insulin-dependent diabetes. Lancet 1993;341:1365–1369.

127. Naquet P, Ellis J, Tibensky D, Kenshole A, Singh B, Hodges R, Delovitch TK. T cell autoreactivity to insulin in diabetic and related non-diabetic individuals. J Immunol 1988;140:2566–2578.

128. Ellis T, Schatz D, Lan M, et al. Relationship between humoral and cellular immunity to IA-2 in IDD Diabetes. 1997;46(suppl 1):195A.

129. Roep BO, Duinkerken G, Schreuder GMT, Kolb H, De Vries RRP, Martin S. HLA-associated inverse correlation between T-cell and antibody responsiveness to islet autoantigen in recent-onset insulin dependent diabetes mellitus. Eur J Immunol 1996;26:1285–1289.

130. Arden SD, Roep B, Neophytou PI, Usac EF, Duinkerken G, De Vries RRP, Hutton JC. Imogen 38: a novel 38-kD islet mitochondrial autoantigen recognized by T cells from a newly diagnosed type 1 diabetic patient. J Clin Invest 1996;97:551–561.

131. Endl J, Otto H, Jung G, Dreisbusch B, et al. Identification of naturally processed T cell epitopes from glutamic acid decarboxylase presented in the context of HLA-DR alleles by T lymphocytes of recent onset IDDM patients. J Clin Invest 1997;99:2405–2415.

132. Lohman T, Leslie RDG, Hawa M, Geysen M, Rodda S, Londei M. Immunodominant epitopes of glutamic acid decarboxylase 65 and 67 in insulin-dependent diabetes mellitus. Lancet 1994;343:1607,1608.

133. Panina-Bordignon P, Lang R, van Endert PM. Cytotoxic T cells specific for glutamic acid decarboxylase in autoimmune diabetes. J Exp Med 1995;181:1923–1927.

134. Rudy G, Stone N, Harrison LC, et al. Similar peptides from two beta cell autoantigens, proinsulin and glutamic acid decarboxylase, stimulate T cells of individuals at risk for insulin-dependent diabetes. Mol Med 1995;1:625–633.

135. Wicker LS, Chen SL, Nepom GT, et al. Naturally processed T cell epitopes from human glutamic acid decarboxylase identified using mice transgenic for the type 1 diabetes-associated human MHC class II allele, DRB1 0401. J Clin Invest 1996;98:2597–2603.

136. Patel SD, Cope AP, Congia M, et al. Identification of immunodominant T cell epitopes of human glutamic acid decarboxylase 65 by using HLA-DR (α1 0101, β1 0401) trangenic mice. Proc Natl Acad Sci USA 1997;94:8082–8087.

137. Abbas AK, Murphy KM, Sher A. Functional diversity of helper T lymphocytes. Nature 1996;383:787–793.

138. Kallman BA et al. Systematic bias of cytokine production toward cell-mediated immune regulation in IDDM and toward humoral immunity in Graves'disease. Diabetes 1997;46:237–243.

139. Pugliese A, et al. HLA DQB1 0602 is associated with dominant protection from diabetes even among islet cell antibody-positive first-degree relatives of patients with IDDM. Diabetes1995;44:608–613.

140. Wilson B, Kent SC, Patton KT, Orbans T, Jackson RA, Exley M, Porcelli S, Schatz D, Atkinson M, Balk SP, Strominger JL, Hafler DA. Extreme Th1 bias of invariant Vα24JαQ T cells in type 1 diabetes. Nature 1998;391:177–181.

141. Makino S, Kunimoto K, Muraoka Y, Mizushima Y, Katagiri K, Tochino Y. Breeding of a non obese, diabetic strain of mice. Exp Anim 1980;29:1–13.

142. Nakhooda AF, Like AA, Chappel CI, Murray FT, Marliss EB. The spontaneous diabetic Wistar rat. Metabolic and morphologic studies. Diabetes 1977;26:100–112.

143. Haskins K, Wegman D, Diabetogenic T-cell clones. Diabetes 1996;45:1299–1305.

144. Bach JF. Insulin-dependent diabetes mellitus as an autoimmune disease. Endocrinol Rev 1994;15:516–542.

145. Ogawa M, Maruyama T, Hasegawa T, Kanaya T, Kobayashi F, Tochino Y, Uda H. The inhibitory effect of neonatal thymectomy on the incidence of insulitis in non-obese-diabetic (NOD) mice. Biomed Res 1985;6:103–105.

146. Dardenne M, Lepault F, Bendelac A, Bach JF. Acceleration of the onset of diabetes in NOD mice by thymectomy at weaning. Eur J Immunol 1989;19:889–895.

147. Gerling IC, Serreze DV, Christianson SW, Leiter EH. Intra-thymic islet cell transplantation reduces beta-cell autoimmunity and prevents diabetes in NOD/Lt mice. Diabetes 1992;41:1672–1676.

148. French MB, Allison A, Crem DS, et al. Transgenic expression of mouse proinsulin II prevents diabetes in nonobese diabetic mice. Diabetes 1997;46:34–39.

149. Thomas-Vaslin V, Damotte D, Coltey M, Le Douarin NM, Coutinho A, Salaun J. Abnormal T cell selection on nod thymic epithelium is sufficient to induce autoimmune manifestations in C57BL/6 athymic nude mice. Proc Natl Acad Sci USA 1997;94:4598–4603.

150. Lund T, O'Reilly L, Hutchings P, Kanagawa O, Simpson E, Gravely R, Chandler P, Dyson J, Picard JK, Edwards A, Kioussis D, Cooke A. prevention of insulin-dependent diabetes mellitus in non-obese diabetic mice by transgenes encoding modified I-A beta-chain or normal I-E alpha-chain. Nature 1990;345:727–729.

151. Boitard C, Bendelac A, Richard MF, Carnaud C, Bach JF. Prevention of diabetes in nonobese diabetic mice by anti-I-A monoclonal antibodies: transfer of protection by splenic T cells. Proc Natl Acad Sci USA 1988;85:9749–9723.

152. Hurtenbach U, Lier E, Adorini L, Nagy ZA. Prevention of autoimmune diabetes in non-obese diabetic mice by treatment with a class II major histocompatibility complex-blocking peptide. J Exp Med 1993;177:1499–1504.

153. Vaysburd M, Lock C, McDevitt H. Prevention of insulin-dependent diabetes mellitus in non obese diabetic mice by immunogenic but not by tolerated peptides. J Exp Med 1995;182:897–902.

154. Wicker LS, Leiter EH, Todd JA, Renjilian RJ, Peterson E, Fisher PA, Podolin PL, Zijlstra M, Jaenisch R, Peterson LB. β2-microglobulin-deficient NOD mice do not develop insulitis or diabetes. Diabetes 1994;43:500–504.

155. Taki T, Nagata M, Ogawa W, et al. Prevention of cyclophosphamide-induced and spontaneous diabetes in NOD/Shi/Kbe mice by anti-MHC class I Kd monoclonal antibody. Diabetes 1991;40:1203–1209.

156. Clare Salzer MJ, Brooks J, Chai A, Van Herle K, Anderson C. Prevention of diabetes in non obese diabetic mice by dendritic cell transfer. J Clin Invest 1992;90:741–748.

157. Schmidt D, Verdaguer J, Averill N, Santamaria P. A mechanism for the major histocompatibility complex-linked resistance to autoimmunity. J Exp Med 1997;186:1059–1075.

158. Chatenoud L, Thervet E, Primo J, Bach JF. Anti CD3 antibody induces long term-remission of overt autoimmunity in non-obese diabetic mice. Proc Natl Acad Sci USA 1993;91:123–127.

159. Koike T, Itoh Y, Ishii T, et al. Preventive effect of monoclonal anti L3T4 antibody on development of diabetes in NOD mice. Diabetes 1987;36:539–541.

160. Hutchings PR, Simpson E, O'Reilly LA, Lund T, Waldmann H, Cooke A. The involvment of Ly2+ T cells in beta cell destruction. J Autoimmun 1990;3(suppl 1):101–109.

161. Sempe P, Bedossa P, Richard MF, Villa MC, Bach JF, Boitard C. Anti alpha/beta T cell receptor monoclonal antibody provides an efficient therapy for autoimmune diabetes in nonobese diabetic (NOD) mice. Eur J Immunol 1991;21:1163–1169.

162. Mori Y, Suko M, Okudaira H, Matsuba I, et al. Preventive effects of cyclosporin on diabetes in NOD mice. Diabetologia 1986;29:244–247.

163. Maki T, Ichikawa T, Blamnco R, Porter J. Long-term abrogation of autoimmune diabetes in nonobese diabetic mice by immunotherapy with anti-lymphocyte serum. Proc Natl Acad Sci USA 1992;89:3434–3438.

164. Kelley VE, Gaulton GN, Hattori M, Ikegami H, Eisenbarth G, Strom TB. Anti-interleukin 2 receptor antibody suppresses murine diabetic insulitis and lupus nephritis. J Immunol 1988;140:59–61.

165. Lenschow DJ, Ho SC, Sattar H, et al. Differential effects of anti B 7.1 and anti B 7.2 monoclonal antibody treatment on the development of diabetes in the nonobese diabetic mouse. J Exp Med 1995;181:1145–1155.

166. Tisch R, McDevitt H. Insulin-dependent diabetes mellitus. Cell 1996;85:291–297.

167. Mueller R, Krahl T, Sarvetnick N. Pancreatic expression of interleukin-4 abrogates insulitis and autoimmune diabetes in Nonobese diabetic (NOD) mice. J Exp Med 1996;184:1093–1099.

168. Wogensen L, Lee MS, Sarvetnick N. Production of interleukin 10 by islet cells accelerates immune-mediated destruction of b cells in non obese diabetic mice. J Exp Med 1994;179:1379–1384.

169. Grewal IS, Grewal KD, Wong FS, Picarella DE, Janeway CA, Flavell RA. Local expression of transgene encoded TNFa in islets prevents autoimmune diabetes in nonobese diabetic (NOD) mice by preventing the development of autoreactive islet-specific T cells. J Exp Med 1996;184:1963–1974.

170. Sarvetnick N, shizuru J, Liggitt D, Martin L, McIntyre B, Gregory A, Parslow T, Stewart T. Loss of pancreatic islet tolerance induced by β cell expression of interferon-γ. Nature 1990;346:844–847.

171. Campbell IL, Kay TW, Oxbrow L, Harrison LC. Essential role for interferon-gamma and interleukin-6 in autoimmune insulin-dependent diabetes in NOD/Wehi mice. J Clin Invest 1991;87:739–742.

172. Yang XD, Tisch R, Singer SM, Cao ZA, Liblau RS, Schreiber RD, McDevitt HO. Effect of tumor necrosis factor a on insulin-dependent diabetes mellitus in NOD mice. I. The early development of autoimmunity and the diabetogenic process. J Exp Med 1994;180:995–1004.

173. Trembleau S, Penna G, Bosi E, Mortara A, Gately MK, Adorini L. Interleukin 12 administration induces T helper type 1 cells and accelerates autoimmune diabetes in NOD mice. J Exp Med 1995;181:817–821.

174. Serreze DV, Hamaguchi K, Leiter EH. Immunostimulation circumvents diabetes in NOD/Lt mice. J Autoimmun 1989;2:759–776.

175. Rappoport MJ, Jaramillo A, Zipris D, et al. Interleukin 4 reverses T cell proliferative unresponsiveness and prevents the onset of diabetes in non obese diabetic mice. J Exp Med 1993;178:87–89.

176. Pennline KJ, Roque-Gaffney E, Monahan M. Recombinant human IL-10 prevents the onset of diabetes in the nonobese diabetic mouse. Clin Immunol Immunopathol 1994;71:169–175

177. Formby B, Jacobs C, dubuc P, Shao T. Exogenous administration of IL-1 alpha inhibits active and adoptive transfer of autoimmune diabetes in NOD mice. Autoimmunity 1992;12:21–27.

178. Jacob CO, Aiso S, Michie SA, McDevitt HO, Acha-Orbea H. prevention of diabetes in nonobese diabetic mice by tumor necrosis factor (TNF): similarities between TNF-alpha and interleukin 1. Proc Natl Acad Sci USA 1990;87:968–972.

179. Areaza GA, Cameron MJ, Jaramillo A, et al. Neonatal activation of CD28 signaling overcomes T cell anergy and prevents autoimmune diabetes by an Il-4 dependent mechanism. J Clin Invest 1997;100:2243–2253.

180. Shehadeh N, Calcinaro F, Bradley BJ, Bruchlim I, Vardi P, Lafferty KJ. Effect of adjuvant therapy on development of diabetes in mouse and man. Lancet 1994;343:706,707.

181. Weiner HL, Oral tolerance: immune mechanisms and treatment of autoimmune diseases. Immunol Today 1997;19:335–342.

182. Ramiya VK, Lan MS, Wasserfall CH, Notkins AL, Maclaren NK. Immunization therapies in the prevention of diabetes. J Autoimmun 1997;10:287–292.

183. Atkinson MA, Maclaren NK, Luchetta R. Insulitis and diabetes in NOD mice reduced by prophylactic insulin therapy. Diabetes 1990;39:933–937.

184. Bowman MA, Campbell L, Darrow BL, Ellis TM, Suresh A, Atkinson MA. Immunological and metabolic effects of prophylactic insulin therapy in the NOD-scid/scid adopitve transfer model of IDDM. Diabetes 1996;45:205–208.

185. Muir A, Peck A, Clare-Salzer M, Song Y, Cornelius J, Luchetta R, Krisher J, Maclaren N. Insulin immunization of nonobese diabetic mice induces a protective insulitis characterized by diminished interferon-g transcription. J Clin Invest 1995;95:628–634.

186. Zhang ZJ, Davidson L, Eisenbarth G, Weiner HL. Suppression of diabetes in non obese diabetic mice by oral administration of porcine insulin. Proc Natl Acad Sci USA 1991;88:10,252–10,256.

187. Bergerot I, Fabien N, Maguer V, Thivolet C. Oral administration of human insulin to NOD mice generates CD4+ T cells that suppress adoptive transfer of diabetes. J Autoimmun 1994;7:655–663.

188. Hancock WW, Polanski M, Zhang J, Blogg N, Weiner HL. Suppression of insulitis in non-obese diabetic (NOD) mice by oral insulin administration is associated with selective expression of interleukin-4 and -10, transforming growth factor-β, and prostaglandin-E. Am J Pathol 1995;147: 1193–1199.

189. Harrison LC, Dempsey-Collier M, Kramer DR, Takahashi K. Aerosol insulin induces regulatory CD8 γδ T cells that prevent murine insulin-dependent diabetes. J Exp Med 1996;184:2167–2174.

190. Tompkins SM, Moore JC, Jensen PE. An insulin peptide that binds an alternative site in class II major histocompatibility complex. J Exp Med 1996;183:857–866.

191. Kaufman DL, Clare-Salzer M, Tian J, et al. Spontaneous loss of T-cell tolerance to glutamic acid decarboxylase in murine insulin-dependent diabetes. Nature 1993;366:69–72.

192. Tisch R, Yang XD, Singer SM, Liblau RS, Fugger L, McDevitt HO. Immune response to glutamic acid decarboxylase correlates with insulitis in non-obese diabetic mice. Nature 1993;366:72–75.

193. Elliott JF, Qin HY, Bhatti S, et al. Immunization with the larger isoform of mouse glutamic acid decarboxylase (GAD$_{67}$) prevents autoimmune diabetes in NOD mice. Diabetes 1994;43:1494–1499.

194. Tian J, Clare-Salzer M, Herschenfeld A, et al. Modulating autoimmune responses to GAD inhibits disease progression and prolongs islet graft survival in diabetes-prone mice. Nature Med 1996;2:1348–1353.

195. Tian J, Atkinson MA, Clare-Salzer M, Herschenfeld A, Forsthuber T, Lehman PV, Kaufman DL. Nasal administration of glutamate decarboxylase (GAD 65) peptides induces Th2 reponses and prevents murine insulin-dependent diabetes. J Exp Med 1996;183:1561–1567.
196. Cetkovic-Cvrlje M, Gerling IC, Muir A, Atkinson MA, Elliott JF, Leiter EH. Retardation or acceleration of diabetes in NOD/Lt mice mediated by intrathymic administration of candidate β-cell antigens. Diabetes 1997;46:1975–1982.
197. Elias D, Markovits D, Reshef T, Van Der Zee R, Cohen IR. Induction and therapy of autoimmune diabetes in the non-obese diabetic (NOD/Lt) mouse by a 65-kDa heat shock protein. Proc Natl Acad Sci USA 1990;87:1576–1580.
198. Elias D, Reshef T, Birk OS, Van Der Zee R, Walker MD, Cohen IR. Vaccination against autoimmune mouse diabetes with a T-cell epitope of the human 65-kDa heat shock protein. Proc Natl Acad Sci USA 1991;88:3088–3091.
199. Zhang ZJ. Insulitis is suppressed in NOD mice by oral administration of insulin peptides and glucagon. FASEB J 1992;6:1693 (abstr)
200. Peterson JD, Haskins K. Transfer of diabetes in NOD-scid mouse by CD4+ T cell clones. Diabetes 1996;45:328–336.
201. Haskins K, Mc Duffie M. Acceleration of diabetes in young NOD mice with a CD4+ islet-specific T cell clone. Science 1990;249:1433–1436.
202. Wong FS, Visintin I, Wen I, Flavell RA, Janeway CA. CD8+T cell clones from young non obese diabetic (NOD) islets can transfer rapid onset of diabetes in NOD mice in the absence of CD4+ cells. J Exp Med 1996;183:67–76.
203. Nagata M, Santamaria P, Kawamura T, Utsigi T, Yoon J. Evidence for the role of CD8+ cytotoxic T cells in the destruction of pancreatic b cells in nonobese diabetic mice. J Immunol 1994;152:2042–2050.
204. Katz JD, Benoist C, Mathis D. T helper cell subsets in insulin-dependent diabetes. Science 1995;268:1185–1188.
205. Zekzer D, Wong FS, Ayalon O, Millet I, Altieri M, Shintani M, Solimena M. GAD-reactive CD4+ Th1 cells induce diabetes in NOD/scid mice. J Clin Invest 1998;101:68–73.
206. Pakala SV, Kurrer MO, Katz JD. T helper (Th2) T cells induce acute pancreatitis and diabetes in immune-compromised nonobese diabetic (NOD) mice. J Exp Med 1997;186:299–306.
207. Boitard C, Yasunami R, Dardenne M, Bach JF. T cell-mediated inhibition of the transfer of autoimmune diabetes in NOD mice. J Exp Med 1989;169:1669–1680.
208. Akhtar I, Gold JP, Pan LY, Ferrara JLM, Yang XD, Kim JI, Tan KN. CD4+ b cell-reactive T cell clones that suppress autoimmune diabetes in Nonobese diabetic mice. J Exp Med 1995;182:87–97.
209. Yang XD, Nathan K, Tisch R, Steinman L, McDevitt H. Inhibition of insulitis and prevention of diabetes in nonobese diabetic mice by blocking L-selectin and very late antigen 4 adhesion receptors. Proc Natl Acad Sci USA 1993;90:10,494–10,498.
210. Hasegawa Y, Yokono K, Taki T, et al. Prevention of autoimmune insulin-dependent diabetes in non-obese diabetic mice by anti LFA-1 and anti ICAM-1 mAb. Int Immunol 1994;6:831–838.
211. Kagi D, Odermatt B, Seiler P, Zinkernagel RM, Mak TW, Hengartner H. Reduced incidence and delayed onset of diabetes in perforin-deficient nonobese diabetic mice. J Exp Med 1997;186:989–997.
212. Larger E, Becourt, Bach JF, Boitard C. Pancreatic islet b cells drive T cell-immune responses in the nonobese diabetic mouse model. J Exp Med 1995;181:1635–1642.
213. Bowman MA, Campbell L, Darrow BL, Ellis TM, Suresh A, Atkinson MA. Immunological and metabolic effects of prophylactic insulin therapy in the NOD-scid/scid adoiptve transfer model of IDDM. Diabetes 1996;45:205–208.
214. Vlahos WD, Seemayer TA, Yale JF. Diabetes prevention in BB rats by inhibition of endogenous insulin secretion. Metabolism 1991;40:825–829.
215. Chernosky AV, Wang Y, Wong FS, Visintin I, Flavell RA, Janeway CA Jr, Matis LA. The role of Fas in autoimmune diabetes. Cell 1997;89:17–24.
216. Reddy S, Bibby NJ, Elliott RB. Ontogeny of islet cell antibodies, insulin autoantibodies and insulitis in the non-obese diabetic mouse. Diabetologia 1988;31:322–328.
217. Daniel D, Wegmann DR. Protection of NOD mice from diabetes by intranasal or subcutaneous administration of insulin peptide B9–23. Proc Natl Acad Sci USA 1996;93:956–960.
218. Tian J, Lehmann PV, Kaufman DL. Determinant spreading of T helper cell 2 (Th2) responses to pancreatic islet autoantigens. J Exp Med 1997;186:2039–2043.

219. Kurrer MO, Pakala SV, Hanson HL, Katz JD. β cell apoptosis in T-cell mediated autoimmune diabetes. Proc Natl Acad Sci USA 1997;94:213–218.
220. Gale EAM. Standardization of IVGTT to predict IDDM. Diabetes Care 1992;15:1313–1316.
221. Vardi P, Crisa L, Jackson RA, Herskowitz RD, et al. Predictive value of intravenous glucose tolerance test insulin secretion less than or greater than the first percentile in islet cell antibody positive relatives of type I (insulin-dependent) diabetic patients. Diabetologia 1991;34:93–102.
222. Carel JC, Boitard C, Bougneres P. Decreased insulin response to glucose in islet cell antibody-negative siblings of type I diabetic children. J Clin Invest 1993;92:509–513.

17 Molecular Basis of Multiple Pituitary Hormone Deficiency

John S. Parks and Milton R. Brown

Contents

DEFINITION

Multiple pituitary hormone deficiency (MPHD) denotes subnormal production of growth hormone (GH) and one or more of the five other peptide hormones that are normally produced by the anterior pituitary. Synonyms for MPHD include combined pituitary hormone deficiency (CPHD) and panhypopituitarism. The latter term can include deficiency of antidiuretic hormone (ADH), which is produced in hypothalamic nuclei and released from the posterior pituitary.

PHENOTYPES

The observed phenotypes depend on which hormones are missing. Deficiency of GH is associated with nearly normal postnatal growth followed by severe postnatal growth failure. Birth lengths are, on average, one standard deviation (SD) below the mean, suggesting an influence of pituitary GH on growth during the third trimester. Lengths at

From: *Molecular and Cellular Pediatric Endocrinology*
Edited by: S. Handwerger © Humana Press Inc., Totowa, NJ

age 1 yr and beyond are generally more than 4 SD below gender- and age-specific norms. Prolactin (Prl) deficiency does not confer a specific phenotype in childhood, but may impair fertility and lactation. Central hypothyroidism caused by deficiency of thyroid stimulating hormone (TSH) can be mild or it can produce cretinism, with severe manifestations of thyroid hormone deficiency evident at birth. Deficiencies of luteinizing hormone (LH) and follicle stimulating hormone (FSH) contribute to micropenis in the newborn male and result in failure of spontaneous pubertal development. Deficiency of corticotropin (ACTH) produces adrenal hypoplasia and contributes to fasting hypoglycemia. Timely recognition of hormone deficiencies and replacement of the missing hormones permits normal growth, development, and reproductive function.

ETIOLOGY

Many cases of MPHD result from processes that damage the pituitary after birth. Craniopharyngiomas and Rathke's pouch cysts are common causes of MPHD in childhood and pituitary adenomas become relatively common in adulthood. In these conditions, the hormone deficiencies may be present before treatment or occur as a consequence of surgery or radiotherapy. Histiocytosis and the acceleration-deceleration trauma of automobile accidents or shaken baby syndrome can damage the pituitary stalk, resulting in deficiencies of GH, TSH, LH, FSH, ACTH and ADH. Secretion of Prl, which is subject to negative hypothalamic control, is usually increased when the portal hypophyseal circulation is disrupted.

The proportion of MPHD cases resulting from genetic causes is fairly large. Autosomal recessive, autosomal dominant, and X-linked recessive forms have been described. Categorization on the basis of family history underestimates genetic contributions to disease. As candidate genes have been identified, the proportion of cases that can be attributed to mutations has increased dramatically. Despite the fact that there is overlap in hypothalamic regulation of anterior pituitary cell types, none of the recognized causes of MPHD involve deficiencies of releasing factors. Instead, the causes reflect mutations in the genes encoding transcriptional activation factors that direct pituitary cell development (Table 1). The differentiation, expansion, and mature function of anterior pituitary cell types depends on the coordinated expression of a spectrum of these factors. They represent a large family of DNA-binding proteins related to the homeobox proteins that were originally discovered in Drosophila. The past decade has brought spectacular advances in understanding of pituitary embryogenesis (1). Most of the work has involved use of murine models (2). Candidate genes have been characterized and in several instances identified as the genes responsible for recognized forms of hypopituitarism in mice. Three pituitary transcription factors, Ptx-1, Prop-1, and Pit-1, have been associated with distinct forms of hypopituitarism in humans. This chapter will consider each of the transcription factors in turn, beginning with those that are expressed at the earliest stages of pituitary development in the mouse.

RPX

The mouse Rpx (Rathke's pouch homeobox) gene appears at embryonic 8.5 (E8.5) in the primordium of the anterior pituitary gland (3). It is expressed in all five anterior pituitary cell types. This paired homeodomain protein competes with Prop-1 for binding to promoter sequences. Expression is normally extinguished by day e13.5. A second

Table 1
Pituitary Transcription Factors: Timing of Appearance in Murine Pituitary and Hormonal Phenotypes Associated with Gene Disruption

Factor	Cells	Appears(E20)	Disappears(E20)	Resulting hormone deficiency phenotype
Rpx	All	8.5	13.5	GH, Prl, TSH, LH, FSH, ACTH (mouse KO)
P-OTX	All	8.5	Persists	GH, Prl, TSH, LH, FSH, ACTH (mouse KO)
P-Lim	All	9.5	Persists	GH, Prl, TSH, LH, FSH (mouse KO)
Ptx-2	S,L,T,G	Before 11	Persists	Variable (Rieger syndrome in humans)
Prop-1	S,L,T,G[a]	10.5	14.5	GH, Prl, TSH, LH, FSH (Ames mouse, human)
Pit-1	S,L,T	14.5	Persists	GH, Prl, TSH (Snell mouse, human)
Gsh-1	Hypothal	8.5	14.5	GH, Prl, LH (mouse KO)

[a]S, somatotrophs expressing GH; L, lactotrophs expressing Prl; T, thyrotrophs expressing α-glycoprotein subunit and β-TSH; G, gonadotrophs expressing α-glycoprotein subunit, β-LH and β-FSH; Hypothal, hypothalamus.

transcription factor, termed Prop-1 appears to be involved in turning off Rpx expression since the protein continues to be expressed in Ames dwarf mice who have deficiencies of GH, Prl, TSH caused by an inactivating mutation of Prop-1. Other mechanisms must be involved in extinction of Rpx expression in corticotropes because Prop-1 is not expressed in these cells. Expression ceases at the normal time in Snell dwarf mice who have a similar spectrum of hormonal abnormalities caused by a mutation in Pit-1 *(4,5)*. There are no known examples of Rpx mutations in humans. The phenotype resulting from Rpx mutations is likely to be complex. It would include pituitary aplasia with complete deficiency of all pituitary hormones and possibly developmental anomalies of other neural structures.

P-OTX

The pituitary OTX or Ptx-1 protein is also expressed at an early stage, beginning at d 8.5. Expression persists in the mature pituitary. This protein was identified in a search for transcription factors that bound to the transcriptional activation domain of Pit-1 *(6)*. It is a 315 amino acid protein with a tryptophan-phenylalanine (WFK) motif in the third alpha helix of the DNA-binding domain. This domain is shared with the other members of the OTX family. It recognizes a TAATCC consensus-binding sequence and it independently activates transcription from the promoter of the alpha-glycoprotein subunit (α-GSU) of TSH, LH, and FSH. The protein also activates the proopiomelanocortin (POMC), GH, and Prl promoters. It acts cooperatively with Pit-1 in activating transcription from the GH and Prl promoters, but not the β-TSH promoter. Thus, P-OTX contributes in different ways to the activation of all 6 anterior pituitary hormones. It is also expressed in the oral epithelium, tongue, mandible, salivary gland, duodenum, and hindlimb. The phenotype produced by inactivating mutations is likely to include hypopituitarism together with developmental abnormalities of these other structures.

P-LIM

The P-Lim transcription factor appears slightly later in development, at dE9.5 in the mouse, and it continues to be expressed in the adult pituitary *(6–9)*. It is a protein of 400 amino acids, with two LIM domains. These are cysteine-rich regions adjacent to two zinc-coordinated structures that mediate protein–protein interactions. Either domain is sufficient for binding to the POU-specific and POU-homeo domains of Pit-1 *(6)*. Like P-OTX, P-Lim independently activates the α-GSU promoter *(10)*. The LIM domains are not required for this activation. P-Lim acts synergistically with Pit-1 in activating transcription from the Prl, β-TSH, and Pit-1 promoters. Targeted gene disruption in mice produces a phenotype of hypopituitarism *(11)*. Rathke's pouch develops normally, but the anterior and intermediate lobes fail to develop. There may be subtle developmental abnormalities of the pons, medulla, and retina, which also express P-Lim So far, no mutations of P-Lim have been described in humans.

PTX-2

Expression of the pituitary homeobox 2 (Ptx-2) gene in the mouse pituitary gland begins before E11 and persists into adulthood *(12,13)*. The gene is also expressed in the brain, eye, kidney, lung, testis, limb mesenchyme, tongue, and umbilicus. It is a "bicoid" homeobox gene. The 60 amino acid homeodomain region differs from that of P-OTX by

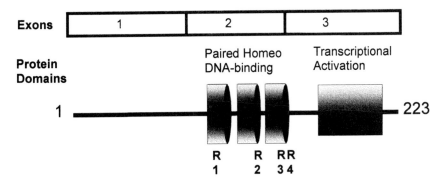

Fig. 1. Prop-1 gene structure and mutations.

only two amino acids *(13)*. Alternative splicing of mRNA produces proteins of 271 (Ptx2a) and 317 (Ptx2b) amino acids that differ in the region preceding the DNA-binding homeodomain *(12)*. There is 99% amino acid homology between the human Ptx-2 gene located on chromosome 4q25 and the mouse gene located on chromosome 3 *(13)*. Rieger syndrome in humans has been mapped to 4q25 *(14)*. This dominantly inherited condition is extremely complex. It includes coloboma of the iris, glaucoma, renal anomalies, anal stenosis, and umbilical hernia as well as variable degrees of hypopituitarism. The recent demonstration of mutations in the human Ptx-2 or RIEG1 gene in six of ten families with Rieger syndrome demonstrates that the condition is caused by haploinsufficiency for this gene and not by deletion of contiguous genes *(13)*.

PROP-1

The "Prophet of Pit-1" (Prop-1) gene is first expressed at E10.5 and expression continues through E14.5. This gene was identified through positional cloning of the gene on mouse chromosome 11 which is responsible for Ames dwarfism *(4)*. It is expressed in somatotrophs, lactotrophs, thyrotrophs, and gonadotrophs. The gene, which consists of three exons, encodes a protein of 223 amino acids that contains a centrally located paired-like DNA-binding domain and a C-terminal transcriptional activation domain (Fig. 1). It binds to promoter sequences containing palindromic TAAT ATTA sequences separated by two or three base-pair spacer sequences. The strongest binding occurs to an ACT<u>AATT</u>GA<u>ATTA</u>GC sequence termed PRDQ9 *(4)*. RPX-1 binds competitively to the same sequence and is capable of forming heterodimers with Prop-1. There are Prop-1 binding sequences in the distal enhancer region of Pit-1 and Prop-1 may act cooperatively with other transcription factors in activating Pit-1.

Ames dwarf mice are homozygous for a missense mutation in codon 83 of Prop-1 that changes serine to proline. The mutant protein retains 20% of wild-type activity in binding to PRDQ9 (Table 2). Transcriptional activation is threefold, compared to 13-fold for the wild-type protein *(4)*. Wu et al. *(15)* described four families with mutations in the Prop-

Table 2
Properties of Mutant Prop-1 Proteins

Protein	Species[a]	Relative binding to PRDQ9	Activation from PRDQ9 promoter
Wild-type	Mouse	100%	13X
Ser83Pro	Ames Mouse	20%	3X
2 bp deletion	Human	<1%	1X
Phe171Ile	Human	<1%	1X
Arg120Cys	Human	10%	1.3X

[a]Mutations observed in humans were expressed in the context of the mouse Prop-1 cDNA sequence.

1 gene located on human chromosome 5. Affected individuals in two families were homozygous for a 2 bp deletion in exon 2. Loss of one of three sequential AG pairs causes a frame shift and results in a truncated protein of 108 amino acids lacking much of the DNA-binding and all of the transcriptional activation domain. When the 2 bp deletion was expressed a mouse Prop-1 background, it did not bind to PRDQ9 and did not activate transcription. The affected individual in a third family was a compound heterozygote for the 2 bp deletion and a missense mutation that substituted isoleucine for phenylalanine at codon 117. The Phe117Ile mutant protein was devoid of DNA-binding and transcriptional activation activities. Two affected individuals in the fourth family were homozygous for a missense mutation that substituted arginine for cysteine at position 120. DNA-binding activity was approx 10% of wild-type and there was a minimal, 1.3-fold, activation of transcription.

The 2 bp deletion in Prop-1 creates a new BcgI restriction site. This makes it easy to screen large numbers of DNA specimens. We found that 31 of a series of 50 MPHD patients treated by Dr. Lenartowska at the Institute of Mother and Child in Warsaw, Poland, were either homozygotes or heterozygotes for the deletion (16). All were deficient in LH and FSH as well as in GH, Prl, and TSH. Roughly one-third of the patients with Prop-1 mutations were deficient in ACTH, compared to two-thirds of those without recognized Prop-1 mutations. Deficiency of ACTH in patients with Prop-1 defects appeared later and was less severe than in patients with other varieties of MPHD.

The phenotype of hormone deficiency in humans with Prop-1 mutations is broader than that in the Ames dwarf mouse. Homozygotes for the Ames Ser83Pro mutations have reduced fertility, but pregnancies have been obtained with combined Prl and thyroid hormone replacement. The difference in degree of gonadotropin deficiency may reflect a species difference or it may be a consequence of the greater severity of the loss of function mutations observed in humans.

All of the Prop-1 mutations that have been observed to date are recessive. Since homodimerization is a prerequisite for transcriptional activation by Prop-1, there is a strong possibility that, as in the case of Pit-1, dominant mutations exist and will be discovered.

PIT-1

Pituitary transcription factor 1 (Pit-1) appears in the mouse pituitary at E14.5 (17). It precedes GH production in somatotrophs and Prl production in lactotrophs, but follows the

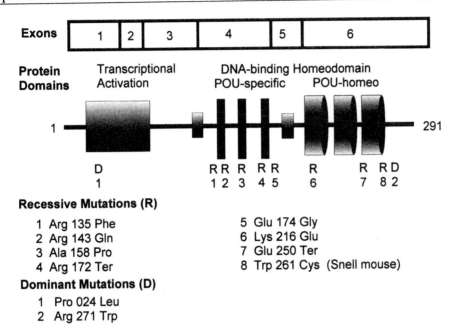

Fig. 2. Pit-1 gene structure and mutations.

appearance of TSH in a small population of thyrotrophs in the rostral tip of the developing pituitary. A larger population of caudomedial thyrotrophs develops after the appearance of Pit-1 and constitutes the permanent population of thyrototrophs in the mouse *(18)*. The mouse Pit-1 protein was identified through a strategy involving affinity purification of nuclear proteins that bound to the GH promoter *(19,20)*. Pit-1 recognizes and activates transcription from promoter sequences in the GH, Prl, β-TSH, and Pit-1 genes *(21,22)*. The protein of 290 amino acids contains an amino terminal transcriptional activation domain and centrally located DNA-binding domains termed the POU-specific and POU-homeo domains *(23–25)*. The mouse Pit-1 gene, located on chromosome 16, and the human Pit-1 gene, located on chromosome 3 *(26)*, each contain six exons (Fig. 2). There is alternative splicing of the pre-mRNA transcript from these exons. Pit-1β and Pit-1T arise by in-frame insertion of 78 and 42 bases, respectively, from the 3' end of exon1 onto the 5' end of exon 2. Both insertions alter the transactivation domain. Pit-1β preferentially activates the GH promoter and shows little activation of Prl. Pit-1T is produced by thyrotropes and exhibits selective activation of TSHβ promoter. Δ4Pit-1 arises by skipping exon 4 and results in loss of the POU-specific domain and loss of binding to the Prl promoter. The splice variants occur at low levels relative to Pit-1 and none of the alternative forms have been associated with MPHD in humans.

Li et al. *(27)* reported that the Jackson dwarf mouse was homozygous for a complex rearrangement of the Pit-1 gene and the Snell dwarf mouse was homozygous for a missense mutation in Pit-1. The Snell mutation involves substitution of cysteine for tryptophan at position 261. This Trp261Cys mutation in the POU-homeo domain eliminates DNA-binding and transcriptional activation. At least ten different Pit-1 mutations have been described in humans with combined GH, Prl, and TSH deficiencies. Most are loss of function mutations that are recessive in their expression. They include a complete deletion of the Pit-1 gene *(28)*, Arg135Phe *(29)*, Arg143Gln *(29)*, Ala158Pro *(28)*, an Arg172Ter nonsense mutation *(30,31)*, Glu174Gly *(31)*, Lys216Glu *(32)*, and a Glu250Ter nonsense mutation *(33)*. Most of these mutations are assumed or have been shown to impair binding of the protein-to-promoter sequences. The Arg158Pro mutant protein showed a 70% reduction in binding, but a complete loss of transcriptional activation activity *(28)*. The Lys216Glu mutant has the very interesting property of being a superactivator at the GH and Prl promoters, but lacks the ability to partner with the retinoic acid receptor at the distal Pit-1 enhancer and upregulate Pit-1 expression *(32)*.

Two Pit-1 mutations, Arg271Trp *(34)* and Pro24Leu *(29)*, confer a dominant negative phenotype. The Arg271Trp mutation is dominant in its expression. The mutant protein has increased DNA-binding activity. Mutant homodimers and heterodimers of mutant and wild-type Pit-1 are transcriptionally inactive. Patients with the dominant Arg271Trp mutation outnumber those with all of the other mutations combined. This reflects the fact that the mutation involves a CpG mutational hot-spot and only one Pit-1 allele needs to be mutated to cause disease *(35)*. The single report of a dominant Pro24Leu mutation did not include studies of DNA-binding or transcriptional activation *(29)*. The proline residue at position 24 is evolutionarily conserved and the leucine substitution does not appear to be a polymorphism.

Virtually all persons with Pit-1 mutations have had complete deficiencies of GH and Prl, with no GH response to GHRH and no Prl response to TRH. The degree of TSH deficiency has been variable. Some patients have had T4 levels within the normal range at presentation, with a decline in T4 after initiation of GH treatment *(36)*. Others have had profound neonatal hypothyroidism with T4 values below the limit of detection *(30)*. One patient, born to a mother with the Arg271Trp mutation who discontinued T4 replacement during pregnancy, was severely affected as a result of combined maternal and fetal hypothyroidism *(37)*. There is also variation in size of the anterior pituitary, as assessed by MRI. Some have had severe hypoplasia and others have had pituitaries of normal volume *(28)*. Factors other than the specific type of Pit-1 mutation seem to be responsible for variation in TSH deficiency and pituitary size.

GSH-1

The Genomic screen homeobox-1 (Gsh-1) gene is expressed very early in the embryonic development of the central nervous system *(38)*. Disrete bands of expression are present by E8.5 in tissues that will form the spinal cord, hindbrain, thalamus, and hypothalamus. Gene structure and organization, with only a single intron, resemble that of clustered homeobox genes *(39)*. The centrally located homeodomain shows a preference for the consensus sequence $GC^T/C^A/CATTA^G/A$. Disruption of Gsh-1 gene in transgenic mice results in pituitary hypoplasia and MPHD with dwarfism and failure to enter puberty *(39)*. The anterior pituitary was reported to be about one-third of normal size with a 95% reduction in GH content, a 75% reduction in Prl content, and a 67% reduction in content of LH per milligram of total protein. 'There was no expression of GHRH in the arcuate nucleus and normal expression of GHRH in neurons of the ventromedial nucleus, which is not involved in regulation of GH secretion. It seems likely that the GHRH gene and Gsh-1 itself are direct targets for activation by Gsh-1. Both promoters contain the Gsh-1 consensus ATTA binding sequences and demonstrate specific binding in gel retardation assays. The lesser degrees of Prl and LH are less easily explained. There is no defect in GnRH expression in the hypothalami of mutant mice.

The Gsh-1 gene is a candidate for mutation in human MPHD with the phenotype of combined GH, Prl, and LH deficiencies. It is not known whether the phenotype could be distinguished from that produced by Prop-1 mutations by virtue of having a positive GH response to short- or long-term stimulation of the pituitary with GHRH.

X-LINKED MPHD

Several families with X-linked MPHD have been described *(40–42)*. The phenotype includes GH and ACTH deficiency with variable expression of TSH and gonadotropin deficiencies. Lagerstrom-Fermer et al. *(43)* have demonstrated linkage to markers for Xq25–26. The gene responsible for this condition has not been cloned and it is not known whether the disorder involves a primary defect at the hypothalamic or at the pituitary level.

CONCLUSION

Basic advances in the understanding of pituitary development, gained through studies of mice, have led to recognition of several distinct forms of hypopituitarism in humans. Autsomal recessive and autosomal dominant disorders have been traced to abnormalities in the genes encoding pituitary transcription factors. Mutations in the Pit-1 gene cause the relatively rare phenotype of combined GH, Prl, and TSH deficiencies. The most common mutation is a single base substitution leading to replacement of arginine with a tryptophan at position 271. It acts in a dominant negative manner. Prop-1 mutations result in central hypogonadism and occasionally ACTH deficiency as well as deficiencies of GH, Prl, and TSH. The most common mutation is a 2 bp deletion leading to a frameshift and production of a truncated peptide. Affected individuals in all but one of the families identified to date have been either homozygotes or compound heterozygotes for this mutant allele. Both Pit-1 and Prop-1 abnormalities lead to Prl deficiency, but neither has been associated with deficiency of ADH. Careful delineation of hormonal phenotype, including measurement of Prl responses to TRH, is crucial in deciding whether to look for abnormalities in these genes in a particular individual or family. Molecular diagnosis is helpful in predicting whether a child will need help in achieving pubertal development. It is also helpful in defining risk factors in subsequent pregnancies and in recognizing the need for treatment of neonatal hypoglycemia and hypothyroidism.

The discovery that Rieger syndrome is caused by haploinsufficiency for the Ptx-2/RIEG1 gene has a different set of implications. The first is that severity of hormonal phenotype may be highly variable and dependent on interaction with variability in other genes. The second is that some transcription factors influencing pituitary development also influence the development of other organ systems. The consequences of disruption of Rpx, P-OTX/Ptx-1, Ptx-2/RIEG1, and a host of yet to be discovered transcription factors are likely to extend far beyond the phenotype of hormone deficiency.

ACKNOWLEDGMENTS

Supported in part by NIH grant DK46312, Genentech Foundation for Growth and Development grant 97-27 and a grant from Pharmacia and Upjohn.

REFERENCES

1. Parks JS, Adess ME, Brown MR. Genes regulating hypothalamic and pituitary development. Acta Paediatr Suppl 1997;423:28–32.
2. Kappen C, Schughart K, Ruddle FH. Early evolutionary origin of major homeodomain sequence classes. Genomics 1993;18:54–70.
3. Hermesz E, Mackem S, Mahon KA. Rpx: a novel anterior-restricted homeobox gene progressively activated in the prechordal plate, anterior neural plate and Rathke's pouch of the mouse embryo. Development 1996;122:41–52.
4. Sornson MW, Wu W, Dasen JS, Flynn SE, Norman DJ, O'Connell SM, Gukovsky I, Carriere C, Ryan AK, Miller AP, Zuo L, Gleiberman AS, Andersen B, Beamer WG, Rosenfeld MG. Pituitary lineage determination by the Prophet of Pit-1 homeodomain factor defective in Ames dwarfism. Nature 1996;384:327–333.
5. Gage PJ, Brinkmeier ML, Scarlett LM, Knapp LT, Camper SA, Mahon KA. The Ames dwarf gene, df, is required early in pituitary ontogeny for the extinction of Rpx transcription and initiation of lineage-specific cell proliferation. Mol Endocr 1996;10:1570–1581.
6. Szeto DP, Ryan AK, O'Connell SM, Rosenfeld MG. P-OTX: a Pit-1-interacting homeodomain factor expressed during anterior pituitary gland development. Proc Natl Acad Sci USA 1996;93:7706–7710.
7. Zhadanov AB, Bertuzzi S, Taira M, Dawid IB, Westphal H. Expression pattern of the murine LIM class homeobox gene Lhx3 in subsets of neural and neuroendocrine tissues. Devel Dynam 1995;202:354–364.
8. Seidah NG, Barale JC, Marcinkiewicz, JC, Mattie MG, Day R, Chretien M. The mouse homoprotein mLIM-3 is expressed early in cells derived from the neuroepithelium and persists in adult pituitary. DNA Cell Biol 1994;13:1163–1180.
9. Bach I, Rhodes SJ, Pearse RV II, Heinzel T, Gloss B, Scully KM, Sawchenko PE, Rosenfeld MG. P-Lim, a LIM homeodomain factor is expressed during pituitary organ and cell commitment and synergizes with Pit-1. Proc Natl Acad Sci USA 1995;92:2720–2724.
10. Roberson MS, Schoderbek WE, Maurer RA. Activation of the glycoprotein hormone alpha-subunit promoter by a LIM-homeodomain transcription factor. Mol Cell Biol 1994;2985–2993.
11. Sheng HZ, Zhadanov AB, Mosinger B Jr, Fujii T, Bertuzzi S, Grinberg A, Lee EJ, Huang SP, Mahon KA, Westphal H. Specification of pituitary cell lineages by the LIM homeobox gene Lhx. Science 1996;272:1004–1007.
12. Gage PJ, Camper SA. Pituitary homeobox 2, a novel member of the bicoid-related family of homeobox genes, is a potential regulator of anterior structure formation. Hum Mol Genet 1997;6:457–464.
13. Semina EV, Reiter R, Leysens NJ, Alward WLM, Small KW, Datson NA, Siegel-Bartlet J, Bierke-Nelson D, Bitoun P Zabel BU, Carey JC, Murray JC. Cloning and characterization of a novel bicoid-related homeobox transcription factor gene, RIEG, involved in Rieger syndrome. Nature Genet 1996;14:392–399.
14. Murray JC, Bennett SR, Kwitek AE, Small KW, Schinzel A, Alward WLM, Weber JL, Bell GI, Buetow KH. Linkage of Rieger syndrome to the region of the epidermal growth factor gene on chromosome 4. Nature Genet 1992;2:46–49.
15. Wu W, Cogan JD, Pfaffle RW, Dasen JS, Frisch H, O'Connell SM, Flynn SE, Brown, MR, Mullis PE, Parks JS, Phillips JA III, Rosenfeld MG. Mutations in PROP1 cause familial combined pituitary hormone deficiency. Nature Genet 1998;18:147–149.
16. Brown MR, Lenartowska I, Oltarzewski M, Wu W, Rosenfeld MJ, Parks JS. Prop-1 mutations and hypopituitarism in Poland. Annual Meeting of The Endocrine Society (Abstract), 1998.
17. Voss JW, Rosenfeld MG. Anterior pituitary development: short tales from dwarf mice. Cell 1992;70:527–530.
18. Li SC, Li S, Drolet DW, Rosenfeld MG. Pituitary ontogeny of the Snell dwarf mouse reveals Pit-1-independent and Pit-1-dependent origins of the thyrotrope. Development 1994;120:515–522.
19. Bodner M, Castrillo J-L, Theill LE, et al. The pituitary-specific transcription factor GHF-1 is a homeobox-containing protein. Cell 1988;55:505–518.
20. LeMaigre FP, Peers B, Lafontaine DA, Mathy-Hartert M, Rousseau GG, Belayew A, Martial JA. Pituitary-specific factor binding to the human prolactin, growth hormone and placental lactogen genes. 1989;8:149–159.
21. Mangalam HJ, Albert VR, Ingraham HA, et al. A pituitary POU domain protein, Pit-1, activates both growth hormone and prolactin promoters transcriptionally. Genes Dev 1989;3:946–958.

22. Fox SR, Jong MTC, Casanova K. et al. Pit-1/GHF-1, is capable of binding to and activating cell-specific elements of both the growth hormone and prolactin gene promoters. Mol Endocr 1990;4:1069–1080.

23. Herr W, Sturm RA, Clerc RG, et al. The POU domain: a large conserved region in the mammalian pit-1, oct-1, oct-2 and Caenorhabditis elegans unc-86 gene products. Genes and Devel 1988;2:1513–1516.

24. Ingraham HA, Flynn SE, Voss JW, et al. The POU-specific domain of Pit-1 is essential for sequence-specific, high affinity DNA binding and DNA-dependent Pit-1-Pit-1 interactions. Cell 1990;61: 1021–1033.

25. Assa-Munt N, Mortishire-Smith RJ, Aurora R, Herr W, Wright PE. The solution structure of the Oct-1 POU-specific domain reveals a striking similarity to the bacteriophage lambda repressor DNA-binding domain. Cell 1993;73:193–205.

26. Raskin S, Cogan JD, Summar ML, Moreno A, Krishnamani MR, Phillips JA 3rd. Genetic mapping of the human pituitary-specific transcriptional factor gene and its analysis in familial panhypopituitary dwarfism. Hum Genet 1996;98:703–705.

27. Li S, Crenshaw EB, III, Rawson EJ, Simmons DM, Swanson LW, Rosenfeld MG. Dwarf locus mutants lacking three pituitary cell types result form mutations in the POU-domain gene Pit-1. Nature 1990;347:528–533.

28. Pfäffle RW, DiMattia G, Parks JS, Brown MR, Wit JM, Jansen M, Van der Nat H, Van den Brande JL, Rosenfeld MR, Ingraham HA. Mutation of the POU-specific domain of Pit-1 as a cause of hypopituitarism without pituitary hypoplasia. Science 1992;257:1118–1121.

29. Ohta K, Nobukuni Y, Mitsubishi H, Fujimoto S, Matsuo N, Inagaki H, Endo F, Matsuda I. Mutations in the Pit-1 gene in children with combined pituitary hormone deficiency. Biochem Biophys Res Comm 1992;89:851–855.

30. Tatsumi K-I, Miyai K, Notomi T, Kaibe K, Amino N, Mizuno Y, Kohno H. Cretinism with combined hormone deficiency caused by a mutation in the PIT1 gene. Nature Genet 1992;1:56–58.

31. Brown MR, Parks JS, Adess ME, Rich BH, Rosenthal IM, Voss TC, VanderHeyden TC, Hurley DL. Central hypothyroidism reveals compound heterozygous mutations in the Pit-1 gene. Horm Res 1998;49:98–102.

32. Cohen LE, Wondisford FE, Radovick S. Role of Pit-1 in the gene expression of growth hormone, prolactin and thyrotropin. Endocrinol Clin North Am 1996;25:523–540.

33. Irie Y, Tatsumi K, Ogawa M, Kamijo T, Preeyasombat C, Suprasongsin C, Amino N. A novel E250X mutation of the PIT1 gene in a patient with combined pituitary hormone deficiency. Endocr J 1995;42:351–354.

34. Radovick S, Nations M, Du Y, Berg LA, Weintraub BD, Wondisford FE. A mutation in the POU-homeodomain of Pit-1 responsible for combined pituitary hormone deficiency. Science 1992;7: 1115–1118.

35. Cohen LE, Wondisford FE, Salvatoni A, Maghnie M, Brucker-Davis F, Weintraub BD, Radovick S. A "hot spot" in the Pit-1 gene responsible for combined pituitary hormone deficiency: clinical and molecular correlates. J Clin Endocr Metab 1995;80:679–684.

36. Wit JM, Drayer NM, Jansen M, et al. Total deficiency of growth hormone and prolactin, and partial deficiency of thyroid stimulating hormone in two Dutch families: a new variant of hereditary pituitary deficiency. Horm Res 1989;32:170–177.

37. de Zegher F, Pernasetti F, Vanhole C, Devlieger H, Van den Rerghe G, Martial JA. A prismatic case: the prenatal role of thyroid hormone evidenced by fetomaternal Pit-1 deficiency. J Clin Endocr Metab 1995;80:3127–3130.

38. Valerius MT, Li H, Stpck JL, Weinstein M, Kaur S, Singh G, Potter SS. Gsh-1: a novel murine homeobox gene expressed in the central nervous system. Devel Dynam 1995;203:337–351.

39. Li H, Zeitler S, Valerius MT, Small K, Potter SS. Gsh-1, an orphan Hox gne, is required for normal pituitary development. EMBO J 1996;15:714–724.

40. Schimke RN, Spaulding JJ, Hollowell JG. X-linked congenital panhypopituitarism. Birth Defects Orig Art Ser 1971;VII(6):21–23.

41. Phelan PD, Connelly J, Martin FIR, Wettenhall HNB. X-linked recessive hypopituitarism. Birth Defects Orig Art Ser 1971;VII(6):24–27.

42. Zipf WB, Kelch RP, Bacon GE. Variable X-linked recessive hypopituitarism with evidence of gonadotropin deficiency in two pre-pubertal males. Clin Genet 1977;11:249–254.

43. Lagerstrom-Fermer M, Sundvall M, Johnson E, Warne GL, Forest SM, Zajac JC, Rickards A, Ravine D, Landegren U, Pettersson U. X-linked recessive panhypopituitarism associated with a regional duplication in Xq25-q26. Am J Hum Genet 1997;50:910–916.

INDEX

ABOUT THE EDITOR

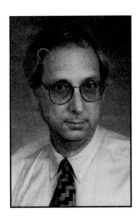

Dr. Stuart Handwerger is the Robert and Mary Shoemaker Professor of Pediatrics and Professor of Anatomy, Neurobiology, and Cell Biology at the University of Cincinnati College of Medicine, where he is Director of the Division of Endocrinology at the Children's Hospital Medical Center. He is board certified in pediatrics and pediatric endocrinology and is an elected member of the Society for Pediatric Research, the American Pediatric Society, the American Federation for Clinical Research, the American Society of Clinical Investigation, and the Association of American Physicians. He is also a member of the Endocrine Society and the Lawson Wilkins Pediatric Endocrine Society and is the author of more than 140 peer-reviewed manuscripts. He served as a member of the National Advisory Council of the National Institute of Child Health and Human Development.